D0070204

Neurological Disorders of Pregnancy

Second Revised Edition

Edited by

Phillip J. Goldstein, M.D.
Obstetrician and Gynecologist-in-Chief, Sinai Hospital of Baltimore, Inc., Associate Professor, Department of Obstetrics/Gynecology, Johns Hopkins University, School of Medicine, Baltimore, Maryland

and

Barney J. Stern, M.D.
Director, Division of Neurology, Sinai Hospital of Baltimore, Inc., Associate Professor of Neurology, Johns Hopkins University, School of Medicine, Baltimore, Maryland

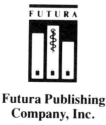

Futura Publishing Company, Inc.
Mount Kisco, NY

Library of Congress Cataloging-in-Publication Data
Neurological disorders of pregnancy / edited by Phillip J.
   Goldstein and Barney J. Stern. — Rev. 2nd ed.
      Includes bibliographical references and index.
      ISBN 0–87993–519–7
      1. Pregnancy, Complications of.   2. Nervous system—
   Disease—Complications and sequelae.   I. Goldstein, Phillip
   J.   II. Stern, Barney J.
      [DNLM: 1. Nervous System Diseases—in pregnancy.   2.
   Pregnancy Complications. WQ 240 N494]
   RG580.N47N48 1992
   618.3'268—dc20
   DNLM/DLC
   for Library of Congress   91–28288

Copyright © 1992

Published by
Futura Publishing Company, Inc.
2 Bedford Ridge Road
Mount Kisco, New York 10549

Every effort has been made to ensure that the information in this book is as up to date and accurate as possible at the time of publication. However, due to the constant developments in medicine, neither the author, nor the editor, nor the publisher can accept any legal or any other responsibility for for any errors or omissions that may occur.

Printed in the United States of America.

Dedication

This book is dedicated to my wife, Sharon for her love, her patience, and her understanding.

Phillip J. Goldstein, M.D.

This book is dedicated to my wife, Elyce; my children Rachel, Melissa, and Jamie; and to my parents, Leo and Henny Stern, for their continuing support and patience in allowing me to develop my career.

Barney J. Stern, M.D.

Contributors

Samuel Adler, M.D.   *Associate Chief of Psychiatry, Sinai Hospital of Baltimore, Inc., Baltimore, Maryland*

Kathy A. Birk, M.D.   *Departments of Obstetrics and Gynecology, Strong Memorial Hospital and Genesee Hospital, Rochester, New York*

Henry Brem, M.D.   *Associate Professor of Neurosurgery, Ophthalmology, and Oncology, Director of Neurosurgical Oncology, Johns Hopkins University, School of Medicine, Baltimore, Maryland*

Rachel F. Brem, M.D.   *Instructor, Department of Radiology, Johns Hopkins University, School of Medicine, Baltimore, Maryland*

Sanjay Datta, M.D.   *Director, Obstetric Anesthesia, Brigham and Women's Hospital, Associate Professor of Anaesthesia, Harvard Medical School, Boston, Massachusetts*

Lois Eldred, MPH   *Director AIDS Professional Education, Johns Hopkins Medical Institutions, Baltimore, Maryland*

Gerald Felsenthal, M.D.   *Chief of Rehabilitation Medicine, Sinai Hospital of Baltimore, Inc., Associate Professor in Rehabilitation Medicine, University of Maryland, School of Medicine, Associate Professor in Rehabilitation Medicine, Johns Hopkins University, Baltimore, Maryland*

Phillip J. Goldstein, M.D.   *Obstetrician and Gynecologist-in-Chief, Sinai Hospital of Baltimore, Inc., Associate Professor, Deparment of Obstetrics/Gynecology, Johns Hopkins University, School of Medicine, Baltimore, Maryland*

Janet Horn, M.D.   *Assistant Professor of Medicine, Johns Hopkins Medical Institutions, Director, Ambulatory Infections, Sinai Hospital of Baltimore, Inc., Baltimore, Maryland*

John Imboden, M.D.   *Psychiatrist-in-Chief, Sinai Hospital of Baltimore, Inc., Associate Professor, Department of Psychiatry, Johns Hopkins University, School of Medicine, Baltimore, Maryland*

Ramesh Khurana, M.D.   *Clinical Associate Professor in Neurology, University of Maryland, School of Medicine, Baltimore, Maryland, Director, Headache Management Center, Columbia, Maryland*

Allan Krumholz, M.D.   *Professor of Neurology, Department of Neurology, University of Maryland, School of Medicine, Baltimore, Maryland*

Roger Kurlan, M.D.   *Associate Professor of Neurology, Department of Neurology, University of Rochester, School of Medicine and Dentistry, Rochester, New York*

Michael L. Levin, M.D.   *Founder, Division of Infectious Diseases, Sinai Hospital of Baltimore, Inc., Assistant Professor of Medicine, Johns Hopkins Medical Institutions, Assistant Professor of Medicine, University of Maryland, Baltimore, Maryland*

Andrew M. Malinow, M.D.   *Director, Obstetric Anesthesia, University of Maryland Medical Centre, Assistant Professor of Anesthesiology, Obstetrics, and Gynecology, Univerity of Maryland, School of Medicine, Baltimore, Maryland*

Robert W. McPherson, M.D.   *Associate Professor, Department of Anesthesiology and Critical Care Medicine, Director, Division of Neuroanesthesia, Johns Hopkins University, School of Medicine, Baltimore, Maryland*

John D. Meyerhoff, M.D.   *Assistant Professor, Division of Rheumatic Diseases, Department of Medicine, University of Maryland, School of Medicine, Baltimore, Maryland*

Christopher F. O'Brien, M.D.   *Instructor and Fellow of Neurology, Department of Neurology, University of Rochester, School of Medicine and Dentistry, Rochester, New York*

Alessandro Olivi, M.D.   *Fellow, Department of Neurosurgery, Johns Hopkins University, School of Medicine, Baltimore, Maryland*

John T. Repke, M.D.   *Associate Professor, Division of Maternal and Fetal Medicine, Department of Gynecology and Obstetrics, Johns Hopkins University, School of Medicine, Baltimore, Maryland*

Richard A. Rudick, M.D.   *Mellen Center for Multiple Sclerosis Treatment and Research, Department of Neurology, Cleveland Clinic Foundation, Cleveland, Ohio*

Baha M. Sibai, M.D.   *Professor and Chief, Division of Maternal-Fetal Medicine, Department of Obstetrics and Gynecology, University of Tennessee, Memphis, Tennessee*

Barney J. Stern, M.D.   *Director, Division of Neurology, Sinai Hospital of Baltimore, Inc., Associate Professor of Neurology, Johns Hopkins Medical Institutions, Baltimore, Maryland*

Gary M. Yarkony, M.D.   *Director, Rehabilitation, Midwest Regional Spinal Cord Injury System, Attending Physician and Director, Spinal Cord Injury Program, Rehabilitation Institute of Chicago, Assistant Professor, Northwestern University Medical School, Adjunct Assistant Professor, Pritzker Institute for Medical Engineering, Illinois Institute of Technology, Chicago, Illinois*

Preface

In an effort to extend the focus of the second edition of *Neurological Disorders of Pregnancy*, we have decided to combine the forces of an obstetrician/gynecologist and a neurologist. Our goal has been to create a resource that is informative both to the obstetrician and family practitioner as well as to the neurologist, internist, neurosurgeon, and other physicians involved in the care of the pregnant patient with neurological disorders. For both of us, this endeavor has been a true learning experience, and we hope our readers will benefit from the expertise of the contributing authors. Many basic science and clinical questions need to be addressed to optimize the care of the pregnant patient with neurological disease. We hope that this edition will stimulate research in the field and provide the impetus for increasing our knowledge as to how to care for the pregnant patient with neurological disease.

Phillip J. Goldstein, M.D.

Barney J. Stern, M.D.

Contents

Eclampsia

Baha M. Sibai, M.D.

Introduction

Eclampsia is defined as the development of convulsions and/or coma during pregnancy or postpartum in patients with signs and symptoms of pre-eclampsia. According to Chesley,[1] a description of the syndrome was mentioned in the ancient writing of both the Egyptians and the Chinese. Eclampsia is a disease that is unique to human pregnancy except for a rare case that has been reported in a subhuman primate.[2] It is mainly a disease of young primigravidas with an increased incidence in single, indigent nonwhite primigravida. In recent years, the reported incidence of eclampsia had ranged from 1 in 110 to 1 in 3,448 pregnancies.[3,4] In twin pregnancies, the reported incidence is 3.5%.[5] The incidence of elampsia or its extent in an individual patient may be reduced by early and adequate prenatal care as well as astute medical judgement.

Pathophysiology

The pathogenesis of pre-eclampsia continues to be the subject of extensive investigation and speculation. Several theories and pathologic mechanisms (Table I) have been implicated as possible etiologic factors, but none of these has been conclusively proven. There is considerable evidence to suggest that the development of pre-eclamp-

From Goldstein PJ, Stern BJ, (eds): *Neurological Disorders of Pregnancy. Second Revised Edition.* Mount Kisco NY, Futura Publishing Co., Inc., © 1992.

Table I.
Mechanisms Suggested as Possible Etiologies for Pre-Eclampsia

- Abnormal placentation
  - abnormal trophoblast invasion
  - increased trophoblast mass
  - abnormal uteroplacental
- Immunological dysfunction
  - primarily a disease of primigradiva
  - immunological complexes in placenta and various organs
  - immunological complexes in maternal serum
  - multisystem involvement
- Coagulation abnormalities
  - abnormal prostaglandin metabolism
  - disseminated intravascular coagulopathy
  - platelet activation and consumption
  - low antithrombin III
- Endothelial damage
  - cytotoxic factors against endothelial cells
  - increased capillary permeability
  - damaged endothelium on electron microscopy
  - increased fibronectin levels
- Dietary factors
  - protein and caloric intake
  - magnesium, calcium, zinc deficiency
  - excessive sodium intake
  - essential fatty acids deficiency
- Endocrine abnormalities
  - activated renin-angiotensin-aldosterone system
  - abnormal catecholamines
  - abnormal progesterone metabolism
  - decreased MCRDS to estradiol
- Genetic predisposition
  - increased incidence in daughter and granddaughters
  - increased incidence in sisters
  - increased incidence in patients with previous disease
- Vasospasm
  - increased sensitivity to vasoactive substances
  - reduced plasma volume in severe disease

---

sia is associated with increased trophoblastic mass (hyperplacentosis) as well as abnormal trophoblast invasion.[6] In addition, there is an increased incidence in patients with previous pre-eclampsia/eclampsia.[7] Moreover, several reports have suggested that abnormal prostaglandin metabolism[8] and endothelium damage[9,10] play a central role in the pathogenesis of pre-eclampsia. The etiologic factors implicated in the pathophysiology of pre-eclampsia have been recently reviewed by Sibai.[11]

The cause of convulsions or coma in eclamptic patients is still open for speculation. Some of the pathologic features that are implicated in the pathogenesis of eclamptic convulsions are listed in Table II.

Eclampsia is a syndrome that may be characterized by functional derangement of multiple organ systems such as cardiovascular, renal, hepatic, hematologic, and central nervous systems. Both pre-eclamptic and eclamptic patients exhibit an increased sensitivity to vasoactive substances such as angiotensin II and catecholamines. Such patients have generalized arteriolar vasospasm resulting in increased peripheral vascular resistance and increased left ventricular stroke work index. Central venous pressure is usually low (0 to 5 cm H_2O) and the pulmonary capillary wedge pressure is in the low normal range (0 to 7 mm Hg).[12,13] The plasma volume is markedly reduced compared to normal pregnancy resulting in hemoconcentration and increased blood viscosity. Renal function is usually characterized by reduced glomerular filtration rate, decreased renal plasma flow, and

---

Table II.
Possible Etiologic Factors Responsible for Convulsions in Eclampsia

- Cerebral Vasospasm
- Cerebral Hemorrhage
- Cerebral Ischemia
- Cerebral Edema
- Metabolic Encephalopathy
- Hypertensive Encephalopathy
  - Microhemorrhages
  - Microinfarcts

reduced uric acid clearance. Liver damage is usually seen as an autopsy finding in patients who die from eclampsia. The typical lesion noted is periportal necrosis with hepatocellular damage.[14] Some other pathophysiological abnormalities seen in eclamptic patients are listed in Table I as etiologic factors in pre-eclampsia.

Diagnosis

The diagnosis of eclampsia is most likely in the presence of hypertension, proteinuria, edema, and convulsions. The clinical course in the development of pre-eclampsia into eclampsia is usually characterized by a prolonged, gradual process that includes excessive weight gain and culminates in generalized convulsions and/or coma. Hypertension is the prerequisite for the diagnosis of eclampsia. The hypertension can be severe (more than 160 mm Hg systolic and/or more than 110 mm Hg diastolic) or mild (systolic blood pressure between 140 and 160 mm Hg or diastolic pressure between 90 and 110 mm Hg). In some cases, the hypertension may be "relative" (120–140/80–90 mm Hg). In this situation, hypertension is signified by any rise in blood pressure that is 30 mm Hg systolic or 15 mm Hg diastolic above first trimester blood pressure readings. Relative hypertension is seen in about 20% of eclamptic patients.[15,16]

The diagnosis of eclampsia is usually associated with significant proteinuria (more than 2+ on dip stick). The degree of proteinuria may fluctuate widely over any 24-hour period, making quantitative 24-hour urine determinations more accurate than random assessment. However, the presence of proteinuria is not required for the diagnosis of eclampsia because approximately 20% of eclamptic patients do not have proteinuria.[15,16] Abnormal weight gain (with or without clinical edema) in excess of 2 pounds per week during the third trimester might be the first warning sign. However, the diagnosis of pre-eclampsia/eclampsia is not always accompanied by excessive weight gain and/or edema during pregnancy.[15,16]

Several other clinical signs and symptoms are potentially helpful in establishing the diagnosis of eclampsia; some occur as clinical warnings even before the onset of convulsion. These include persistent occipital headache, blurred vision, photophobia, epigastric and/or right upper quadrant pain, and hyperactive deep tendon reflexes, especially with clonus.

Laboratory Findings

The diagnosis of eclampsia is not dependent on any specific laboratory data. The frequency of abnormal findings (renal, hepatic, coagulation) is influenced by multiple factors such as the presence of associated medical or obstetric complications, quality of obstetric care, and adequacy of compensatory physiological mechanisms.[17] Serum uric acid is usually elevated (> 6.2 mg/dL) in most cases of eclampsia (69%). Other renal function tests such as serum creatinine and creatinine clearance are abnormal in about 50% to 70% of the cases.[18]

Hemoconcentration (increased hematocrit and reduced plasma volume) and increased blood viscosity are seen in most cases of eclampsia. Thrombocytopenia (platelet count < 150,000 per mm^3) is seen in approximately 15% to 30% of eclamptic patients. This complication can be life-threatening in some cases. The full picture of disseminated intravascular coagulopathy may be seen in neglected cases of eclampsia and/or association with abruptio placentae and fetal demise.[17,18]

Conventional liver function tests such as alkaline phosphatase, lactic dehydrogenase, serum transaminases, and bilirubin may be elevated in 20% to 74% of eclamptic patients.[18] A syndrome of hemolysis, elevated liver enzymes, and low platelets (HELLP syndrome) is encountered in approximately 10% of eclamptic patients. This syndrome is usually seen after prolonged disease and in those patients with associated medical disease.[19]

Cerebral Pathology

Cerebral pathology in the form of edema and/or petechial hemorrhage is a common autopsy finding in patients who died from eclampsia.[20] The diagnosis of eclampsia is not dependent on any single clinical or diagnostic neurological finding. Focal neurological signs such as hemiparesis are rare. Neurodiagnostic tests such as electroencephalography (EEG), computed axial tomographic scan, lumbar puncture, and cerebral arteriography are rarely used for the diagnosis of eclampsia.

The EEG is acutely abnormal in the majority of eclamptic patients.[21-24] The EEG pattern during eclampsia is usually that of diffuse slow activity (θ or δ waves), occasionally with focal slow activity and occasional paroxysmal spike activity.[24] None of these EEG findings is pathognomonic of eclampsia.

The introduction of computed tomographic (CT) scan has provided an opportunity to investigate the nature of cerebral abnormalities in eclamptic patients. This technique is considered safe in pregnancy when performed after the first trimester. There are several reports describing the CT scan findings in complicated cases of eclampsia (patients with focal neurological signs, sudden loss of vision, and/or coma). The abnormal patterns found were either edema, hemorrhage, or infarcts. Cerebral edema was reported to be either diffuse, patchy, or localized (mostly to the occipital lobes).[25–30] The CT findings have included reversible diminished density of white matter scattered throughout the brain with or without reduced lateral ventricle size. These authors recommend using fluid restriction, dexamethasone and/or mannitol to treat such patients. Devitt et al.[31] described a case of eclampsia with acute hydrocephalus in which the CT scan evaluation demonstrated the presence of posterior fossa edema leading to obstructive hydrocephalus. The patient was treated with a ventriculoperitoneal shunt to relieve the obstruction.

Cerebral hemorrhage is a common autopsy finding in patients who died from eclampsia; however, it is an unusual finding on CT scanning. Beck and Menezes[32] reported a case of eclampsia in which CT scan evaluation demonstrated periventricular subependymal hemorrhage. Colosimo et al.[33] reported abnormal CT scan findings in five eclamptic women, one of whom demonstrated the presence of intracerebral hemorrhage. Will et al.[34] reported on three patients with eclampsia who developed acute neurological deterioration in the postpartum period. Two patients had subarachnoid hemorrhage and one had residual neurological deficit. A CT scan demonstrated the presence of infarcts in two cases and intracerebral hemorrhage in a third case. In all three cases, cerebral angiography revealed widespread arterial vasoconstriction. In the case demonstrating hemorrhage on CT scan, a magnetic resonance imaging (MRI) examination performed 1 week later was reported normal.

Sibai et al.[35] studied the CT scan findings in 20 patients with atypical eclampsia. Six patients had transient neurological deficit including three with transient cortical blindness, one was in a coma, and the others had either late postpartum eclampsia or early onset eclampsia. The CT scan findings were normal in all 20. Similar findings were also reported by Pritchard and associates.[36] In contrast, Richards et al.[37] reported abnormal CT scan findings in 15 (75%) of 20 unconscious eclamptic patients. A brain stem hemorrhage was diagnosed in 1 patient; the remaining 19 demonstrated the presence of cerebral edema of varying degrees. In addition, abnormal CT scan findings were found in 14 (29%) of 49 eclamptic patients studied by Brown and associates.[37] These authors noted that the incidence of abnormal CT scan findings significantly increased with the recent use of high-resolution CT scan equipment The CT scans were performed over a 6-year period with the highest incidence of abnormal findings (50%) being present during the final year of the study. The reported CT scan abnormalities ranged from occipital hypodensities to diffuse cerebral edema. The authors noted that CT scan findings altered the clinical management in only one patient.

Crawford et al.[38] described abnormal MRI findings in one eclamptic patient. The study was performed 48-hours postpartum and the findings were consistent with focal edematous changes. The CT scan in this patient was normal. Fredriksson et al.[39] studied repeated CT scan and MRI findings in two eclamptic women. Computed tomograms showed decreased attenuation, and T2 weighted MRI showed increased signal intensity focally in the cerebral cortex and the deep gray and white matter. Repeat CT scan and MRI studies revealed complete resolution. Although more studies are needed, MRI holds promise as a useful diagnostic technique in understanding the pathophysiology of eclamptic convulsions.

During the past 12 years, 265 eclamptic women were managed at this institution. Sixty-six patients underwent CT scanning: in 6 (9%) the scans demonstrated the presence of edema. Eighteen patients had MRI evaluation; 5 (22%) were abnormal. The characteristic abnormality seen on MRI was multiple areas of increased signal on T2 images in the border zones between the major cerebral arteries. The CT scan was also abnormal in only one of these five patients. Cerebral angiography was performed in five patients, one of whom demonstrated the presence of diffuse vasospasm. Thus, it is the author's opinion that neurodiagnostic tests should be restricted to evaluation of eclamptic patients with focal neurological deficits or with atypical onset (early onset, late onset, refractoriness to magnesium sulfate) to rule out the presence of potential cerebrovascular pathology such as ischemic or hemorrhagic stroke. The differential diagnosis of convulsions during pregnancy and the puerperium includes a list of med-

Table III.
Differential Diagnosis of Eclampsia

   I. Stroke
      1. cerebral venous thrombosis
      2. cerebral arterial occlusion
      3. intracerebral hemorrhage
      4. subarachmoid hemorrhage
  II. Hypertensive disease
      1. hypertensive encephalopathy
      2. phoechromocytoma
 III. Space-occupying central nervous system lesions
      1. brain tumor
      2. brain abscess
 IV. Infectious diseases
      1. meningitis
      2. encephalitis
  V. Metabolic diseases
      1. hypoglycemia
      2. hypocalcemia
      3. water intoxication
 VI. Epilepsy
VII. Drug effects

ical and central nervous system disorders (Table III). Specific topics are discussed elsewhere in this book.

Clinical Course

The onset of eclamptic convulsions can be ante partum, intra-partum, or postpartum. About 75% of eclampsia cases develop before delivery, while 25% occur after delivery. Although most cases of post-partum eclampsia appear within the first 24 hours, some cases can develop beyond 48-hours postpartum and have been reported as late as 2-weeks postpartum.[40] In such cases, an extensive neurological evaluation should be performed to rule out the presence of other cerebral pathology.

Almost all cases (95%) of ante partum eclampsia develop during the third trimester.[41] The remaining cases occur between 21 to 27 weeks gestation. In rare instances, eclampsia has been reported to occur before 20 weeks gestation.[42]

Management

The basic principles in the management of eclampsia involve the following measures:

1. Maternal support of vital functions
2. Control of convulsions and prevention of recurrent convulsions
3. Correction of maternal hypoxemia and/or acidemia
4. Control severe hypertension within a safe range
5. Initiate process of delivery.

Eclamptic convulsions constitute a life-threatening emergency. The cardinal steps in management are to prevent maternal injury during the convulsive episode, such as insertion of a padded tongue blade between the teeth and to safeguard against potential maternal morbidity following the convulsions. The most urgent part of therapy is to insure maternal oxygenation and to minimize the risk of aspiration.

Parenteral magnesium sulfate ($MgSO_4$ $7H_2O$ USP) is the drug of choice to control and prevent eclamptic convulsions. The drug does not cause any significant maternal-neonatal central nervous system depression when used properly. During its administration, the mother is awake and alert and laryngeal reflexes are intact, which helps to protect against aspiration. Fetal magnesium levels tend to equilibrate with maternal levels following prolonged administration; however, neuromuscular depression in the newborn is rarely seen with proper use of the drug.[43] In contrast, the use of other anticonvulsants such as narcotics, sedatives (diazepam), tranquilizers (phenothiazine), and barbiturates can cause significant maternal-neonatal central nervous system and respiratory depression.[44] The use of the agents may depress the laryngeal reflexes and allow aspiration.

The usual anticonvulsive dose of magnesium sulfate to arrest eclamptic convulsions is 4 to 6 g given intravenously over 5 to 10 minutes. This dose is followed by one of three commonly used regimens as recommended in Table IV. If a patient develops recurrent convulsions after the administration of magnesium sulfate, then another bolus dose of 2 to 5 g can be given over 3 to 5 minutes. If convulsions recur, then a short-acting barbiturate such as sodium

Table IV.
Specific Recommended Regimens of Magnesium Sulfate to Treat Eclamaptic Convulsions

I. Pritchard's IM regimen
   4 grams IV over 3 to 5 minutes + 10 grams IM as loading dose
   Maintenance dose of 5 grams IM every 4 hours
II. Zuspan's IV regimen
   4 grams IV over 5 to 10 minutes as loading, maintenance dose of 1 to 2 grams per hour
III. Sibai's IV regimen
   6 grams IV over 120 minutes as loading, maintenance dose of 2 to 3 grams per hour

amobarbital should be given in a dose of up to 250 mg intravenously over 3 minutes to control the seizures.

Maternal plasma levels of magnesium (Mg) after parenteral administration of $MgSO_4$ depend on the volume of distribution and renal clearance of the magnesium ion. The volume of distribution is usually increased during pregnancy, and more so in eclamptic patients due to extracellular fluid retention. In contrast, renal clearance is usually decreased in eclamptic patients. The usual loading dose of 4 g given intravenously is likely to result in instant maternal Mg plasma levels of 5 to 8 mg/dL. This increase is transient and plasma levels fall rapidly within the first 60 minutes. The regimen recommended by Pritchard[45] will ordinarily keep maternal plasma Mg levels between 5 and 8 mg/dL. The maintenance dose of 1 g/h recommended by Zuspan[46] will produce plasma levels between 3 and 4 mg/dL, but even the dose of 2 g/h has been demonstrated to produce plasma levels below mg/dL in approximately 50% of patients.[43] The recommended "therapeutic" levels of magnesium range from 4.8 to 8.4 mg/dL, however, the acutal therapeutic level is unknown. An occasional patient might develop convulsions at plasma magnesium levels that are well in the therapeutic range (Fig. 1).

The first sign of magnesium toxicity is loss of patellar reflexes that occurs at plasma magnesium levels of 10 to 12 mg/dL. Hence, any order for administration of the drug should include checking patellar reflexes before continuing the maintenance dose. Other early signs and symptoms of magnesium toxicity include nausea, a feeling of warmth, flushing, slurred speech, and somnolence, that occur at

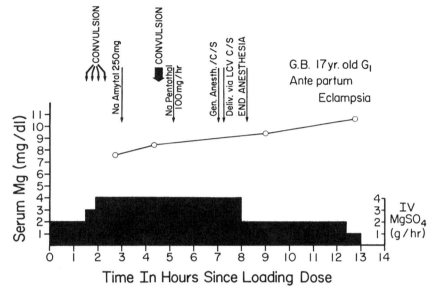

Figure 1: A seventeen-year-old G_1 (gravida 1) who continued to have convulsions despite adequate serum magnesium levels. The patient had to be intubated and maintained on sodium pentothal drip to control convulsions. The mother was neurologically intact following delivery. An EEG performed then revealed diffuse encephalopathy, and CT scan was normal. She had normal findings on follow-up and has had a normotensive pregnancy since then.

plasma levels of 9 to 12 mg/dL. Respiratory difficulty will develop at plasma levels of 15 to 17 mg/dL, while total paralysis and cardiac arrest develop at plasma levels of 30 to 35 mg/dL.[47] It is important to keep an ampule containing 1 g of calcium gluconate at the bedside to be used as an antidote in case of magnesium toxicity.

The anticonvulsant mechanism of action of magnesium ion is unknown. There is considerable controversy surrounding its peripheral versus central nervous system effects. This subject was recently reviewed by Sibai et al.[24] Some authors suggest that magnesium sulfate is a poor anticonvulsant because it controls convulsions by blocking peripheral neuromuscular transmission because it interferes with the liberation of acetylcholine and reduces the sensitivity to acetylcholine at the motor end plate. This view is supported by the experimental work of Hilmy and Somjen in both animals[48] and humans.[49]

The authors induced hypermagnesemia sufficient to paralyze skeletal muscles in two males, but they were unable to induce significant depression of the central nervous system. Based on these findings, these authors suggested that the central nervous system is protected from high levels of serum magnesium by a barrier mechanism that keeps the concentration of magnesium in the brain within physiological limits. On the other hand, a reduction in electroencephalographic neuronal burst firing and interictal spike generation was demonstrated in animals made epileptic by topical application of penicillin-G to the cerebral cortex of dogs, cats, and subhuman primates.[50] In these experiments, Borges and Gucer[50] demonstrated that the degree of suppression was directly proportional to maternal serum magnesium levels, was reversible, and occurred at magnesium levels well below those required for complete neuromuscular blockade. However, the technique used in such experiments is known to alter the permeability of the brain to magnesium ion, and the authors did not study a control group of animals made epileptic who did not receive magnesium sulfate. In addition, large clinical studies using magnesium sulfate in patients with severe pre-eclampsia/eclampsia have suggested that magnesium presents convulsions through a central nervous system effect because the therapeutic levels of magnesium reported as being adequate to control convulsions are well below the levels needed to produce complete neuromuscular blockade.[45]

Sibai et al.[24] studied the EEG findings in 36 eclamptic patients during the administration of magnesium sulfate (serum magnesium levels 4.5–11.0 mg/dL) and after magnesium sulfate was discontinued (serum magnesium levels 1.8–2.5 mg/dL). Seventy-five percent of the eclamptic patients had abnormal EEG findings despite adequate serum magnesium levels. In addition, there was no difference in EEG findings recorded during the magnesium sulfate administration and the EEG findings following the discontinuance of magnesium sulfate. Moreover, four of the patients demonstrated paroxysmal spike activity with two of them having evidence of seizure activity recorded on the EEG despite adequate magnesium levels. The authors concluded that abnormal EEG findings in eclamptic patients are not altered by serum magnesium levels achieved in the clinical management of these patients. It is important to emphasize that adequate therapeutic levels of magnesium do not influence the abnormal EEG patterns recorded in eclamptic patients (Fig. 2).[24] Other actions of magnesium ion might include a transient and mild hypotensive effect when given as an

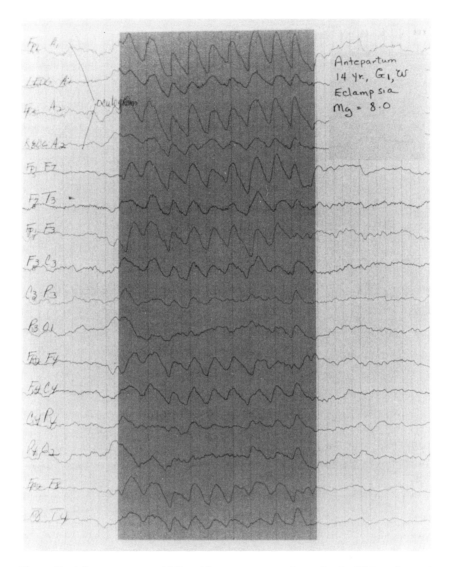

Figure 2: A fourteen-year-old G₁ with ante partum eclampsia. An EEG performed at serum magnesium level of 8.0 mg/dL reveals diffuse encephalopathy with marked slowing in the form of δ waves.

intravenous bolus, mild reduction in uterine activity during active labor, and variable effects on beat-to-beat fetal rate variability.[45]

Other Anticonvulsants

In many centers outside the United States, magnesium sulfate is rarely used to prevent or treat eclamptic convulsions.[51,52] During the past 60 years, numerous anticonvulsive drugs have been used for this indication. Some of these drugs have included bromethol, chloral hydrate, paraldehyde, phenothiazines, lytic cocktails, barbiturates, diazepam, chlordiazepoxide, and clonazepam. The use of large doses of diazepam (> 30 mg) intravenously during labor is associated with loss of beat-to-beat fetal heart rate variability and significant neonatal morbidity (respiratory depression, apnea, hypotonia). The use of chlormethiazole in anticonvulsive doses has been associated with maternal respiratory depression and even death.[53] The use of intravenous phenobarbitone has the potential of producing laryngospasm and circulatory and respiratory depression. It is important to note that none of these drugs has been proven to be superior to or as effective as magnesium sulfate in treating eclamptic convulsions.

Recently, phenytoin has been advocated for the prevention and treatment of convulsions in the United Kingdom, Australia, and Canada.[53,54] In addition, its use for this indication has been recommended by some internists and neurologists in the United States.[55-57] These latter authors criticized the wide use of magnesium sulfate as being empiric and dogmatic, and the drug was labelled as being "a poor anticonvulsant" and "a bad medicine". Slater et al.[53] evaluated a regimen of phenytoin based on maternal weight in only 26 patients (7 had severe pre-eclampsia, 17 had mild disease, and 2 had eclampsia). They reported no seizures after the phenytoin was begun (750 mg top 1250 mg intravenously at a rate of < 25 mg/min). In addition, the authors noted no major maternal or neonatal side effect. Moosa and El-Zayat[58] used phenytoin (100 mg three times a day) in 50 pre-eclamptic women and compared the pregnancy outcome to that in another 50 patients who received similar management except for phenytoin. They suggested that phenytoin had a favorable effect on maternal blood pressure and fluid balance in addition to its anticonvulsive effects. On the other hand, Tuffnell et al.[59] reported that 3 of

18 (17%) pre-eclamptic/eclamptic women developed further convulsions after the administration of the recommended dose. A similar experience was also reported by Slater et al.[60] in their subsequent report in which 2 of 8 (25%) eclamptic patients developed another seizure following the initiation of the phenytoin infusion. Ryan et al.[54] reported their clinical experience with phenytoin prophylaxis in 104 patients with severe pre-eclampsia/eclampsia, 5 of whom had eclampsia. The authors evaluated phenytoin serum levels and maternal side effects using four different regimens. The final regimen (15 mg/kg intravenously, given as 10 mg/kg initially, then 5 mg/kg 2 hours later) provided adequate therapeutic levels and had minimal maternal perinatal side effects. Eighty patients received this regimen with one (1.25%) developing convulsions after this regimen. In their discussion, the authors noted another patient who developed convulsions after an adequate dose of phenytoin. In addition, the authors suggested obtaining serum albumin and phenytoin levels during the administration of this drug.

Friedman and associates[61] reported a prospective randomized clinical trial comparing a standardized regimen of intravenous phenytoin (n = 45) to intravenous magnesium sulfate (n = 60), as seizure prophylaxis, in pre-eclampsia/eclampsia. No seizures occurred in pre-eclamptic patients who received either drug, but subsequent convulsions developed in the two eclamptic patients assigned to the phenytoin group. The authors noted lower maternal side effects, shorter duration of the active phase of labor, and a lower amount of estimated blood loss at vaginal delivery in the phenytoin group.

In summary, there is limited experience with the use of phenytoin in pre-eclampsia/eclampsia. The data comparing the efficacy and safety of magnesium sulfate to phenytoin have been recently reviewed by Sibai.[62] Until a clinical trial is conducted, comparing the safety and efficacy of magnesium sulfate and phenytoin for the treatment of eclamptic seizures, a definitive recommendation for a change in medical management cannot be made.

Following control of convulsions and adequate maternal oxygenation, the next step in management should involve keeping maternal blood pressure within a reasonably safe range (systolic blood pressure below 160 mm Hg and/or diastolic pressure below 110 mm Hg). The objective of treating severe hypertension is to prevent stroke without compromising uteroplacental blood flow that is already reduced in eclampsia. Hydralazine is a safe and effective drug to use in the management of severe hypertension during pregnancy. The drug should be administered intravenously as intermittent bolus injections of 5- to 10-mg doses every 20 minutes. Frequent and close monitoring of maternal blood pressure is necessary to titrate the dose of hydralazine against maternal blood pressure. The ultimate goal of therapy is to keep systolic blood pressure between 140 and 150 mm Hg and/or diastolic pressure between 90 and 100 mm Hg. Other potent antihypertensive medications such as sodium nitroprusside or nitroglycerine are rarely needed in eclampsia. Diuretics are not indicated except in the presence of pulmonary edema.

Donaldson[55] claims that eclamptic convulsions are secondary to cortical lesions developing after a sudden increase in blood pressure in a previously normotensive patient. He attributes these cortical lesions to failure of cerebral autoregulation resulting in rupture of capillary junctions with leakage of both plasma and red blood cells. Consequently, he believes that lowering of maternal blood pressure is essential to the prevention of eclamptic seizures. Hence, he suggests that "magnesium sulfate is a poor anticonvulsant" because it is not an antihypertensive agent. Jost[21] studied the EEG findings in nine eclamptic patients and reported that the EEG abnormalities are directly related to the severity of maternal hypertension and that these abnormalities will resolve following lowering of maternal blood pressure to the normotensive range. However, Kolstad[23] and Sibai et al.[24] did not find any correlation between the degree of maternal blood pressure elevation and the presence of an EEG abnormality. Additionally, Sibai et al.[24] did not find any correlation between the percentage rise in mean arterial blood pressure from the last prenatal visit to blood pressure reading at the time of EEG recording and the subsequent EEG findings. Such findings do not suggest any relationship between eclamptic convulsions and degree of maternal hypertension.

As stated earlier, the EEGs were acutely abnormal in approximately 75% of eclamptic patients studied. Some of these abnormalities persisted for up to 6 months following eclampsia. However, all of them gradually returned to normal on follow-up. It is also important to note that such EEG abnormalities were recorded at a time when these patients were normotensive at 6-weeks postpartum. Again, this tends to emphasize the lack of relationship between the patient's blood pressure and EEG findings. Computed tomographic scans were performed in 26 patients who had complicated and/or typical presentation of eclampsia (three patients had transient neurological deficit and three patients had transient cortical blindness). The CT scans were normal in all. Cerebral arteriograms were performed in three patients to rule out the presence of associated cerebrovascular pathology, and likewise were normal. Transient neurological deficits were observed in a few patients, but none of them had residual neurological deficit on follow-up. Likewise, most patients were normotensive within 6 weeks after delivery and several patients had one or more uneventful normotensive pregnancies following the eclamptic episode.

Labor and Delivery

Delivery of the fetus and placenta is the definitive treatment of eclampsia. Once convulsions and severe hypertension are well controlled and the patient has been stabilized, preparation for delivery should be initiated. All patients should have continuous fetal observation. Intravenous oxytocin may be used to induce labor. Severe fetal bradycardia and late decelerations are frequently seen during and immediately following eclamptic convulsions that may be secondary to maternal hypoxia and acidosis. Management of such patterns should involve correcting maternal hypoxia and acidosis, which is commonly followed by gradual recovery of the fetal heart rate pattern.[63,64]

Maternal analgesia can be provided by the intermittent use of small doses (25–50 mg) of intravenous meperidine. Local infiltration anesthesia with pudendal block may be used in most cases of vaginal delivery. A balanced general anesthesia can be used for abdominal deliveries, but probably the anesthesia of choice is an epidural. There has been controversy regarding the use of epidural analgesia-anesthesia with some authors[65] against its use because of the potential maternal hypotension and reduced uteroplacental blood flow, but other authors[66] reported no adverse maternal or fetal outcome when epidural analgesia was used in such patients. This subject was recently reviewed by Jones and Joyce.[67] It must be emphasized that the use of epidural analgesia in such patients requires the availability of central hemodynamic monitoring and personnel with special expertise in obstetrical anesthesia.

All patients should have laboratory evaluation of urine protein and specific gravity, creatinine, electrolytes, platelet count, and liver enzymes. The patient should be monitored very closely during labor and delivery with special attention to fluid intake and output. Such patients are at increased risk for pulmonary edema from fluid overload and compromised renal function. Urinary output should be monitored every hour and fluid administration should not exceed 150 cc/h. Parenteral magnesium sulfate should be continued throughout labor and delivery and for at least 24-hours postpartum. If the patient has oliguria (less than 100 mL/4 hours), the rate of both fluid administration and dose of $MgSO_4$ should be reduced. It is advisable that all such patients, especially those of less than 36 weeks gestation, should be managed at tertiary care centers.

Following delivery, the patient should be monitored in the recovery room, with evaluation of reflexes included, for at least 24 hours during which time maternal vital signs and intake-output should be monitored hourly. Some of these patients might even require intensive and invasive hemodynamic monitoring during labor and postpartum. Most patients will show evidence of resolution of the disease process within 24 hours after delivery. However, some patients might require intensive monitoring for several days. Such eclamptic patients might require $MgSO_4$ treatment for more than 24-hours postpartum. Some authors recommend the use of short-term phenobarbital therapy when parenteral magnesium sulfate is discontinued in hospitalized eclamptic patients during the immediate postpartum period. This recommendation would appear to be reasonable in view of the persistent EEG abnormalities in some of these patients. However, such therapy will prevent early ambulation, and its efficacy has not been studied in a controlled manner. In addition, some internists and neurologists prescribe long-term anticonvulsive therapy (as for epilepsy) for the majority of patients with postpartum eclampsia. This therapy is unwarranted because most patients will have normal EEGs within 6 weeks after delivery. Most patients will be normotensive at the time of discharge from the hospital, and no patient should have any neurological deficit at that time. Some patients might continue to have severe hypertension that can be controlled with a variety of antihypertensives. Such patients should be reevaluated within 1 week after discharge from the hospital. Most of these patients will be normotensive on follow-up, at which time antihypertensive medications can be discontinued.

Pregnancy Outcome

Eclampsia is associated with increased perinatal mortality and morbidity. The reported perinatal mortality varies between 10% and 28%. For fetuses alive on admission to perinatal centers, the neonatal mortality rate is approximately 4%.[68] The recent advances in obstetrics and neonatal intensive care units are responsible for the improved perinatal outcome. Most of the perinatal deaths are related to prematurity, severe fetal growth retardation, and increased incidence of abruptio placentae.[68] These same factors are responsible for the increased neonatal morbidity encountered in infants of eclamptic mothers.

Eclampsia continues to be a major cause of maternal mortality and is associated with significant maternal morbidity. The reported maternal mortality rate varies between 0% and 14%.[16,36,69,70] Most cases of maternal mortality are associated with complicated or mismanaged cases or eclampsia.[69,70] Potential maternal complications are summarized in Table V. Some of them are iatrogenic (pulmonary edema or aspiration) while others are unavoidable (retinal detachment). Abruptio placentae is the most frequent complication while intracerebral hemorrhage is the most serious.

The long-term prognosis of both mother and infant of well managed cases of eclampsia suggests normal growth and development for infants[68] and no residual neurological deficit for the mothers.[7,71] The long-term follow-up of patients following eclampsia was the subject of a remarkable study by Chesley and associates.[71] The authors

---

Table V.
Maternal Complications in Eclampsia

Abruptio placentae
Disseminated intravascular coagulopathy
Intracerebral hemorrhage
Pulmonary edema
Aspiration pneumonia
Acute renal tubular necrosis
Retinal detachment
Ruptured liver
Transient cortical blindness

studied 267 women for up to 40 years following eclampsia. They found that the incidence of chronic hypertension and remote mortality was increased among women who had eclampsia as multiparas, but not among those who had eclampsia during the first pregnancy. Sexton[72] reported on six patients who developed epilepsy several years following eclampsia and concluded that eclampsia may result in long-term neurological deficit. The patients in that report, however, were apparently selected from a group of cases of eclampsia that were complicated by hemorrhage, shock, and sepsis.

Sibai and associates[7] compared the subsequent pregnancy outcomes and remote prognosis in 406 young women who had either severe pre-eclampsia (n = 287) or eclampsia (n = 119) during their first pregnancies to a matched control group of 409 women who remained normotensive throughout their first pregnancies, and found an increased incidence of pre-eclampsia/eclampsia (14% vs. 5.6%). In the subgroup that was followed ten years or longer, the incidence of subsequent chronic hypertension among the pre-eclamptic group was 51%. None of the eclamptic women had subsequent seizures or neurological deficit on follow-up.

The incidence of eclampsia (1:320) at the University of Tennessee, Memphis, a tertiary referral center for five states, has not changed over the past 30 years. During the last 12 years, 265 cases of eclampsia were managed. The incidence of eclampsia in women registered in the prenatal clinics is about one in 620 deliveries. Analysis of all cases suggests that earlier diagnosis, adequate prenatal care, and appropriate management of pre-eclampsia might have prevented eclampsia in about two thirds of the cases.[16,41] The total perinatal mortality in that group of patients was approximately 10%. The majority of perinatal deaths was due to either extreme prematurity (< 700 g), congenital anomalies, or congenital infections. For those fetuses alive on admission to the perinatal center, the perinatal mortality was approximately 5%. One maternal death in a patient who was moribund on admission was recorded; however, maternal morbidity was frequent. Abruptio placentae occurred in 10% of cases, while pulmonary edema developed in 4.2% and acute renal failure developed in 4.5%. Eight patients (3%) had cardiorespiratory arrest and 5 (2%) had aspiration pneumonia (all of them were maternal transport patients). Almost all cases of cardiorespiratory arrest and/or aspiration pneumonia were seen in patients who received multiple pharmacotherapy (phenytoin, phenobarbital, phenothiazines, or diazepam). Several of these patients developed convulsions while receiving the above drugs as prophylaxis against convulsions when pre-eclamptic. In addition, 4 of 7 eclamptic women who received phenytoin developed subsequent convulsions despite adequate therapeutic levels. During the past 12 years, more than 10,000 woman received intravenous magnesium sulfate for pre-eclampsia/eclampsia. The incidence of eclampsia in women receiving intravenous magnesium sulfate for pre-eclampsia was about 0.3%. Additionally, approximately 13% of the eclamptic women developed one or more convulsions after instituting magnesium sulfate. The majority remained free of seizures after an additional 2–4 g of intravenous bolus of magnesium sulfate. Only two patients required muscular paralysis with intubation to control further seizures.

Transient neurological deficit developed in 8 (3.1%) and transient cortical blindness occurred in 6 (2.3%) of these patients. Three patients were comatose and no patient developed intracerebral hemorrhage. In addition, none of these patients had any residual neurological deficit or seizures on long-term follow-up.

References

1. Chesley LC: History. In: *Hypertensive Disorders in Pregnancy.* Edited by LC Chesley New York, NY: Appleton-Century Crofts; 1978:17–34.
2. Baird JM Jr: Eclampsia in a lowland gorilla. *Am J Obstet Gynecol* 141:345, 1981.
3. Richards AM, Moodley J, Graham DI, et al: Active management of the unconscious eclamptic patient. *Br J Obstet Gynecol* 93:554, 1986.
4. Moller B, Lindmark G: Eclampsia in Sweden, 1976–1980. *Acta Obstet Gynecol Scand* 65:307, 1988.
5. Long PA, Oats JN: Pre-eclampsia in twin pregnancy—severity and pathogenesis. *Aust NZ J Obstet Gynecol* 27:1, 1987.
6. Khong TY, DeWolf F, Robertson WB, et al: Inadequate maternal vascular response to placentation in pregnancies complicated by pre-eclampsia and by small-for-gestational age infants. *Br J Obstet Gynecol* 93:1049, 1986.
7. Sibai BM, El-Mozer A, Gonzalez-Ruiz A: Severe pre-eclampsia/eclampsia in young primigravid women: subsequent pregnancy outcome and remote prognosis. *Am J Obstet Gynecol* 155:1011, 1986.
8. Friedman SA: Pre-eclampsia: a review of the role of prostacyclins. *Obstet Gynecol* 71:122, 1988.
9. Roberts JM, Taylor RN, Rodgers GM, et al: Pre-eclampsia: an endothelial cell disorder. *Am J Obstet Gynecol* 161:1200, 1989.
10. Shanklin DR, Sibai BM: Ultrastructural aspects of pre-eclampsia. I. Pla-

cental bed and uterine boundary vessels. *Am J Obstet Gynecol* 161:735, 1989.

11. Sibai BM: Pre-eclampsia/eclampsia. *Curr Prob Obstet Gynecol Fertil* 13(1):1–45.

12. Hankins GVD, Wendel GD, Cunningham FG, et al: Longitudinal evaluation of hemodynamic changes in eclampsia. *Am J Obstet Gynecol* 150:506, 1984.

13. Mabie WC, Ratts T, Sibai BM: The central hemodynamics of severe pre-eclampsia. *Am J Obstet Gynecol* 161:1443, 1989.

14. Sheehan JL, Lynch JB: *Pathology of Toxemia of Pregnancy.* Baltimore, MD: Williams & Wilkins, 1973.

15. Sibai BM, McCubbin JH, Anderson GD, et al: Eclampsia I. Observations from 67 recent cases. *Obstet Gynecol* 58:609, 1981.

16. Sibai BM: Eclampsia VI. Maternal-perinatal outcome in 254 consecutuive cases. *Am J Obstet Gynecol* 163(3):1049–1054, 1990.

17. Lopez-Llera M, Espinsoa MD, Deleon MD, et al: Abnormal coagulation and fibrimolysis in eclampsia. *Am J Obstet Gynecol* 124:681, 1976.

18. Sibai BM, Anderson GD, McCubbin JH: Eclampsia II. Clinical significant of laboratory findings. *Obstet Gynecol* 59:153, 1982.

19. Sibai BM, Taslimi MM, El-Nazer A, et al: Maternal-perinatal outcome associated with the syndrome of hemolysis, elevated liver enzymes, and low platelets in severe pre-eclampsia/eclampsia. *Am J Obstet Gynecol* 155:501, 1986.

20. Hibbard LT: Maternal mortality due to acute toxemia. *Obstet Gynecol* 42:263, 1973.

21. Jost H: Electroencephalographic records in relation to blood pressure changes in eclampsia. *Am J Med Sci* 216:57, 1948.

22. McIntosh RR: The significance of fits in eclampsia. *J Obstet Gynaecol Br Emp* 59:197, 1952.

23. Kolstad P: The pratical value of electro-encephalography in pre-eclampsia and eclampsia. *Acta Obset et Gynec Scandinav* 40:127, 1961.

24. Sibai BM, Spinnato JA, Watson DL, et al: Effect of magnesium sulfate on electroencephalographic findings in pre-eclampsia/eclampsia. *Obstet Gynecol* 64:261, 1984.

25. Beeson JH, Duda EE: Computed axial tomography scan demonstration of cerebral edema in eclampsia preceded by blindness. *Obstet Gynecol* 60:529, 1982.

26. Benedetti TJ, Quilligan EJ: Cerebral edema in severe pregnancy-induced hypertension. *Am J Obstet Gynecol* 137:860, 1980.

27. Kirby JC, Jaindl JJ: Cerebral CT findings in toxemia of pregnancy. *Radiology* 151:114, 1984.

28. Gaitz JP, Bamford CR: Unusual computed tomographic scan in eclampsia. *Arch Neurol* 39:66, 1983.

29. Naheedy MH, Biller J, Schiffer M, et al: Toxemia of pregnancy: cerebral CT findings. *J Comput Assist Tomogr* 9:497, 1985.

30. Dunn R, Lee W, Cotton DB: Evaluation by computerized axial tomography of eclamptic women with seizures refractory to magnesium sulfate therapy. *Am J Obstet Gynecol* 155:267, 1986.

31. Devitt JH, Noseworthy TW, Shustack A, et al: Acute hydrocephalus and eclampsia. *Can Med Assoc J* 134:370, 1986.
32. Beck DW, Menezes AH: Intracerebral hemorrhage in a patient with eclampsia. *JAMA* 246:1492, 1981.
33. Colosimo C, Fileni A, Moschini M, et al: CT findings in eclampsia. *Neuroradiology* 27:313, 1985.
34. Will AD, Lewis KL, Hinshaw DB, et al: Cerebral vasoconstriction in toxemia. *Neurology* 37:1555, 1987.
35. Sibai BM, Spinnato JA, Watson DL, et al: Eclampsia IV. Neurological findings and future outcome. *Am J Obstet Gynecol* 152:184, 1985.
36. Pritchard JA, Cunningham FG, Pritchard SA: The Parkland Memorial Hospital protocol for treatment of eclampsia: evaluation of 245 cases. *Am J Obstet Gynecol* 148:951, 1984.
37. Brown CEL, Purdy P, Cunningham FG: Head computed tomographic scans in women with eclampsia. *Am J Obstet Gynecol* 159:915, 1988.
38. Crawford S, Varner MW, Digre KB, et al: Cranial magnetic resonance imaging in eclampsia. *Obstet Gynecol* 70:474, 1987.
39. Fredriksson K, Lindvall O, Ingemarsson I, et al: Repeated cranial computed tomographic and magnetic resonance imaging scans in two cases of eclampsia. *Stroke* 20:547, 1989.
40. Watson DL, Sibai BM, Shaver DV, et al: Late postpartum eclampsia: an update. *S Med J* 76:1487, 1983.
41. Sibai BM, Abdella TN, Spinnato JA, et al: Eclampsia V. The incidence of non-preventable eclampsia. *Am J Obstet Gynecol* 154:581, 1986.
42. Sibai BM, Abdella TN, Taylor HA: Eclampsia in the first half of pregnancy. *J Rep Med* 27:706, 1982.
43. Sibai BM: Reassessment of intravenous $MgSO_4$ therapy in pregnancy preeclampsia/eclampsia. *Magnesium Bull* 4:81, 1982.
44. Hibbard BM, Rosen M: The management of severe pre-eclampsia and eclampsia. *Br J Anesthesiol* 49:3, 1977.
45. Pritchard JA: The use of magnesium sulfate in pre-eclampsia/eclampsia. *J Reprod Med* 23:107, 1979.
46. Zuspan FP: Problems encountered in the treatment of pregnancy-induced hypertension. *Am J Obstet Gynecol* 131:591, 1978.
47. McCubbin JH, Sibai BM, Abdella TN, et al: Cardiopulmonary arrest due to acute maternal hypermagnesemia. *Lancet* 9:1058, 1981.
48. Hilmy MI, Somjen GG: Distribution and tissue uptake of magnesium related to its pharmacological effects. *Am J Physiol* 214:406, 1968.
49. Somjen G, Hilmy M, Stephen CR: Failure to anesthetize human subjects by intravenous administration of magnesium sulfate. *J Pharmacol Exp Ther* 154:652, 1966.
50. Borges LF, Gucer G: Effect of magnesium on epileptic foci. *Epilepsia* 19:81, 1978.
51. Lewis PG, Bulpitt CJ, Zuspan FP: A comparison of current British and American practice in the management of hypertension in pregnancy. *J Obstet Gynecol* 1:78, 1980.
52. Trudinger BJ, Parik I: Attitudes to the management of hypertension in

pregnancy: a survey of Australian fellows. *Aust NZ Obstet J Gynecol* 22:191, 1982.

53. Slater RM, Wilcox FL, Smith WF, et al: Phenytoin infusion in severe pre-eclampsia. *Lancet* 1:1417, 1987.
54. Ryan G, Lange IR, Naugerl MA: Clinical experience with phenytoin prophylaxis in severe pre-eclampsia. *Am J Obstet Gynecol* 161:1297, 1989.
55. Donaldson JO: Does magnesium sulfate treat eclamptic convulsions? *Clin Neuropharmacol* 9:37, 1986.
56. Kaplan PW, Lesser RP, Fisher RS, et al: No, magnesium sulfate should not be used in treating eclamptic convulsions. *Arch Neurol* 45:1361, 1988.
57. Hachinski V: Magnesium sulfate in the treatment of eclampsia. *Arch Neurol* 45:11364, 1988.
58. Moosa SM, El-Zazat SG: Phenytoin infusion in severe pre-eclampsia. *Lancet* 2:1147, 1987.
59. Tuffnell D, O'Donovan P, Lilfard RF, et al: Phenytoin in pre-eclampsia. *Lancet* 2:273, 1989.
60. Slater RM, Wilcox FL, Smith WD, et al: Phenytoin in pre-eclampsia. *Lancet* 2:1224, 1989.
61. Friedman SA, Lim KH, Baker CA, et al: A comparison of intravenous phenytoin sodium and magnesium sulfate in pre-eclampsia. Abstract #12. Proceedings of the 10th Annual Meeting of the Society of Perinatal Obstetricians. Houston, Texas, January 23–27, 1990.
62. Sibai BM: Magnesium sulfate is the ideal anticonvulsant in pre-eclampsia/eclampsia. *Am J Obstet Gynecol* 162:1141–1145, 1990.
63. Boehm, FH, Growdon JH: The effect of eclamptic convulsions of the fetal heart rate. *Am J Obstet Gynecol* 120:851, 1974.
64. Paul RH, Kee SK, Bernstein SG: Changes in fetal heart rate: uterine contraction patterns associated with eclampsia. *Am J Obstet Gynecol* 130:165, 1978.
65. Lindheimer MD, Kata AL: Hypertension in pregnancy. *N Engl J Med* 313:675, 1985.
66. Benedetti TJ, Benedetti JK, Stenchiver MA: Severe pre-eclampsia: maternal and fetal outcome. *Clin Exp Hypertens* 1(2–3):401–416, 1982.
67. Jones MM, Joyce TH: Anesthesia for the parturient with pregnancy induced hypertension. *Clin Obstet-Gynecol* 30:591, 1987.
68. Sibai BM, Anderson DG, Abdella TN, et al: Eclampsia III. Neonatal outcome, growth, and development. *Am J Obstet Gynecol* 146:307, 1983.
69. Lopez-Leera MM: Complicated eclampsia: ifteen years experience in a referral medical center. *Am J Obstet Gynecol* 142:28, 1982.
70. Adetoro OO: A sixteen year survey of maternal mortality associated with eclampsia in Llorin, Nigeria. *Int J Gynecol Obstet* 30:117, 1989.
71. Chesley LC, Annitto JE, Casgrove RA: The remote prognosis of eclamptic women: sixth periodic report. *Am J Obstet Gynecol* 124:446, 1976.
72. Sexton JA: Epilepsy as a sequel of obstetrical complications. *J Kentucky Med Assoc* 74:595, 1976.

2

Epilepsy in Pregnancy

Allan Krumholz, M.D.

Introduction

Epilepsy is the most frequent serious neurological syndrome encountered by obstetricians and is among the most common disorders treated by neurologists.[1] Epilepsy is estimated to affect approximately 4% of the population, and approximately 10% of people may have a seizure at some time in their lives.[2]

Seizures and epilepsy in pregnancy pose numerous problems for patients and their doctors. For example, pregnancy may adversely influence seizure control for women with epilepsy. Furthermore, seizures occurring during pregnancy and antiepileptic drugs (AEDs) used to treat seizures have the potential to harm the development of the fetus and the outcome of the pregnancy.[1] Consequently, an understanding of the relationship of seizures, AEDs, and pregnancy is important for physicians who care for women of childbearing potential with seizures.

Definition of Epilepsy

Epilepsy is a disorder of the central nervous system characterized by recurrent seizures. In general, epilepsy is diagnosed only after two or more seizures have occurred and are attributed to a brain disorder. Seizures are the product of abnormal electrical discharges in the brain

From Goldstein PJ, Stern BJ, (eds): *Neurological Disorders of Pregnancy. Second Revised Edition.* Mount Kisco NY, Futura Publishing Co., Inc., © 1992.

and manifest as episodic disorders of motor, sensory, or conscious function. Epilepsy may be acquired or secondary to specific brain disorders or injuries. However, most epilepsy is idiopathic, meaning that it has no clearly determined cause.

Seizure Classification

There are many different types of epileptic seizures (Table I). An international commission has developed a standard classification that has been widely adopted,[3,4] and divides seizures into those that are "partial" because they are localized or originate in a focal portion of the brain, and those that are "generalized" because they involve the entire brain simultaneously. The most common type of partial seizure is the complex partial (psychomotor or temporal lobe) seizure. The two major types of generalized seizures are tonic-clonic (grand mal) and absence (petit mal) seizures. Seizure classification is important

---

Table I.
Classification of Epileptic Seizures*

I. Partial (focal, local) Seizures
   A. Simple partial seizures (consciousness not impaired)
      1. With motor signs
      2. With sensory symptoms
      3. With autonomic symptoms (e.g., epigastric sensation)
      4. With psychic symptoms (e.g., deja-vu, macropsia)
   B. Complex partial seizures (consciousness is impaired)
   C. Partial seizures evolving to secondary generalized seizures†
II. Generalized Seizures
   A. 1. Absence seizures
      2. Atypical absence seizures
   B. Myoclonic seizures
   C. Tonic seizures†
   D. Tonic-clonic seizures†
   E. Atonic seizures
III. Unclassified Epileptic Seizures (e.g., due to inadequate or incomplete data)

---

* Adapted from the Commission on the Classification and Terminology of the International League Against Epilepsy: *Epilepsia* 22:501, 1981.[4]
† More dangerous in pregnancy.

for proper AED selection so it is necessary to appreciate how various seizures manifest.

Seizure Manifestations

The manifestations of partial seizures vary depending on what local area of the brain is involved. For example, partial motor seizures originate in motor cortex and manifest with contralateral convulsions in an extremity. An important distinction for classification depends on whether consciousness is preserved: when consciousness is spared, partial seizures are designated as "simple partial seizures," but if consciousness is impaired the seizure is termed a "complex partial seizure." Complex partial seizures are also associated with stereotyped and often repetitive movements termed automatisms.

The most dramatic and well recognized type of seizure is the generalized tonic-clonic convulsion. This is characterized by generalized, often violent, convulsions of the trunk and extremities and is associated with loss of consciousness. Another generalized form of seizure is the absence or petit mal seizure. Typical absence seizures are brief and consist of short (usually less than 15 seconds) lapses of consciousness that may occur many times in the course of a day and are associated with a characteristic EEG pattern of 3 per second spike and wave discharges. Absence seizures are most common among children and are rare as the only seizure type in adults. Myoclonic seizures are a type of generalized seizure that typically manifests as very rapid and brief muscle jerks that are often most prevalent upon awakening from sleep.

Seizures that begin as partial seizures may secondarily generalize or progress into other types of seizures. Furthermore, many individuals with epilepsy are subject to a variety of seizure types rather than just a single, limited form of seizure. For the pregnant individual with epilepsy, generalized tonic-clonic or similar severe convulsive seizures cause the greatest concern because of their potential harmful effects on the fetus.

Inheritance of Epilepsy

Parents with epilepsy have an increased risk of having children with epilepsy.[5,6] It is difficult to give precise figures for the risk of inheriting epilepsy because epilepsy is a heterogeneous disorder. However it is possible to offer some comparative statistics and general guidelines. The prevalence of epilepsy in the general population before the age of 40 is 1% to 2%.[2] The relatives of an individual with epilepsy may have a two to four times higher risk, with the highest risk for nearer relations.[5,6] Still, the risk of epilepsy for the children of individuals with epilepsy remains relatively low, probably below 5% to 10% in most instances.[7] This risk is higher when the mother, rather than the father, has epilepsy.[5,6]

The nature and cause of a seizure disorder may also be of value for predicting the risks for seizures in offspring. For example, acquired epilepsy, manifesting as complex partial seizures, is probably less likely to be genetically transmitted than idiopathic forms of epilepsy, such as those characterized by typical absence seizures.[5-7] In general, however, the inheritance of epilepsy is difficult to predict because epilepsy seems to be a polygenic disorder, the expression of which is dependent on multiple risk factors and manifests when those factors combine to reach a critical cumulative level.

Diagnostic Procedures

When epilepsy is clinically suspected, several neurodiagnostic tests should be considered to establish the diagnosis, determine the etiology, and guide future therapy. The diagnosis of epilepsy is most secure when a characteristic clinical syndrome is associated with supporting abnormal EEG findings.

Computed tomographic (CT) scanning and magnetic resonance imaging (MRI) provide effective, relatively noninvasive methods of diagnosing structural brain lesions. For individuals with seizures, MRI has a greater sensitivity than CT scanning and is becoming the imaging procedure of choice. Neither a CT scan nor MRI is contraindicated during pregnancy. Indeed the radiation risks associated with properly shielded CT scans are minimal. There are no established harmful effects on the fetus from MRI. When indicated, lumbar puncture remains an essential and irreplaceable testing procedure for the diagnosis of inflammatory or infectious neurological disorders that can cause seizures. In general, the scope of the diagnostic evaluation of seizures during pregnancy should be individualized to the specific clinical situation.

Prognosis

Fortunately, over 50% of individuals with epilepsy have their seizures completely controlled. An additional 30% achieve control adequate to avoid substantial functional impairment. Unfortunately, nearly 20% of epilepsy patients have seizures so frequently that their ability to function is significantly impaired; nearly 5% of individuals with epilepsy have incapacitating seizures.[8]

The long-term prognosis for many patients with epilepsy is also fairly good; about 80% achieve seizure remissions lasting 5 years or longer.[9] For many of these individuals, particularly women of childbearing potential, the discontinuation of all AEDs deserves consideration.

Antiepileptic Drugs for Epilepsy

When choosing an AED for epilepsy, the type of seizure disorder involved is among the first considerations. Because no AED is uniformly safe in pregnancy, this should also be the first consideration when treating women of childbearing potential. In general, it is best to use a single AED (monotherapy) when pregnancy is an issue. The use of multiple AEDs (polypharmacy) appears to contribute to the toxic effects of AEDs and is usually of limited value for improving seizure control.[10] In some cases more than one AED may be necessary for seizure control. However, multiple AED therapy is of special concern in women of childbearing potential because of its higher teratogenic potential. [11]

Indeed, management of the pregnant female with epilepsy is one of the most difficult problems in epilepsy care. Basically, the two major issues are: (1) the effects of pregnancy on seizures in the mother and (2) risk of seizures and AEDs for the fetus.

Effects of Pregnancy on Epilepsy

Seizure Frequency

Although the findings of early studies on the effect of pregnancy on seizure frequency differ substantially,[12] recent reviews have come

Table II.
Changes in Seizure Frequency During Pregnancy

Authors	Number of Pregnancies	Seizure Frequency (%)		
		Unchanged	Increased	Decreased
Knight (1975)	84	50%	45%	5%
Schmidt (1982)*	2,165	53%	24%	23%
Schmidt (1983)	136	50%	37%	13%

* A large review series with pooled data form several studies.

to rather similar conclusions (Table II).[12,14] For most women with epilepsy, there is likely to be no significant increase in seizure frequency during pregnancy, with seizure frequency remaining unchanged in about 50% and actually decreasing in almost 25% of women (Table II). Although an increase in seizure frequency is reported in 24% to 45% of patients, some studies suggest that this increase occurs mostly at the beginning or the end of pregnancy,[12,13] and relates principally to AED noncompliance, low AED blood levels, and maternal sleep deprivation, the last of which often occurs when the newborn is first brought home.[12–14] When such problems are identified and corrected, the seizures are reported to be substantially reduced.[12,14]

The psychological stress and physical fatigue of pregnancy are hypothesized to be major factors contributing to an increase in seizure frequency.[12,14] Other pregnancy-related events such as anemia may further increase fatigue and lower seizure threshold.[12–14] Therefore, the stress, fatigue, and anxiety of pregnancy may indeed account for some of the increase in seizure frequency,[12] and are particularly important factors to identify because they may be correctable.

The frequency of patient's seizures prior to pregnancy may be predictive of seizures during pregnancy. Knight[13] reported that almost all patients who had seizures more frequently than once a month suffered more seizures during pregnancy, while of those with a seizure frequency of less than one every 9 months, only one quarter (25%) demonstrated an increase in seizures during pregnancy.

There is no consistent correlation between the type of seizure and seizure frequency during pregnancy. Also, the seizure course during one pregnancy does not predict seizure frequency or severity in subsequent pregnancies.[12]

Gestational Epilepsy

Gestational epilepsy is the term used for a seizure disorder occurring only during pregnancy and unrelated to eclampsia. Approximately 13% of all women with epilepsy first begin having seizures during pregnancy.[12] About 40% of these woman only have seizures during pregnancy and have true "gestational" seizures or epilepsy.[12,13] In other women, seizures recur outside of pregnancy, so their onset of seizures during pregnancy may simply be a coincidence, reflecting overlap between the usual age of onset for epilepsy and the childbearing years.

Also it is not entirely clear that gestational epilepsy should be considered a distinct clinical entity. For example, there is no specific trimester of pregnancy or type of epilepsy that is associated with gestational seizures. A number of factors have been suggested that may lower the seizure threshold during pregnancy and precipitate seizures.[15]

Hormonal Influences on Seizures

The influence of specific hormones on the nervous system is considered one mechanism that may account for the increase in seizures sometimes observed during pregnancy. However, in pregnant women correlations of serum estrogen and progesterone or other hormone levels to seizures have not demonstrated convincing relationships.[15] Confirmation of the seizure influencing effects of sex hormones in women might be expected from studies of catamenial epilepsy, the frequently described occurrence of seizure in relation to menses; however studies have failed to demonstrate this influence.[16]

During pregnancy, progesterone and estrogen plasma concentrations increase to maximum values in the last trimester of pregnancy, while chorionic gonadotropin peaks early in the first trimester and then descends to a plateau that is maintained until the end of pregnancy.[12,15] Support for the hypothesized influence of estrogen and progesterone on seizures during pregnancy comes primarily from animal models and experiments. Estrogen has been associated with an increased frequency and severity of seizures and epileptiform spikes in animals.[12,15] In contrast, progesterone has been related to a reduction in seizure susceptibility, and has been shown in animal models to increase the seizure threshold.[12,15] In animal experiments, gonadotropin levels have been directly related to the presence of paroxysmal epileptiform discharges.[12]

Despite the lack of clinical evidence, it seems likely, based mainly on experimental data, that some of the apparent lowering of seizure threshold during pregnancy may relate to the effects of estrogen or chorionic gonadotropin, and that progesterone, by raising the seizure threshold, may in part counterbalance this effect. The relative ratio of these hormones varies among individuals during pregnancy, which may be a factor accounting for the variability in seizure frequency observed during pregnancy.

Effects of Metabolic Factors and Antiepileptic Drug Disposition on Seizures

Certain metabolic factors are thought to worsen seizures during pregnancy. Of major concern is the often noted fall in AED blood levels during pregnancy.[12] Low serum AED levels may be a consequence of increased body weight and fluid volume, impaired AED absorption, accelerated drug metabolism, and decreased drug protein binding,[12,17] all of which are seen in pregnancy.

Protein binding of AEDs is reduced in pregnancy. This is probably related to hormonal effects and may account for the accelerated metabolism of some AEDs, particularly those that are normally largely protein bound such as phenytoin.[17] Standard serum AED levels measure the total amounts of AED, both free and protein bound. However, the efficacy of an AED such as phenytoin actually depends mostly on the free rather than the bound fraction of drug. Consequently, in pregnant women with reduced protein binding, standard serum AED levels may not be a reliable measure of the effectiveness of a drug.[17,18] Recently, free AED levels have become more available and may prove clinically useful for monitoring AED levels during pregnancy.[18]

Other pregnancy-associated factors that might contribute to increasing seizure frequency include alterations of serum electrolytes, such as sodium, calcium, or magnesium.[12] Furthermore, pregnancy is associated with a mild, compensated respiratory alkalosis related to progesterone-dependent hyperventilation; alkalosis has been associated with a lowered seizure threshold.[12]

Antiepileptic Drug Noncompliance

Generally in seizure patients, and particularly in pregnant women noncompliance is a major reason for a decrease in AED plasma levels and seizure breakthrough.[12–14] One major cause for noncompliance during pregnancy is that pregnant women may decrease their AED dosage on their own for fear of harming the fetus.[14] Therefore, to prevent seizure breakthrough, with its potentially serious consequences for both mother and fetus, the importance of taking AEDs properly should be stressed early in the care of women of childbearing potential. Importantly, it has been demonstrated that better compliance improves seizure control during pregnancy.[14]

Neurologic and Other Disorders Related to Epilepsy and Seizures

Proper management of seizures during pregnancy requires not only the treatment of seizures but also consideration of their causes. For example, certain neurological disorders such as brain tumors, arteriovenous malformations, or stroke[12,19,20] (see Chapter 3) may first present with seizures.

Also, the new onset of seizures late in pregnancy should always suggest the possibility of eclampsia.[20] Eclampsia is usually not difficult to distinguish from the other causes of seizures because of its characteristic features (Chapter 1). In the United States, therapy for eclampsia has traditionally been centered on the parenteral administration of magnesium sulfate[21] and when necessary, the addition of antihypertensives such as hydralazine, sedatives, or AEDs. However, because magnesium is not an established AED,[20,22] if eclampsia is not clearly established as the cause of seizures in a pregnancy, or if seizures persist after initial treatment, therapy with standard AEDs should be considered. Optimal therapy for eclampsia is yet to be established.[20]

Status epilepticus in pregnancy is generally rare, but it is also potentially very dangerous for both the mother and fetus. Treatment is similar to the standard management of status epilepticus, with the added precaution that the fetus' condition should also be carefully monitored.[23]

Effects of Epilepsy and Antiepileptic Drugs on the Mother and Fetus

Perinatal Complications

Pregnant women with epilepsy have been estimated to have twice the incidence of unfavorable outcomes than the general population.[24,25] The specific findings of one such study are described in Table III.[24] Conclusions from other studies vary and the incidence of complications remains controversial.[24,26] In one recent study, neither epilepsy nor exposure to AEDs was associated with a significantly higher incidence of fetal loss.[27]

Risk of Seizures

Many factors may contribute to the complications associated with seizures. Antiepileptic drugs are one such factor, while convulsive seizures themselves may be another. Patients with frequent seizures have a higher risk of poor outcomes in pregnancy, but it is unclear whether this reflects the effects of seizures or the influence of more AEDs or higher dosages used for such frequent seizures.[25] Adverse genetic and social factors, as well as underlying medical or neurological disorders associated with epilepsy, may also contribute to the incidence of unfavorable outcomes.[25,26]

Furthermore not all seizures have the same risks. Although generalized convulsive seizures are reported to produce hypoxia in the fetus, other types such as partial or absence seizures may not have

Table III.
Frequency of Maternal Complications and Fetal Outcomes for Pregnancies of Women with Epilepsy in Norway

Maternal Complications	Epilepsy	No Epilepsy
Total pregnancies	372	125,423
Hyperemesis gravidarum	1.3%	0.8%
Vaginal hemorrhage	5.1%*	2.2%
Toxemia	7.5%*	4.7%
Birth by		
Cesarean section	3.2%*	1.1%
Forceps/vacuum extractor	6.3%*	2.4%
Gestation less than 37 weeks	8.9%*	5.0%
Birth weight below 2,500 g	7.4%*	3.7%
Hypoxia at birth	1.9%	0.7%
Any congenital malformation	4.5%	2.2%
Infant Mortality Rates (per 1,000 births)		
Stillbirth	5.3	7.8
Perinatal	31.8*	14.6
Neonatal death	29.3*	8.0
Postnatal death	5.3	3.4

* p value is less than 0.01.

Adapted from Bjerkedal T, Bahana SL The course and outcome of pregnancy in women with epilepsy. *Acta Obstet Gynecol Scand* 52:245, 1973.[24]

adverse effects.[28] Consequently, for individuals with partial or non-convulsive seizures, seizure control may not be as critical as for individuals with forms of generalized convulsive seizures.

Generalized tonic-clonic seizures, especially when prolonged, have marked cardiovascular and metabolic effects. Although there is little direct knowledge about placental blood flow during maternal seizures, fetal lactic acidosis and hypoxia have been documented in a few instances.[28]

Although seizures may produce fetal hypoxia and cause fetal compromise, AEDs that are necessary to control seizures have themselves been implicated as a cause of malformations in the fetus. The clinician caring for a pregnant woman with epilepsy is thus confronted with the dilemma of trying to prevent seizures by using drugs that can cause fetal malformations.

Antiepileptic Drug Teratogenicity

The teratogenicity of AEDs is a major concern.[23,29,30,31] "Minor" congenital malformations, or congenital anomalies, may be defined as deviations from normal morphology that do not require intervention and do not impair function. In contrast, "major" congenital malformations are physical defects that warrant medical or surgical intervention and cause major functional problems.[31] The incidence of both minor and major malformations is reported to be higher in infants of mothers with epilepsy who are on AEDs.[1,11,25,31] The most commonly reported minor malformations (Table IV) include superficial skin and skeletal disorders such as distal digital hypoplasia, simian creases, V-shaped eyebrows, hypertelorism, epicanthal folds, low-set ears, and a broad nasal bridge.[31] Although such fetal abnormalities are probably more common in the children of women on AEDs, neither has the exact incidence of such minor malformations been established nor has it been confirmed that they have any serious consequences.[31,32] The more serious congenital malformations associated with AEDs (Tables V and VI) do have long-term consequences and include cleft palate, cleft lip, and cardiac septal defects.[11]

Estimates of risks for congenital malformations in pregnant women with epilepsy are listed in Table IV, V, and VI. In general, the risks are about twice that for women without epilepsy, but the incidence has varied among studies.[32] Malformations are known to occur in 1% to 3% of control populations (Table V). For women with

Table IV.
Frequency of Congenital Anomalies (or Minor Malformations) in Children of Mothers Taking Antiepileptic Drugs (AEDs)

Congenital Anomaly	Mothers Taking AEDs	Mothers Not Taking AEDs
Epicanthal folds	58%	45%
Depressed nasal bridge	27%	16%
Hypertelorism	17%	12%
Fingernail hypoplasia	14%	0.5%

Adapted from Janz D: Antiepileptic drugs and pregnancy: altered utilization patterns and teratogenesis. *Epilepsia* 23(Suppl 1):S60, 1982.

Table V.
Frequency of Major Malformations in Children of Mothers with Epilepsy Treated During Pregnancy with Antiepileptic Drugs (AEDs)

Source	Mothers With Epilepsy Taking AEDs Malformations	Mothers With Epilepsy Not Taking AEDs Malformations	Mothers Without Epilepsy Malformations
Janz (1975)	88 (6.0%) of 1,461 live births	19 (4.2%) of 455 live births	2,940 (2.5%) of 117,176 live births

Table VI.
Relative Frequency of "Major" Malformation in the Children of Mothers Treated with Antiepileptic Drugs (AEDs) During Pregnancy

Malformation	Incidence*
Orofacial clefts	1.8%
Congenital heart lesions	1.5%
Skeletal abnormalities	1.0%
Hypospadias	0.5%
Anencephaly	0.3%
Microcephaly	0.3%
Neural tube defects	0.3%
Intestinal atresia	0.3%
Hydrocephalus	0.1%
Total malformations (101 live births)	5.8%

* Pooled data from several series. From Janz D: The teratogenic risk of antiepileptic drugs. *Epilepsia* 16:162, 1975.[1]

epilepsy it is difficult to separate the influence of hereditary factors, the consequences of seizures, and the effects of AEDs without a large prospective controlled study. Current analyses are based on population studies that, although sometimes prospective, are not controlled.[19] Still, evidence supports that AEDs are teratogenic. For instance, the incidence of fetal malformations has been directly correlated with the number of AEDs taken during pregnancy and their dosage.[11] Also animal studies support the teratogenicity of AEDs.[31] Importantly, women with epilepsy who are not taking AEDs, even if they are having seizures, have a lower incidence of children with congenital malformations than women taking AEDs (Table V).[1,11]

Teratogenicity of Specific Antiepileptic Drugs

All AEDs have been associated with teratogenicity. Although congenital malformations were initially emphasized with phenytoin, as the "fetal hydantoin syndrome," more recent evidence suggests that all currently used AEDs have risks and that the adverse effects may be cumulative.[11,31,33] Indeed the appropriate emphasis should be on a "fetal AED syndrome". Trimethadione (Tridione® [Abbot Laboratories, North Chicago, IL, USA]) is the AED with the most well established teratogenic effect.[34] Trimethadione is an oxazolidine derivative. This category of drugs also includes paramethadione (Paradione® [Abbot Laboratories, North Chicago, IL, USA]), which is subject to the same concerns and restrictions. Trimethadione has been convincingly associated with a malformation syndrome which includes heart and genitourinary defects, cranial facial anomalies, hypoplasia of the fingers and nails, mild to moderate mental retardation, and intrauterine growth retardation in 80% of exposed individuals.[11,29,34] Fortunately both trimethadione and paramethadione, which are used primarily for absence seizures, can be substituted by other, safer AEDs.

Concern about valproic acid (Depakote®, Depakene® [Abbot Laboratories, North Chicago, IL, USA]) has centered on the occurrence of congenital neural tube defects[35–37] that occurs in 1% to 2% of all valproic acid exposures during pregnancy. This is an incidence tenfold higher than for the general population.[36,38] Other malformations and anomalies have also been reported with valproic acid use in human pregnancies,[39] and valproic acid has also been shown to cause congenital malformations in experimental animals.[37] The exact teratogenic risk of valproic acid is not firmly established, but the malformations are so severe that some experts have suggested avoiding this drug in pregnancy unless absolutely necessary for seizure control.[23] For women exposed to valproic acid in the first trimester of pregnancy, an ultrasound evaluation of the fetus at 16- to 20-weeks gestation is what I recommend to determine the presence of a neural tube defect.[38] If a neural tube defect is not found, amniocentesis and determination of α-fetoprotein (AFP) and acetycholinesterase before the twentieth week of gestation is still advised.[38] The combined use of ultrasound and amniocentesis is estimated to detect 92% to 95% of all neural tube defects.[38] Maternal serum α-fetoprotein (MSAFP) assay alone is not adequately sensitive to serve as the sole screening test in this situation, but an approach combining MSAFP and ultrasonography performed with high-quality equipment by someone experienced in the identification of congenital anomalies is more sensitive and avoids the risk of amniocentesis, which may be as high as 0.5% for pregnancy loss, so this approach has recently been recommended as an alternative to amniocentesis in such situations.[40] More data on the teratogenic effects of valproic acid are necessary before any final conclusions are justified as to both the risk of malformations and the optimal strategy for managing this serious problem.

Phenytoin (Dilantin® [Parke-Davis, Morris Plains, NJ, USA]) is the AED most frequently associated with fetal malformations.[32,41] However, this probably relates more to the high frequency of phenytoin use than its teratogenic potential.[11,32,42] Characteristically, the fetal hydantoin syndrome is reported to exhibit craniofacial anomalies including dysmorphic nasal features, epicanthal folds, wide mouth, and prominent lips. Limb defects, including hypoplasia of the fingers and nails, are also described. Intrauterine growth retardation, microcephaly, mild to moderate mental retardation, and major congenital malformations described in Table VI have also been proposed as part of this syndrome.[32] Although phenytoin is not established to be more dangerous than other standard AEDs, because of the numerous reports of phenytoin associated fetal anomalies and malformations, many physicians are anxious to use other AEDs during pregnancy.

One alternative AED for patients with generalized tonic-clonic or complex partial seizures has been carbamazepine (Tegretol® [Geigy Pharmaceuticals, Ardsley, NY, USA]). However, recent studies question the safety of carbamazepine in pregnancy and suggest its risks are similar to phenytoin or valproic acid.[11,42,43] Indeed, one recent study reports that the carbamazepine-related risk of neural tube defects may be approximately 1% and suggests prenatal detection measures for women taking carbamazepine similar to those recommended for women on valproic acid.[43] However, in my opinion, because the evidence for neural tube defects with carbamazepine is not as compelling as with valproic acid, I do not at present routinely recommend amniocentesis for pregnant women exposed to carbamazepine, but instead suggest screening with MSAFP and high-quality ultrasound between 16- and 20-weeks gestation.[40] However, for carbamazepine, as well as for valproic acid, the optimal screening strategies for neural tube detects and other malformations remain to be established, so managing these individuals requires particularly careful consideration of the risks and benefits of these various diagnostic approaches, reevaluation of options as new information becomes available, and coordination of efforts by neurologists and obstetricians.

Other AEDs considered for use in pregnancy include phenobarbital, primidone (Mysoline® [Wyeth-Ayerst, Philadelphia, PA, USA]), ethosuximide (Zarontin® [Parke-Davis, Morris Plains, NJ, USA]), and benzodiazepine derivatives such as clonazepam (Klonopin® [Roche Laboratories, Nutley, NJ, USA]). It remains unclear that any one of these AEDs is substantially safer than other AEDs in pregnancy. What is well established is that all AEDs have substantial teratogenic risks and that individuals taking multiple AEDs and higher doses of AEDs are at the greatest risk.[11]

Postulated Mechanisms of Antiepileptic Drug Teratogenicity

No single mechanism of AED teratogenicity has been established but several mechanisms have been proposed. Indeed exact mechanisms of teratogenicity may vary between AEDs because the drugs themselves fall into many different pharmacological categories.

One of the first mechanisms proposed for AED teratogenicity was folate deficiency. Several AEDs have been associated with low levels of folic acid (see below).[44] Of particular importance however are some clinical studies[45,46] and one animal study[47] suggesting that folic acid therapy may prevent AED induced teratogenic effects.

Recent interest has focused on the possibility that some AED metabolites, particularly epoxides, may be responsible for teratogenicity. Both carbamazepine and phenytoin are metabolized through the arene oxide pathway to form epoxide intermediates.[47] These epoxide intermediates are then detoxified by the enzyme epoxide hydrolase. The risk of congenital malformations has been predicted prenatally by measurement of epoxide hydrolase activity.[48,49] It has been suggested that the lower the level, and the less the activity, of epoxide hydrolase in the fetus exposed to these AEDs, the greater the buildup of epoxide teratogens, and the more likely and severe the associated congenital malformations.[42,48,49] Furthermore, the higher risks for malformations found with multiple AED usage in pregnancy may also be related to interactions in this arene oxide metabolic pathway due to the simultaneous use of multiple AEDs.[50]

There are other postulated mechanisms for AED teratogenicity. For example, weak acids in general, and particularly valproic acid and ethosuximide, may act as teratogens by altering the acid-base milieu of the early mammalian embryo.[51] Despite many theories, the precise mechanisms of AED teratogenicity are still not established.

Antiepileptic Drug Recommendations

Since all AEDs appear to have teratogenic potential, the first consideration when evaluating antiepileptic therapy for women of childbearing potential is to determine whether any drug at all is necessary. This is a critical but often unemphasized option. Nearly 80% of people with epilepsy achieve remission of their seizures for many years.[9] In such situations discontinuation of AEDs should be considered. Recent studies indicate that the risk of seizure recurrence for such individuals may be in the range of 20% to 60%,[52,53] depending on such factors as the seizure type and its cause, the age of the individual, the presence of associated neurological problems, EEG abnormalities, and the duration of the seizure-free interval.[52,53]

Furthermore, some individuals on AEDs may not really require them. For example, individuals with a single seizure may have no more than a 20% to 60% chance of seizure recurrence, depending on defined risk factors.[54] Therapy with an AED in such cases is not always necessary because of the relatively low recurrence rate of seizures for many of these individuals. Moreover, many episodic disorders may be mistaken for epilepsy including syncope, migraine, and various behavioral or psychological disturbances; these individuals may be unnecessarily treated for epilepsy. Antiepileptic drugs are also widely used for disorders other than epilepsy such as migraine, depression, or other behavioral disorders; in such situations discontinuation of AEDs may be possible with little risk.

Discontinuing AED therapy or not using AEDs is the most effective way to avoid the known teratogenic risks of AEDs. However, this is a complex decision, one that should consider the risks of continued AED therapy, such as fetal malformations, against the potential danger of discontinuing AEDs.

Even for the individual with active seizures, there may be reasons for altering AEDs when pregnancy is at issue. It is important that whatever AED is used that it be effective in controlling seizures, particularly the most dangerous types of seizures, generalized tonic-clonic seizures. To minimize the AED teratogenic risk, it is safer to use AED monotherapy rather than therapy with multiple drugs.

Some seizures may not have much risk for the fetus or mother.[28] Simple partial, complex partial, and absence seizures (Table I) have not been associated with serious effects on the fetus unless they progress to generalized convulsive seizures. Some individuals with these types of seizures may want to consider avoiding the teratogenic risk of AEDs by discontinuing medications under a physician's supervision.

Another practical consideration that can help reduce the teratogenic effects of AEDs is the careful monitoring of AED blood levels in pregnancy. Unless absolutely necessary to control convulsive seizures, very high levels of AEDs should be avoided because the teratogenic risks appear dose dependent.[11] In particular it is important to measure serum AED levels early in the pregnancy and, if possible, prior to conception. After the first trimester, the teratogenic susceptibility of the fetus decreases substantially. Because seizures tend to worsen toward the end of the pregnancy, higher AED levels, which may be necessary to control seizures late in pregnancy, should be of less teratogenic risk at this time.

Folate Deficiency

Folic acid depletion has been described in individuals taking AEDs and may be a possible causative factor for the teratogenic effects of these drugs.[44] Several AEDs, particularly phenytoin, phenobarbital, and primidone, have been associated with low folate levels, possibly due to their effects on the intestinal absorption of folate.[32,44] Although folate deficiency has been hypothesized as a possible mechanism for the malformations in children of mothers with epilepsy who take AEDs, this has not been conclusively established.[32] Still, because of this possibility, and animal experiments suggesting that this adverse effect may be prevented with vitamin supplementation,[47] it seems advisable to provide folate and other vitamin supplements to pregnant women receiving AEDs. Prenatal vitamin preparations typically contain about 500 μg of folic acid, which should be adequate to maintain a normal serum level. However, the exact dosage that should be used is not established, and if such therapy is likely to be of benefit, it seems advisable to begin therapy prior to conception.

Clotting Disorders in the Neonate

Some AEDs, notably phenobarbital, phenytoin, and primidone, are known to interfere with vitamin K metabolism.[55–59] This may explain an AED induced hemorrhagic disorder in the newborn that has been observed with a variety of AEDs and can have serious consequences including death. Bleeding in AED induced hemorrhagic disorders usually occurs within the first 24 hours after birth and consists of hemorrhage from internal sites such as the lung, abdomen, and brain. The exact incidence of this syndrome is not established, but it is reported in 7% of pregnancies in women receiving phenobarbital or phenytoin.[58] This AED induced disorder should be distinguished from the more common neonatal disorder, hemorrhagic disease of the newborn, which typically develops from the second to the fifth day of life, is associated with more superficial and less severe bleeding, and is probably caused by immature hepatic enzyme function or the presence of clotting-inhibiting factors.[55–58]

Studies of coagulation factors in newborns born to epileptic mothers taking AEDs demonstrate coagulation defects in up to 50% of infants. The clotting parameters show a decrease in vitamin K-dependent factors and a prolonged prothrombin time. Although the pathophysiology of this AED related coagulation defect is unknown, it is postulated to relate to a deficiency of vitamin K, probably caused by AED induction of fetal microenzymes responsible for vitamin K catabolism[55-59] Displacement of vitamin K from binding proteins may also occur.[55] Administration of vitamin K may prevent these AED induced clotting disorders.[57] It is recommended that vitamin K_1 phytonadione therapy be given to mothers taking AEDs, particularly those taking AEDs known to interfere with clotting mechanisms. Prophylactic administration of vitamin K_1 prior to delivery can reverse clotting abnormalities.[58] The maternal dosage recommended is 20 mg of oral vitamin K_1 daily for 2 weeks before the expected date of delivery.[56] Alternatively 10 mg of vitamin K_1 has been given to the mother a few hours prior to delivery, but it is not established whether either of these regimens is effective.[59] Because of concerns about possible adverse effects in pregnancy, I do not recommend using vitamin K_3 (menadione). After delivery, an infant's clotting factors, including prothrombin time, partial thromboplastin time, and specific vitamin K dependent clotting factor assays, if available, should be studied from cord blood. The infant should be given 1 mg of vitamin K_1 intramuscularly or intravenously.[56,59] Clotting factors should be checked again 2 to 4 hours later and additional injections of vitamin K_1 or fresh frozen plasma infusions administered as necessary.[55,56,58,59]

Parturition

The management of delivery presents some special problems for women with epilepsy. In general, it is wise to avoid nonessential medications during labor so as to be prepared for the possibility that general anesthesia and intubation may be necessary. Still, even when general anesthesia and intubation may be needed, the anesthetist may permit the patient to take essential medications such as AEDs along with small amounts of liquid.[60] This will lower the risk of seizures due to withdrawal from AEDs. Even though there is decreased gastric emptying during labor, there seems to be little risk of aspiration or other difficulties with judicious administration of oral medications.

When it is not considered reasonable to allow oral medications, parenteral AEDs may be given. The standard AEDs available for parenteral administration include phenytoin and phenobarbital. Phenytoin is effective intravenously but is not predictably effective when given intramuscularly.[61] Phenobarbital is well absorbed either intravenously or intramuscularly. The benzodiazepines, such as diazepam (Valium®) or lorazepam (Ativan®), can also be given parenterally but are less often used for seizure prophylaxis because of their sedating effects on the neonate.

Postnatal Considerations

Antiepileptic drugs have been associated with neonatal depression, which may manifest as sedation, hypotonia, and poor breathing or sucking.[57] The clinical picture, which usually appears at birth, disappears within 2 to 8 days. It occurs in 5% to 10% of newborns born to mothers treated with AEDs, mostly phenobarbital, phenytoin, and primidone. Drug withdrawal symptoms develop in 20% to 65% of the newborns and are associated with a postnatal fall of plasma drug concentrations. Clinical signs and symptoms include hyperactivity, excessive crying, disturbed sleep, tremors, myoclonic jerks, hypertonia, hyperreflexia, hyperventilation, hyperphagia, vomiting, sneezing, and yawning.[57]

Postpartum Antiepileptic Drug Considerations

Following pregnancy, major shifts occur in the mother's fluid and electrolyte balance and body weight. These changes can effect AEDs pharmacology. After delivery, AED dosage may initially be maintained at prepartum levels, but AED blood levels should be measured within the first few weeks of delivery to determine whether adjustments of AED doses are necessary. Serum AED levels and the mother's clinical condition should be used to determine the proper AED dosage.

Breast Feeding

Breast feeding is a concern for the pregnant female with epilepsy. Many AEDs are excreted in breast milk. The exact concentration depends to some degree on protein binding. Feeding difficulties have been described in the breast-fed children of mothers who are taking sedative AEDs such as phenobarbital. However, in general, breast feeding can be continued during the neonatal period in most mothers on AEDs. Still, caution is advised and the neonate should be observed for unusual symptoms.[29,57]

Contraception

Pregnancy and epilepsy should be considered in one other context: birth control. Antiepileptic drugs and oral contraceptives may interfere with each other's effectiveness.[15] This probably relates to hepatic microsomal enzyme induction and drug metabolism. Antiepileptic drug dosage can usually be adjusted depending on clinical symptoms and serum AED levels. An early sign of oral contraceptive failure in a woman taking an AED may be breakthrough bleeding. Such bleeding may be corrected by the use of an oral contraceptive containing higher hormone concentrations.[15] Birth control pills, although possibly somewhat less effective in patients on AEDs remain an effective birth control method for individuals with epilepsy.[15]

Summary

Women with epilepsy who are of childbearing potential or become pregnant should be advised of the risks involved (Table VII) for the mother and the fetus. To lessen the risk of AED teratogenicity and optimize the potential for an uncomplicated pregnancy several measures should be considered (Table VII).

Pregnancy for the great majority of women with epilepsy is a safe and fulfilling experience with a happy outcome. However, there are important medical issues that require early and careful consideration by the physician who cares for the pregnant woman with epilepsy. Thoughtful review of current literature and communication

Table VII.
Recommendations for Care of the Pregnant Woman With Epilepsy

I. Prior to conception:
  A. Determine whether antiepileptic (AED) drug therapy is really needed
  B. If needed, determine whether AED therapy is appropriate
    1. Avoid trimethadione and paradione
    2. Use single AED therapy whenever possible
    3. Minimize total AED dosage
  C. Other
    1. Discuss risk of congenital anomalies and malformation
    2. Discuss hereditary risk for epilepsy
    3. Provide vitamin (folate) supplementation
II. During pregnancy:
    1. Use a single AED whenever possible
    2. Minimize AED dosage, particularly in the first trimester
    3. Emphasis of AED therapy should be on preventing generalized convulsive seizures
    4. AED therapy is best guided by monitoring AED blood levels
    5. For patient exposed to valproic acid consider ultrasound evaluation of fetus and amniocentesis prior to 20 weeks gestation
    6. For patient exposed to carbamazepine, I consider MSAFP and ultrasound evaluation of the fetus prior to 20-weeks gestation.
    7. Provide vitamin (folate) supplementation
    8. Give the mother 20 mg of vitamin K_1 daily for two weeks prior to expected date of delivery
III. At delivery:
    1. Infant should be given 1 mg of vitamin K_1
    2. Infant should be carefully observed for bleeding problems
    3. Attention should be given to maternal AED requirements
IV. Postpartum:
    1. Follow mother's AED blood levels and adjust AED doses as necessary
    2. Monitor breast-fed infants for AED effects or withdrawal symptoms
    3. Examine infants carefully for congenital malformations or anomalies

between obstetrician and neurologist are necessary to maximize the potential for a successful pregnancy.

References

1. Janz D: The teratogenic risk of antiepileptic drugs. *Epilepsia* 16:159, 1975.
2. Hauser WA, Annegers JF: Epidemiologic measurements for the determination of genetic risk. In *Genetics of the Epilepsies*. Edited by G Beck-

Mannagetta, VE Anderson, H Doose, et al: Berkin-Heidelberg. Springer-Verlag, 1989, pp. 7–12.

3. Commission on Classification and Terminology of the International League Against Epilepsy: Proposal for classification of epilepsies and epileptic syndromes. *Epilepsia* 26:268, 1985.
4. Commission on Classification and Terminology of the International League Against Epilepsy: Proposal for revised clinical and electroencephalographic classification of epileptic seizures. *Epilepsia* 22:501, 1981.
5. Annegers JF, Hauser WA, Anderson VE, et al: The risks of seizure disorders among the relatives of patients with childhood onset epilepsy. *Neurology* 32:174, 1982.
6. Annegers JF, Hauser WA, Elveback LR, et al: Seizure disorders in the offspring of parents with a history of seizures: A maternal-paternal difference. *Epilepsia* 17:1, 1976.
7. Janz D, Beck-Mannagetta G, Scheffner D, et al: Epilepsy in the children of epileptic parents. In *Epilepsy, Pregnancy and the Child*. Edited by D Janz, M Dam, A Richens, et al: New York, NY. Raven Press, 1982, pp. 527–534.
8. Rodin E: Medical and social prognosis in epilepsy. *Epilepsia* 13:121, 1972.
9. Annegers JF, Hauser WA, Elveback LR: Remission and relapse in patients with epilepsy. *Epilepsia* 20:729, 1979.
10. Mattson RH, Cramer JA, Collins JF, et al: Comparison of carbamazepine, phenobarbital, phenytoin, and primidone in partial and secondarily generalized tonic-clonic seizures. *N Engl J Med* 313:145, 1985.
11. Nakane Y, Okum T, Takahashi R, et al: Multi-institutional study on the teratogenicity and fetal toxicity of antiepileptic drugs: A report of a collaborative study group in Japan. *Epilepsia* 21:663, 1980.
12. Schmidt D: The effect of pregnancy on the natural history of epilepsy: Review of the literature. In *Epilepsy, Pregnancy, and the Child*. Edited by D Janz, M Dam, A Richens, et al: New York, NY. Raven Press, 1982, pp. 3–14.
13. Knight AH, Rhind EG: Epilepsy and pregnancy: A study of 153 pregnancies in 59 patients. *Epilepsia* 16:99, 1975.
14. Schmidt D, Canger R, Avanzini G, et al: Changes of seizure frequency in pregnant epileptic women. *J Neurol Neurosurg Psychiatry* 46:751, 1983.
15. Mattson RH, Cramer JA: Epilepsy, sex hormones, and antiepileptic drugs. *Epilepsia* 26(Suppl 1):S40, 1985.
16. Newmark ME, Penry JK: Catamenial epilepsy: A review. *Epilepsia* 21:281, 1980.
17. Levy RH, Yerby MS: Effects of pregnancy on antiepileptic drugs utilization. *Epilepsia* 26(Suppl 1):S52, 1985.
18. Levy RH, Schmidt D: Utility of free level monitoring of antiepileptic drugs. *Epilepsia* 26(Suppl 1):S52, 1985.
19. Donaldson JO: Epilepsy. In *Neurology of Pregnancy*. Philadelphia, PA. WB Saunders Company, 1989, pp. 229–267.
20. Donaldson JO: Eclampsia and other causes of peripartum convulsions. In *Neuroloqy of Pregnancy*. Philadelphia, PA. WB Saunders Company, 1989, pp. 269–310.

21. Pritchard JA, Cunningham FG, Pritchard SA: The Parkland Memorial Hospital protocol for treatment of exlampsia: Evaluation of 245 cases. *Am J Obstet Gynecol* 148:951, 1984.
22. Fisher RS, Kaplan PW, Krumholz A, et al: Failure of high-dose intravenous magnesium sulfate to control myoclonic status epilepticus. *Clin Neuropharm* 11:537, 1988.
23. Dalessio DJ: Seizure disorders and pregnancy. *N Engl J Med* 1312:559, 1985.
24. Bjerkedal T, Bahana SL: The course and outcome of pregnancy in women with epilepsy. *Acta Obstet Gynecol Scand* 52:245, 1973.
25. Nelson KB, Ellenberg JH: Maternal seizure disorder, outcome of pregnancy, and neurologic abnormalities in the children. *Neurology* 32:1247, 1982.
26. Anderman E, Dansky L, Kinch RA: Complications of pregnancy, labour and delivery in epileptic women. In *Epilepsy, Pregnancy, and the Child.* Edited by D Janz, M Dam, A Richens, et al. New York, NY. Raven Press, 1982, pp. 61–74.
27. Annegers JF, Baumgartner KB, Hauser WA, et al: Epilepsy, antiepileptic drugs, and the risk of spontaneous abortion. *Epilepsia* 29:451, 1988.
28. Teramo K, Hiilesmaa MA, Bardy A, et al: Fetal heart rate during a maternal grand mal epileptic seizure. *J Perinat Med* 7:3, 1979.
29. American Academy of Pediatrics Committee on Drugs: Anticonvulsants and pregnancy. *Pediatrics* 63:331, 1979.
30. Commission on Genetics, Pregnancy, and the Child, International League Against Epilepsy: Guidelines for the care of epileptic women of childbearing age. *Epilepsia* 30:409, 1989.
31. Yerby MS: Problems and management of the pregnant woman with epilepsy. *Epilepsia* 28(Suppl 3):S29, 1987.
32. Janz D: Antiepileptic drugs and pregnancy: Altered utilization patterns and teratogenesis. *Epilepsia* 23(Suppl 1):S53, 1982.
33. Smithells RW: Environmental teratogens of man. *Br Med Bull* 32:27, 1976.
34. German I, Ehlers KH, Kowal A: Trimethadione and human teratogenesis. *Teratology* 3:349, 1976.
35. Tein I, MacGregor DL: Possible valproate teratogenicity. *Arch Neurol* 42:291, 1985.
36. Robert E, Guibaud P: Maternal valproic acid and congenital neural tube defects. *Lancet* 2:1096, 1982.
37. Brown NA, Kao J, Fabros S: Teratogenic potential of valproic acid. *Lancet* 1:660, 1980.
38. Weinbaum PJ, Cassidy SB, Vintzileos AM, et al: Prenatal detection of a neural tube defect after fetal exposure to valproic acid. *Obstet Gynecol* 67:31S, 1986.
39. DiLiberti JH, Farndon PA, Dennis NR, et al: The fetal valproic acid syndrome. *Am J Med Genet* 19:473, 1984.
40. Nadel AS, Green JK, Holmes LB, et al: Absence of need for amniocentesis in patients with elevated levels of maternal serum α-fetoprotein and normal ultrasonographic examinations. *N Engl J Med* 323:557, 1990.

41. Hanson JW: Teratogen update: Fetal hydantoin effects. *Teratology* 33:349, 1986.
42. Jones KL, Lacro RV, Johnson KA, et al: Pattern of malformations in the children of women treated with carbamazepine during pregnancy. *N Engl J Med* 320:1661, 1989.
43. Rosa FW: Spina bifida in infants of women treated with carbamazepine during pregnancy. *N Engl J Med* 324:674, 1991.
44. Malpas JS, Spray GH, Witts LJ: Serum folic acid and vitamin B12 levels in anticonvulsant therapy. *Br Med J* 1:955, 1966.
45. Dansky LV, Andermann E, Sherwin AI, et al: Maternal epilepsy and congenital malformations: A prospective study with monitoring of plasma anticonvulsant levels during pregnancy. *Ann Neurol* 21:176, 1987.
46. Biale Y, Lewenthal H, Ben Aderet N: Congenital malformations due to anticonvulsant drugs. *Obstet Gynecol* 215:439, 1975.
47. Zhu M, Zhou S: Reduction of the teratogenic effects of phenytoin by folic acid and a mixture of folic acid, vitamins, amino acids: a preliminary trial. *Epilepsia* 30:246, 1989.
48. Strickler SM, Dansky LV, Miller MA, et al: Genetic predisposition to phenytoin-induced birth defects. *Lancet* ii:746, 1985.
49. Buehler B, Delimont D, van Waes M, et al: Prenatal prediction of the risk of the fetal hydantoin syndrome. *N Engl J Med* 322:1567, 1990.
50. Lindhout D, Hoppener RJ, Meinardi H: Teratogenicity of antiepileptic drug combinations with special emphasis on epoxidation (of carbamazepine). *Epilepsia* 25:77, 1984.
51. Nau H, Scott WJ Jr: Weak acids act as teratogens by accumulating in the basic milieu of the early mammalian embryo. *Nature* 323:276, 1986.
52. Emerson R, D'Souza BJ, Vining PE, et al: Stopping medication in children with epilepsy. *N Engl J Med* 304:1125, 1981.
53. Callaghan N, Garret A, Goggi: Withdrawal of anticonvulsant drugs in patients seizure free for two years. *N Engl J Med* 318:942, 1988.
54. Hauser WA, Anderson VE, Lowenson RB, et al: Seizure recurrence after a first unprovoked seizure. *N Engl J Med* 307:522, 1982.
55. Solomon GE, Higartner MW, Kutt H: Coagulation defects caused by diphenylhydantoin. *Neurology* 22:1165, 1972.
56. Bleyer WA, Skinner AL: Fetal neonatal hemorrhage after maternal anticonvulsant therapy. *JAMA* 235:626, 1976.
57. Bossi L: Neonatal period including drug disposition in newborns: Review of the literature. In *Epilepsy, Pregnancy, and the Child*. Edited by D Janz, M Dam, A Richens, et al: New York, NY. Raven Press, 1982, pp. 327–341.
58. Deblay MF, Vert P, Andre M, et al: Transplacental vitamin K prevents hemorrhagic disease of infants of epileptic mothers. *Lancet* 1:1247, 1982.
59. Srinivasan G, Seeler RA, Tiruvury A, et al: Maternal anticonvulsant therapy and hemorrhagic disease of the newborn. *Obstet Gynecol* 59:250, 1982.
60. Roizen MF: Preoperative evaluation of patients with diseases that require special preoperative evaluation and intraoperative management. In *Anesthesia*. Edited by RD Miller. New York, NY. Churchill Livingstone, 1981, p. 48.
61. Serrano EE, Roye DB, Hammer RH, et al: Plasma diphenylhydantoin. *Neurology* 23:311, 1973.

3

Cerebrovascular Disease and Pregnancy

Barney J. Stern, M.D.

Introduction

Neurological illness often results from diseases of the heart and vascular system. Systemic conditions, especially hematologic diseases, can also cause neurological problems. The resulting neurological deficit may be permanent or transient, depending on the severity of the insult to the central nervous system (CNS). Management of the pregnant stroke patient is a unique medical challenge, because the needs of both mother and fetus must often be considered. Furthermore, the common causes of stroke are less likely to occur in young women and therefore relatively obscure etiologies of stroke must be considered by the clinician.

The average annual initial stroke incidence rate for women is 4.1 per 100,000 under age 35 and 25.7 per 100,000 for ages 35– 44.[1] Stroke mortality has decreased from the 1950s through the 1970s, probably because of better control of hypertension.[2,3] However, in the early 1980s the declining incidence rate for stroke seems to have stabilized at approximately 10 per 100,000 for individuals less than 45 years of age.[3] Pregnancy has been said to increase the risk of ischemic infarction thirteenfold over the expected rate for young women.[4] However, a recent study in Rochester, Minnesota found 5.1 cerebral infarctions per 100,000 person years of observation during pregnancy

From Goldstein PJ, Stern BJ, (eds): *Neurological Disorders of Pregnancy. Second Revised Edition.* Mount Kisco NY, Futura Publishing Co., Inc., © 1992.

compared to 3.5 per 100,000 for all women aged 15–39 years.[5] A survey in Wisconsin demonstrated only a relative risk of 1.16 for stroke during pregnancy.[6] From 1982–1985, the maternal mortality rate for CNS disorders (excluding hemorrhage) in Massachusetts was 0.3 per 100,000 live births and 0.9 per 100,000 live births for intracranial hemorrhage.[7]

Optimal management of the stroke patient involves determination of the etiology of the stroke, minimizing the neurological deficit, prevention of subsequent events, and rehabilitation. The first three issues will be discussed in this chapter.

Thorough evaluation of the patient with a suspected stroke is necessary to define the pathophysiology of the neurological problem.[8] After a thorough history and physical examination, an imaging study of the brain is usually indicated. Both computed tomography (CT) and magnetic resonance imaging (MRI) can define CNS hemorrhage, edema, mass effect, and ventricular size.[9] Although there is exposure to ionizing radiation when a brain CT scan is done, with proper abdominal shielding, this test may be done during pregnancy. A CT scan is usually readily available and is the preferred test for the rapid detection of CNS hemorrhage, especially subarachnoid hemorrhage (SAH). Computed tomographic scan image acquisition time is rapid, which is advantageous when evaluating a critically ill or agitated patient. An MRI scan does not expose the patient to ionizing radiation and is a very sensitive method for detecting cerebral edema resulting from brain injury. However, scan acquisition time is relatively long and critically ill patients are technically difficult to manage during scanning.

A precise definition of cerebrovascular anatomy is desirable for the evaluation of the young stroke patient. Conventional arterial angiography can be done, but technological advances now permit excellent visualization of the vascular anatomy with intra-arterial digital subtraction angiography. Development of MRI angiography will allow the intra- and extracranial vessels to be seen noninvasively without exposure to ionizing radiation.[10]

If there is no contraindication, an examination of the cerebrospinal fluid (CSF) can provide useful diagnostic information such as documentation of subarachnoid blood or a CSF pleocytosis suggesting infection or inflammation. Cerebrospinal fluid should be sent for appropriate cultures or immunological assays.

Physiological alterations, including changes in blood viscosity and coagulability, occur during pregnancy and puerperium and may predispose to stroke or affect patient management once a stroke has occurred. A rise in fibrinogen concentration[11-13] as well as in the levels of clotting factors VII, VIII, IX, and X occurs.[14-16] Some studies have demonstrated a decrease in fibrinolytic activity during pregnancy;[12,17] other data reveal enhanced fibrinolysis,[11] that presumably helps maintain homeostasis.[18] During pregnancy there is a decrease in tissue-type plasminogen activator and an increase in tissue plasminogen inhibition.[17] Beginning at 12–14 weeks of pregnancy there is an increase in plasma fibrinopeptide A that reflects increased thrombin formation.[13] During the second and third trimesters there is decreased activity of the clotting inhibitor antithrombin III with a modest increase in protein C, another anticoagulant.[13,19] Protein S, yet another clot inhibitor, decreases during pregnancy.[19,20] β-Thromboglobulin, a measure of platelet-activation, increases during pregnancy[21] and platelets become more aggregable in the second and third trimesters and the puerperium.[13,22] An increase in fibrinogen, factor VIII:C, and platelets occurs from the third to fifth day postpartum.[23] Overall, there is a hypercoagulable state during pregnancy[13,20] and for approximately 2 to 3 weeks postpartum.[24] A high fibrinogen level is associated with increased blood viscosity and a decrease in cerebral blood flow that may predispose to stroke during times of low flow.[25] Elevated levels of factor VIII, fibrinopeptide A, and β thromboglobulin have been associated with hypercoagulability in both acute ischemic and hemorrhagic strokes.[26]

During pregnancy there is an expansion of plasma volume and a decrease in hematocrit resulting in decreased blood viscosity.[27-29] This may improve cerebral perfusion and help prevent stroke.[25] Ideally, cerebral vascular autoregulation should maintain normal blood perfusion. The stress of labor may temporarily change cerebral hemodynamics: during phase II of a Valsalva maneuver there is a 21% decrease in internal carotid artery blood flow.[30] If cerebral blood flow decreases during labor and delivery, in the setting of a hypercoagulable state, a situation conducive to venous thrombosis in the brain might exist.[31]

The role of prostaglandins in pregnancy and labor and in vascular disease is under great scrutiny. Prostacyclin, a vasodilator and platelet antiaggregant, is not as effective a platelet antiaggregant during pregnancy as compared to the nonpregnant state.[32] As labor proceeds, plasma levels of prostaglandin $F_{2\alpha}$ progressively increase.[33,34] Pros-

Table I.
Potential Risk Factors and Causes for Stroke in Pregnancy and the Puerperium

Vasculopathy
  aneurysm
  arteriovenous malformation
  venous thrombosis
  atherosclerosis
  vasculitides
    systemic lupus erythematosis,
    polyarteritis nodosa,
    syphilis, etc.
  Takayasu's disease
  fibromuscular dysplasia
  arterial dissection
    spontaneous
    traumatic
  carotid cavernous sinus fistula
  Moyamoya disease
  pregnancy associated intimal hyperplasia
  reversible cerebral segmental vasoconstriction
  transient emboligenic aortoarteritis
Embolism
  paradoxical embolus
  peripartum cardiomyopathy
  nonbacterial thrombotic endocarditis
  fat or air embolism
  mitral valve prolapse
  valvular heart disease
  infective endocarditis
  atrial fibrillation
  sick sinus syndrome
  left atrial myxoma
  cardiomyopathy
Hematologic conditions
  hemoglobin SS and SC disease
  thrombotic thrombocytopenia purpura
  antiphospholipid
  paroxysmal nocturnal hemoglobinuria
  antithrombin III deficiency
  Protein C deficiency
  Protein S deficiency
  factor VIII elevation
Miscellaneous
  migraine
  alcohol abuse
  drug use and abuse
  metastatic trophoblastic carcinoma
  human immunodeficiency virus infection and associated conditions
  eclampsia

taglandin $F_{2\alpha}$ is a cerebral vasoconstricting agent[35] and potentiator of (peripheral) adrenergic stimulation.[36] In one experimental model, infusion of subarachnoid blood and prostaglandin $F_{2\alpha}$ increased the likelihood of cerebral vasospasm compared to administration of blood alone.[35] However, a more recent study did not demonstrate an elevation of prostaglandin $F_{2\alpha}$ following experimental SAH in dogs; only prostaglandin $F_{2\alpha}$ levels were increased in the CSF.[37] Fluctuation in prostaglandin levels during pregnancy and the peripartum period might have an effect on ischemic infarction and subarachnoid hemorrhage.

The causes of stroke in young patients are extensive,[8,38] but if only the pregnant or puerperal patient is considered, the diagnostic classification may be somewhat more limited (Table I). Although some causes of stroke are unique to pregnancy, other conditions, such as migraine and mitral valve prolapse, occur commonly in young women and must be considered as possible etiologies of stroke during pregnancy or the puerperium.

Vasculopathy

Subarachnoid hemorrhage is a serious problem; bleeding from aneurysms or arteriovenous malformations (AVM) accounts for one half of maternal deaths due to cerebral hemorrhage. Subarachnoid hemorrhage is the third most common cause of nonobstetric maternal death.[39] The severity of this condition is further emphasized by the fact that about one half of patients with SAH die within 3 months of presentation.[40]

Intracranial aneurysms are an important consideration during pregnancy and the puerperium for several reasons: (1) patients can develop an aneurysmal SAH; (2) patients with a documented aneurysm may become pregnant or desire information of the risks involved in becoming pregnant; and (3) patients who have known risk factors for harboring an aneurysm can become pregnant or desire information regarding the risk of becoming pregnant.

Aneurysmal SAH can occur at any time during pregnancy,[40a] though the last trimester seems to carry an extra risk.[39,41] A period up to 6-weeks postpartum is also particularly associated with SAH. Occasionally, SAH may occur during labor or delivery.[39]

A patient presenting with the abrupt onset of severe headache, especially if the quality of the headache is unique in the patient's experience, should be suspected of having a SAH.[42] If meningismus or focal neurological signs, such as a third nerve palsy with impaired ocular motility and a nonreactive, dilated pupil are present, the likelihood of hemorrhage is increased. As many as one half of patients with a ruptured intracranial aneurysm will have a "warning hemorrhage" 7 to 10 days prior to a major bleed.[43–45] Although eclampsia can cause some of the same manifestations (such as headache and hypertension) as SAH, the absence of proteinuria and presence of meningismus should direct attention to a consideration of SAH.[42,46] A patient's prognosis is dependent on the neurological "grade," and detection of a warning hemorrhage allows prompt intervention to prevent subsequent deterioration.[47]

If a patient is suspected of having an SAH, a CT scan without contrast enhancement should be obtained to try to identify subarachnoid and/or ventricular blood. If blood is imaged, a contrast agent is administered if there is no contraindication, to attempt to visualize the source of the hemorrhage. Magnetic resonance images can also reveal a SAH. If blood is seen on CT scan or MRI, a lumbar puncture (LP) is not necessary because the diagnosis of SAH has already been made by an imaging technique. However, if the CT scan or MRI does not demonstrate blood, a LP should be performed to detect a small SAH missed by these imaging modalities.[47,48]

The patient with an SAH is at risk for numerous complications. These include hyponatremia, intravascular volume depletion, cardiac arrhythmias and infarction, seizures, increased intracranial pressure, hydrocephalus, aneurysmal rebleeding, and vasospasm causing delayed ischemic stroke. The management of patients with aneurysmal SAH is complex and beyond the scope of this chapter.[40,49] Prevention of rebleeding with early aneurysm surgery and the likelihood, prevention, and treatment of vasospasm are important concepts that should be considered in each patient.[50] However, the decision to use any therapeutic intervention should be tempered by possible obstetrical complications. For instance, the teratogenic potential of nimodipine, a calcium channel blocker that decreases the likelihood of vasospasm-associated delayed ischemic deficits, has not been assessed in humans and should be used in pregnancy only "if the potential benefit justifies the potential risk to the fetus."[51,52] Calcium channel blocking agents can have tocolytic activity.[53,54] Expansion of the intravascular volume, another effective means of treating vasospasm, should be carefully done in pregnant patients with already expanded intravascular fluids.[42]

Once a pregnant woman is identified as having an aneurysmal SAH, her obstetrical and neurological needs must be considered.[40a] Surgical treatment of an intracerebral aneurysm is possible during pregnancy and should be considered if the fetus is immature.[40a,42,55–58] Neurosurgical intervention can be combined with cesarean section if the fetus is mature.[42,59–61] The major neurosurgical modification imposed by pregnancy is the choice of anesthetic agents and techniques to lower intracranial pressure.[58–60,62] The overall management of the patient's pregnancy should be guided by obstetrical concerns, especially after the aneurysm is successfully treated with surgery. Modern neurosurgical and obstetrical anesthesia techniques allow close monitoring of maternal blood and intracranial pressures and fetal heart rate to minimize maternal and fetal risk.[57]

Various conditions are known to predispose to cerebral aneurysms. Identification of patients with these risk factors allows for early detection and successful treatment of an aneurysm while it is asymptomatic.[63] Aneurysms may occur on a familial basis[64] or may be associated with AVM,[65,66] moyamoya disease,[67] fibromuscular dysplasia, polycystic kidneys, coarctation of the aorta, pseudoxanthoma elasticum, and Ehlers-Danlos and Marfan's syndromes.[47] Interestingly, pregnancy-associated hypertension is a risk factor for the development of an aneurysm.[68]

Optimal management of patients at risk of harboring an aneurysm is dependent on a multifactorial analysis of the natural history of unruptured aneurysms coupled with the risks of intervention.[69–71] There seems to be a consensus that asymptomatic aneurysms greater than 7–10 mm in diameter should be treated surgically because of the relatively high risk of SAH.[72,73] Some investigators consider aneurysms greater than 5 mm in diameter deserving of surgical intervention.[74] A reasonable initial approach to the problem would seem to be identification of the high-risk patient, careful questioning to define prior events suggestive of a warning hemorrhage, and an attempt to visualize an aneurysm with MRI scanning and digital subtraction angiography.

The mode of delivery of a patient harboring an aneurysm that has not been surgically treated is controversial, with both cesarean section[62,75,76] and vaginal delivery[41,56,77–79] having advocates. Wiebers[80] has suggested that cesarean section be performed at 38 weeks if SAH occurred in the last trimester and vaginal delivery be allowed if SAH occurred in the first or second trimesters. Epidural anesthesia and forceps are recommended if vaginal delivery is elected.[58,79] Fetal well being seems to be preserved equally by either route of delivery.[40a] If surgical treatment of an aneurysm is not elected, the management of labor and deliver may have to be modified to minimize undue hemodynamic stress.[40a]

Arteriovenous malformations are another cause of intracranial hemorrhage.[56] The patient with an AVM tends to bleed during the 16th to the 24th week of pregnancy, shortly before labor, during delivery, or early in the puerperium.[41] The overall risk of bleeding from an AVM during pregnancy is 87%.[41] If a patient does have a hemorrhage during pregnancy due to an AVM, the risk of rebleeding during that pregnancy is 27%.[41] Patients with SAH due to an AVM tend to do better than those with SAH due to an aneurysm.[41]

Optimal management of an AVM has yet to be defined.[40a,80a] Embolization and/or surgical resection[81] can be attempted during pregnancy. Stereotactic radiosurgery, using the gamma knife or linear accelerators, can be used to treat an AVM[82–84b] and can be combined with surgery and/or embolization. Proton beam therapy may also be used to treat an AVM.[85] However radiosurgery does not protect against hemorrhage in the first year or so following therapy;[85] therefore, radiosurgery would not be effective in preventing hemorrhage within the time frame of a pregnancy if initiated during that pregnancy.

A spinal AVM can cause SAH[86] or intramedullary hematoma.[87] Symptoms due to a spinal AVM may fluctuate during pregnancy.[88] A spinal AVM should be considered as a possible cause of SAH if there is no obvious intracranial source of bleeding and no hematologic abnormality. A history of back pain or symptoms and signs referable to the spinal cord increase the likelihood of a spinal AVM.[88] Magnetic resonance imaging is an ideal technique for visualizing a spinal AVM during pregnancy.[89]

Because an AVM is liable to bleed during labor, patients harboring an AVM should be considered for elective cesarean section prior to the onset of labor.[80,80a,90] Presumably, the fragile vessels of an AVM cannot withstand the hemodynamic stress of labor and delivery.[41] However, vaginal delivery is possible and has been advocated.[40a]

Intracranial *venous thrombosis*, particularly superior sagittal sinus thrombosis, has a predilection for the puerperium. Patients typically present in the first 2-weeks postpartum,[91–93] but may become ill in the first[94,95] or last trimester.[91] Symptoms include headache, vomiting, convulsions, hemiparesis, blurred vision,[96] and altered mentation. Papilledema, meningismus, and fever may occur.[91–93,97] Typically there is thrombosis of the superior sagittal sinus with extension of clot into cortical veins producing hemorrhagic infarctions. The CSF may be bloody because of this hemorrhagic tendency.[98] Historically, the diagnosis was made by angiography but now CT scan and MRI[98a] can noninvasively confirm the diagnosis. A CT scan may reveal multiple parasagittal hemorrhages,[99] (Fig. 1) increased density of the tor-

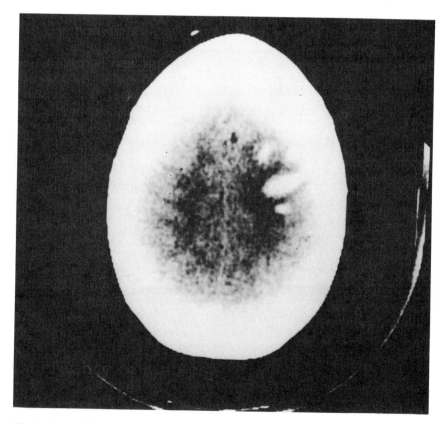

Figure 1: A CT scan without contrast administration demonstrates multiple venous thromboses with surrounding edema. (Courtesy of Robin Yu, M.D.)

cular herophili,[100] thrombosed veins,[99] small ventricles[101,102] and an "empty triangle" sign.[101]

The cause of the association of venous thrombosis with pregnancy is unknown. A hypercoagulable state has been blamed for the association,[91,93] but when clotting parameters of patients are compared to appropriate control groups, there is no significant difference between patients with venous thrombosis and healthy postpartum women.[92] Hematologic disorders such as paroxysmal nocturnal hemoglobinuria and hemoglobin SS disease are associated with venous thrombosis (see below), as are various causes of hyperviscosity such as dehydration.

The prognosis for patients with intracranial venous thrombosis is usually good and most recover without serious sequelae.[91–93,97,103–105] In life-threatening disease, however, control of increased intracranial pressure is critical.[92,94,103,106] Care should be exercised to avoid excessive dehydration and subsequent exacerbation of the thrombotic condition.[98] Anticonvulsants can be used to prevent seizures. Heparin has been administered successfully to some patients,[93,97,106,107] whereas other authors counsel against anticoagulation because of the risk of hemorrhage.[98,103] Although the presence of hemorrhagic lesions on CT scan would seem to prohibit the use of anticoagulants, heparin has been used safely in this setting,[97,97a] especially if intracranial hypertension is controlled.[106] Antiplatelet therapy has been suggested[92] and urokinase infusion has been used in a single patient with a postpartum thrombosis.[107] Thrombectomy of the superior sagittal sinus has been advocated for severe disease.[92]

Atherosclerosis is relatively rare in young women but does occur. Conditions predisposing to atherosclerosis such as hypertension and hyperlipidemia[108] would make a diagnosis of atherosclerotic cerebrovascular disease more likely in a young patient. Hypertension would also predispose to lacunar infarction due to arteriolar degeneration. Patients with homocystinuria,[109] as well as heterozygotes for homocystinuria,[110] are at increased risk for premature atherosclerosis and ischemic stroke.

Vasculitides cause stroke. The diagnosis is hastened by documentation of systemic disease and confirmatory serologic findings. A single patient with an isolated angiitis of the brain presenting with an intense headache during labor has been described.[111] Syphilis and other chronic meningitides should be considered if a CSF pleocytosis is present.

Takayasu's disease[112,113] is a chronic inflammatory arteriopathy that predisposes to stroke. The presence of bruits and diminished or absent pulses in a young patient are suggestive of the diagnosis. Takayasu's disease can be asymptomatic and initially discovered during a routine prenatal examination. Hypertension during pregnancy and especially during labor is the most common complication.[114,115] Intracerebral hemorrhage secondary to severe hypertension and antecedent cerebral ischemia may occur during labor.[114] With appropriate central hemodynamic monitoring, vaginal delivery can be accomplished[115,116] although cesarean section has been advised for women with severe Takayasu's disease.[114] The erythrocyte sedimentation rate is often elevated during the acute inflammatory stage of the illness. Corticosteroid therapy has been used to decrease the inflammatory reaction and can lead to reversal of arterial stenosis.[113,117,118]

Fibromuscular dysplasia of arteries supplying the brain is generally associated with a good prognosis[119] but stroke does happen.[119–121] Intracranial aneurysms can occur with fibromuscular dysplasia and, if present, can represent a significant risk to the pregnant patient. Fibromuscular dysplasia is also associated with arterial dissection and carotid-cavernous sinus fistula.[122,123] Management of fibromuscular dysplasia is controversial;[119] anticoagulation or antiplatelet therapy has been advocated to prevent a stroke or its recurrence.[120,121,124] Dilatation of affected arteries and direct surgical repair of diseased vessels may be considered.[120,121,125]

Internal carotid artery dissection is spontaneous or secondary to trauma.[126] Dissections can be accompanied by ipsilateral hemicrania and Horner's syndrome[127] and lead to stroke. Besides being associated with fibromuscular dysplasia, arterial dissections have been noted to occur in patients with cystic medial necrosis and Marfan's syndrome. A patient with carotid artery dissection 6 days following labor has been described.[128] Carotid duplex testing and MRI can suggest a diagnosis of carotid dissection[129] but the definitive diagnostic test is angiography. Therapeutic interventions include heparin administration[130] or surgery.[131] Initial medical therapy seems appropriate since many patients do well and recanalization does occur.[126,130]

Blunt cervical trauma can cause a carotid dissection and a delayed neurological deficit. Frequently a history of neck trauma is not available or attention may be diverted from the cervical carotid artery by other concomitant injuries.[132,133] Vertebral artery dissection can also occur spontaneously or following relatively extreme neck motion.[126]

A *carotid cavernous sinus fistula* can occur spontaneously during pregnancy or the puerperium. Patients present with unilateral exophthalmos, conjunctival hyperemia, retinal venous distention, an ocular bruit, or oculomotor disturbances. Intracranial hemorrhage has been rarely reported as a complication of these fistulae.[134] The fistula can heal spontaneously,[135,136] although usually transarterial balloon occlusion, or occasionally surgery, is indicated.[134,137–140] Ocular pneumoplethysmography may be a noninvasive technique to support the diagnosis pending definitive angiographic confirmation.[141]

Moyamoya disease can present with intracranial hemorrhage or ischemic stroke.[142] Moyamoya disease is characterized by progressive stenosis of the rostral internal carotid artery with development of an extensive collateral network. Aneurysms, pseudoaneurysms, and dilated vessels occur in association with moyamoya disease and predispose to intracerebral hemorrhage. Both cesarean section and vaginal delivery have been performed safely in women with moyamoya disease; careful control of blood pressure is warranted.[143–145] Optimal therapy for moyamoya disease is not defined; extracranial-intracranial anastomosis and encephaloduroarteriosynangiosis have been considered to improve cerebral blood flow[67,143,144] and antiplatelet therapy is often given.[142]

Pregnancy-associated arterial *intimal hyperplasia* has been implicated as a cause of transient cerebral ischemia.[146] This vasculopathy, which is hypothesized to be hormonally dependent, resolves following pregnancy. A postpartum *"reversible cerebral segmental vasoconstriction"* syndrome characterized by headache and focal neurological deficits has been described, as well as a patient with persistent vasospasm.[147a]

Transient emboligenic aortoarteritis describes an inflammatory focus in the media of the aorta and its major branches. A mural thrombus may develop over the inflamed area and give rise to an embolus. The erythrocyte sedimentation rate is elevated during the active inflammatory stage of the lesion.[148]

Cardiogenic Embolism

A *paradoxical embolus* should be considered as a possible cause of stroke in a patient with a venous thrombosis or right sided cardiac lesion.[149] Deep venous thrombosis is not uncommon during pregnancy and can be the source of an embolus reaching the brain via a patent foramen ovale, atrial septal defect, pulmonary arteriovenous malformation, or ventricular septal defect.[150] Air contrast echocardiography can demonstrate a patent foramen ovale and should be done during a Valsalva maneuver that causes hemodynamic changes that predispose to paradoxical emboli.[149,151,152] An overt leg venous thrombosis may not be present, but a noninvasive vascular examination such as a Doppler study can detect a blood clot. Puerperal ovarian vein thrombosis can be another source of paradoxical emboli.[153–155] Patients developing venous thrombosis should be evaluated for hypercoagulable syndromes (see below).

Peripartum cardiomyopathy is an uncommon disorder associated with mural thrombi.[156] A cerebral embolism can arise and even be the presenting feature of the cardiac disease.[156–158] *Puerperal nonbacterial thrombotic endocarditis* has been associated with hypercoagulability and may lead to cerebral emboli.[159]

Other rare causes of stroke during pregnancy are fat and air emboli. A *fat embolus* can develop after injury to adipose tissue.[160] Degenerating placental and decidual tissue was the apparent source of fat emboli in a single patient.[160] As will be discussed, maternal bone marrow can be the source of fat emboli in patients with hemoglobin SS or SC disease. *Air embolus* has been associated with abortion, cesarean section, vaginal trauma, and vaginal insufflation during pregnancy.[161–163] Air may gain access to uterine veins after entering the cervix and dissecting to the subplacental sinuses.[164,165] An air embolus can be visualized on CT scan[166] and treated with hyperbaric oxygenation.[162,165,167]

Mitral valve prolapse (MVP) has been associated with an increased likelihood of cerebral embolism in young patients.[168] Recent comments[149] have emphasized the infrequency of stroke, only 1 in 11,000 per year, in young individuals with MVP and recommend that other causes of stroke be evaluated before assigning blame to prolapsing mitral valves. Infective endocarditis and arrhythmias should be considered as causes of cardiogenic emboli in patients with MVP,[149,169,170] as well as prothrombotic conditions (see below).[171] There seems to be no undue risk of stroke during pregnancy and the puerperium, though MVP has been associated with stroke during these periods.[172–174] Emboli are usually due to sterile thrombi on the abnormal valves. Mitral valve prolapse deserves consideration as a cause of stroke even if appropriate cardiac auscultatory findings are absent.[175] The diagnostic yield of echocardiography is low in patients without clinical signs unless the patient has a first-degree relative with MVP.[169] The prognosis of MVP-associated stroke is generally good and therapy can consist of antiplatelet agents,[175] or occasionally anticoagulation.[168,176]

Patients with *artificial cardiac valves* can tolerate the hemodynamic demands of pregnancy.[177,178] Patients have a systemic embolic complication at a rate of 4.2% per "pregnant patient years".[178] The maternal risk of stroke must be balanced against the effects upon the mother and fetus of anticoagulants.[179–181] To avoid the fetal complications of coumadin, heparin therapy has been advocated.[182] However, heparin may not prevent thrombosis of the cardiac valve prosthesis or embolic stroke in all patients, and its use is associated with greater technical difficulties and expense than oral anticoagulants.[183–186] Heparin therapy has been associated with stillbirth or prematurity in one third of the pregnancies during which it is administered.[179]

An optimal anticoagulation protocol has yet to be devised.[178,181,187] Ginsberg and Hirsch conclude that, overall, heparin is safer for the fetus than oral anticoagulants, but carries a risk of osteoporosis for the mother when used for more than 6 months.[181] They propose using heparin during the first 12 weeks of gestation, coumadin from week 13 to 32, and heparin till term. Alternatively, heparin might be used throughout pregnancy.

Other causes of cardiogenic embolus include *infective endocarditis*,[188] *valvular heart disease, atrial fibrillation*, and *left atrial myxoma*, as well as *cardiomyopathies* and *nonbacterial thrombotic endocarditis* not etiologically associated with pregnancy.[149]

Echocardiography is indicated for young stroke patients with possible cardiogenic emboli.[149,189–191] Although small thrombi may not be detected on echocardiography, chamber size and valvular disease are well documented. Two-dimensional transesophageal echocardiography seems to provide a higher diagnostic yield than two dimensional transthoracic echocardiography.[192] Continuous ambulatory electrocardiography (Holter monitoring) can be used in selected patients to detect arrhythmias that predispose to emboli.[149,189,193]

Anticoagulation is commonly used prophylactically in patients with artificial cardiac valves and selected individuals with rheumatic heart disease to decrease the risk of systemic embolization. Most other conditions associated with cardiogenic embolism are not treated expectantly with anticoagulants although such treatment is a consideration at times depending on the underlying problem.[149] If the cardiac disease itself is treatable or resolves, anticoagulation can be discontinued.[194]

Because cardiogenic emboli can cause strokes that evolve from ischemic to hemorrhagic infarcts, the optimal time after a stroke to initiate anticoagulation to prevent a recurrent embolus has been under careful scrutiny.[149] In general, patients who suffer an embolic stroke that compromises a relatively small volume of brain can begin heparin therapy after 48 hours if a CT scan does not show a hemorrhagic infarct. Large embolic infarcts should be observed for 5 to 7 days prior to anticoagulation; if no blood is seen on CT scan after 1 week, anticoagulation should be relatively safe. In either event, a loading dose of heparin should not be used.[195] Immediate anticoagulation for a cerebral embolus should be deferred if a hemorrhagic infarct is demonstrated by CT scan. The agent of choice for long-term anticoagulation in pregnancy remains controversial; as discussed, coumadin and heparin each offer advantages and disadvantages.[179,181,182] A decision as to which agent to use is dependent, in part, on the nature of the specific problem, the stage of pregnancy, and the wishes and expected compliance of the patient.

Hematologic Conditions

Many hematologic diseases such as *thrombotic thrombocytopenic purpura* are associated with stroke but *hemoglobin SS* and *SC diseases* are among those conditions most likely to be associated with stroke in young women.[196] Pregnancy may be an added risk factor for neurological complications in patients with these hemoglobinopathies.[197] Hemoglobin SS disease is associated most commonly with ischemic infarction but can also cause hemorrhagic infarction, intraparenchymal and subarachnoid hemorrhage, and sinus and cortical vein thrombosis.[198] Large vessel occlusive disease is thought to follow proliferation of arterial intima and media damaged by ischemic insults to the vessel wall due to occlusion of the vasa vasorum.[198] Intracerebral and subarachnoid hemorrhage may follow ischemia to arterioles and capillaries.[198] Chronic exchange transfusion therapy seems to decrease the risk of recurrent stroke and slow the progression of the arterial lesion.[196,199] Hemoglobin SC disease predisposes to stroke in rare instances.[196,200] Both hemoglobin SS and SC disease have been associated with bone marrow-derived fat emboli, particularly during pregnancy.[201–203] The fat emboli cause an altered mental status, bone pain, pulmonary distress, or fever.[201]

Antiphospholipid (aPL), such as the lupus anticoagulant (LA) and anticardiolipin antibodies (aCL), are immunoglobulins associated with CNS and ocular ischemic events.[204] The LA can be an isolated finding or occur in the setting of systemic lupus erythematosus or phenothiazine, phenytoin, and penicillin use.[204] Ischemic stroke can be caused by in situ thrombosis, cardiogenic emboli, and potentially, paradoxical emboli from venous thrombosis.[204–206] A history of prior stroke, deep venous thrombosis, and spontaneous abortion suggests the presence of aPL. A false-positive venereal disease reasearch laboratory (VDRL) test for syphilis, thrombocytopenia, and an activated partial thromboplastin time (APTT) prolonged 5 seconds or more over the normal range suggest the presence of aPL.[207] An enzyme-linked immunosorbent assay (ELISA) or radioimmunoassay (RIA) for aCL and the Russell Viper venom and kaolin clotting times for the LA are some of the other tests available.[204] Optimal therapy for the aPL syndromes remains unknown; anticoagulants, antiplatelet agents, and immunosuppressive techniques have been used. [207,208]

Paroxysmal nocturnal hemoglobinuria (PNH) is a hypercoagulable disorder predisposing to cerebral venous thrombosis, especially in the postpartum period.[196,209,210] Anticoagulants have been suggested to treat CNS venous thrombosis and can be used with care if a hemorrhagic venous infarction is present.[97a,196,211] Patients with PNH can tolerate pregnancy but need to be carefuly monitored.[212–214]

Antithrombin III, protein C, and *protein S* are endogenous anticoagulants.[215,216] Deficiency of these proteins is associated with venous thrombosis, [217–219] although arterial thrombosis and stroke are particularly associated with antithrombin III deficiency.[220] Deficiency of protein C[220a] and free protein S[221] have been found in young stroke patients. An elevated plasma *factor VIII* level has been associated with multiple cerebral arterial thromboses.[222] Factor VIII is normally elevated during pregnancy[14] and patients with a preexisting chronic elevation of factor VIII might be at particularly high risk during pregnancy. As a better understanding of hypercoagulable states develops, a hematologic evaluation should be considered a part of the assessment of young stroke patients with otherwise unexplained ischemic stroke syndromes.[38,222a]

Miscellaneous

Migraine can cause ischemic stroke[223–226a] and may develop during pregnancy.[227–229] Elicitation of a prior history of migraine helps to support a diagnosis of stroke due to migraine. Migraine-like headaches occur in individuals with antiphospholipid antibodies; patients with migraine and stroke should be evaluated for aPL.[204] The relationship of migraine to pregnancy is discussed in depth in Chapter 5.

Alcohol consumption is a risk factor for subarachnoid and intracerebral hemorrhage.[230–233] The pathophysiology accounting for this relationship is yet to be determined.[234] Although alcohol intoxication has been indicated as a risk factor for ischemic stroke in young patients,[235,236] this finding remains controversial.[231] Current evidence suggests that "moderate" alcohol intake results in a "J"-shaped pattern of risk for ischemic stroke in whites.[232,233] The relative risk for ischemic stroke from alcohol in blacks and Orientals is minor or absent.[232,233]

Drug abuse can lead to hemorrhagic or ischemic strokes. A variety of drugs has been implicated including heroin, amphetamines, cocaine, phencyclidine, Talwin and pyribenzamine (T's and blues), and lysergic acid diethylamide (LSD). Routes of drug administration vary from individual to individual and therefore the pathophysiology of drug-associated stroke is varied. Potential mechanisms include endocarditis, embolization of foreign matter, drug-induced changes in hemodynamics such as hypertension or vasoconstriction, and immunological alterations leading to vascular injury.[237,238] A careful history and physical examination, together with appropriate toxicological tests, is often necessary to define the role of drug abuse in a stroke victim. Evidence for multiple drug use is frequent.[239]

Cocaine, and especially "crack" cocaine, has been implicated as the cause of various types of stroke.[238–239b] Snorted cocaine and "crack" smoking are particularly associated with stroke. Intracerebral and subarachnoid hemorrhage can occur in patients without an underlying vascular lesion or in patients harboring an aneurysm or

AVM.[240,241] Large or small artery occlusions are seen in some individuals with ischemic infarction. Patients, especially those suffering a hemorrhagic event, should have angiography to define the vascular anatomy.

Choriocarcinoma can cause a multitude of neurological problems.[242,243] Transient symptoms and signs develop from tumor emboli and permanent deficits can occur. Emboli can also lead to intraparenchymal and subarachnoid hemorrhage; aneurysmal dilatation of arteries may be present.[244-248] Mass lesions may develop from the hematogenous spread of trophoblastic tumors and be associated with hemorrhagic events. Patients with appropriate findings following a pregnancy or abortion should have serum chorionic gonadotropin assayed to screen for the presence of trophoblastic disease.

Human immunodeficiency virus (HIV) infected patients with the acquired immunodeficiency syndrome (AIDS) can develop ischemic and hemorrhagic stroke.[249] Ischemic infarction is associated with nonbacterial thrombotic endocarditis, cerebral vasculitis,[250] and the vasculopathies linked to lymphoma, syphilis,[251] cryptococcal and tuberculous meningitis, and herpes zoster. The lupus anticoagulant is found in AIDS patients. Central nervous sytem toxoplasmosis can cause transient neurological deficits. Hemorrhagic strokes are caused by thrombocytopenia, mycotic aneurysm rupture, and hemorrhage into metastatic Kaposi sarcoma.

Eclampsia, as discussed in Chapter 1, causes multiple neurological problems including CNS hemorrhage.

Summary

The causes of stroke during and after pregnancy are many. A systematic and thorough analysis of the patient is often required for a precise diagnosis. Elicitation of a key historical fact or a simple laboratory test can provide a critical clue.[38] For instance, several conditions present at characteristic times during pregnancy and the puerperium and knowledge of these relationships may simplify the path to a diagnosis (Table II).[4] Likewise, the presence of a hemorrhage on CT scan or MRI allows the clinician to direct attention to several important stroke syndromes that are particularly likely to occur with this finding (Table III).

Table II.
Major Risk Periods for Selected Syndromes

	Trimester			Labor/Delivery	Postpartum
	1	*2*	*3*		
Intracranial hemorrhage					
Subarachnoid bleed					
aneurysm			*	*	*
arteriovenous malformation		*		*	*
Takayasu's disease				*	
Moyamoya disease		*	*		*
Venous thrombosis					*
Cardiogenic embolus					
Peripartum cardiomyopathy			*		*
Nonbacterial thrombotic endocarditis					*
Fat embolus				*	
Trophoblastic disease					*
Eclampsia			*	*	*
Arterial occlusions	*	*			*

Table III.
Some Causes of Hemorrhagic Lesions in Pregnancy and the Puerperium

Intracranial hemorrhage
  aneurysm
  arteriovenous malformation
Venous thrombosis
Takayasu's disease (with hypertension)
Moyamoya disease
Cerebral embolism
Drug use and abuse
Trophoblastic carcinoma
Kaposi sarcoma
Eclampsia

The optimal management of cerebrovascular disease is predicated on a precise knowledge of the underlying pathophysiological processes. This knowledge is expanding rapidly and therefore new therapeutic strategies are evolving.[252,253] For instance, proper indications and methods for anticoagulation are still being defined. Even the optimal aspirin dose during pregnancy needs to be addressed.[254] Another area of controversy is the role of intracranial pressure (ICP) monitoring for acute stroke syndromes. Elevated ICP is a "final common pathway" for many types of CNS disease and often can be controlled by conventional measures such as hyperventilation, judicious dehydration, and corticosteroid therapy. Barbiturate therapy can lower ICP refractory to conventional measures[255,256] and holds promise in the care of selected stroke patients.[257,258]

Many issues concerning ICP reduction need to be studied further. For instance, high dose bolus therapy with mannitol is known to decrease ICP but can cause marked changes in fetal fluid balance.[259,260] Low doses of mannitol, administered as needed to control the ICP, may be used but the effect of low dose mannitol on the fetus is not well known.[58]

The implications of these comments are obvious. Stroke care is changing and optimal management of the stroke victim requires consultation with neurologists and neurosurgeons having up-to-date knowledge.[261] Physicians need to be cognizant of the many controversies still unresolved.

References

1. Robins M, Baum HM: Incidence. *Stroke* 12(Suppl 1):I45-I57, 1981.
2. Whisnant JP: The decline of stroke. *Stroke* 15:160–168, 1984.
3. Broderick JP, Phillips SJ, Whisnant JP, et al: Incidence rates of stroke in the eighties: the end of the decline in stroke? *Stroke* 20:577–582, 1989.
4. Wiebers DO: Ischemic cerebrovascular complications of pregnancy. *Arch Neurol* 42:1106–1113, 1985.
5. Wiebers DO, Whisnant JP: The incidence of stroke among pregnant women in Rochester, Minn, 1955 through 1979. *JAMA* 254:3055–3057, 1985.
6. Sandmire HF: Maternal mortality in Wisconsin: cerebral vascular accident. *Wis Med J* 88:23–24, 1989.
7. Sachs BP, Brown DAJ, Driscoll SG, et al: Maternal mortality in Massachusetts. *N Engl J Med* 316:667–672, 1987.

8. Hart RG, Miller VT: Cerebral infarction in young adults: a practical approach. *Stroke* 14:110–114, 1983.
9. Ramadan NM, Deveshwar R, Levine SR: Magnetic resonance and clinical cerebrovascular disease. *Stroke* 20:1279–1283, 1989.
10. Ross JS, Masaryk TJ, Modic MT, et al: Magnetic resonance angiography of the extracranial carotid arteries and intracranial vessels. *Neurology* 39:1369–1376, 1989.
11. Fletcher AP, Alkjaersig NK, Burstein R: The influence of pregnancy upon blood coagulation and plasma fibrinolytic enzyme function. *Am J Obstet Gynecol* 134:743–751, 1979.
12. Bonnar J, McNicol GP, Douglas AS: Fibrinolytic enzyme system and pregnancy. *Br Med J* 3:387–389, 1969.
13. Pinto S, Abbate R, Rostagno C, et al: Increased thrombin generation in normal pregnancy. *Acta Eur Fertil* 19:263–267, 1988.
14. Nilsson IM, Kullander S: Coagulation and fibrinolytic studies during pregnancy. *Acta Obstet Gynecol Scand* 46: 273–285, 1967.
15. Whitfield LR, Lele AS, Levy G: Effect of pregnancy on the relationship between concentration and anticoagulant action of heparin. *Clin Pharmacol Ther* 34:23–28, 1983.
16. Chan SYW, Chan PH, Ho PC, et al: Factor VIII-related antigen levels in normal pregnancy and puerperium. *Eur J Obstet Gynecol Reprod Biol* 19:199–204, 1985.
17. Wright JG, Cooper P, Astedt B, et al: Fibrinolysis during normal human pregnancy: complex inter-relationships between plasma levels of tissue plasminogen activator and inhibitors and the euglobulin clot lysis time. *Br J Hematol* 69:253–258, 1988.
18. Ballegeer V, Mombaerts P, Declerck PJ, et al: Fibrinolytic response to venous occlusion and fibrin fragment D-dimer levels in normal and complicated pregnancy. *Thromb Haemostasis* 58:1030–1032, 1987.
19. Malm J, Laurell M, Dahlback B: Changes in the plasma levels of vitamin K-dependent proteins C and S and of C4b-binding protein during pregnancy and oral contraception. *Br J Haematol* 68:437–441, 1988.
20. de Boer K, ten Cate JW, Sturk A, et al: Enhanced thrombin generation in normal and hypertensive pregnancy. *Am J Obstet Gynecol* 160:95–100, 1989.
21. Pekonen F, Rasi V, Ammala M, et al: Platelet function and coagulation in normal and preeclamptic pregnancy. *Thromb Res* 43:553–560, 1986.
22. Lewis PJ, Boylan P, Friedman LA, et al: Prostacyclin in pregnancy. *Br Med J* 280:1581–1582, 1980.
23. Tooke JE, McNicol GP: Thrombotic disorders associated with pregnancy and the pill. *Clin Hematol* 10:613–630, 1981.
24. Dahlman T, Hellgren M, Blomback M: Changes in blood coagulation and fibrinolysis in the normal puerperium. *Gynecol Obstet Invest* 20:37–44, 1985.
25. Thomas DJ: Whole blood viscosity and cerebral blood flow. *Stroke* 13:285–287, 1982.
26. Landi G, D'Angelo A, Boccardi E, et al: Hypercoagulability in acute stroke: prognostic significance. *Neurology* 37:1667–1671, 1987.

27. Ueland K, Novy MJ, Peterson EN, et al: Maternal cardiovascular dynamics. IV. The influence of gestational age on the maternal cardiovascular response to posture and exercise. *Am J Obstet Gynecol* 104:856–864, 1969.

28. Sullivan JM, Ramanathan KB: Management of medical problems in pregnancy: severe cardiac disease. *N Engl J Med* 313:304–309, 1985.

29. Wood JH, Kee DB Jr: Hemorheology of the cerebral circulation in stroke. *Stroke* 16:765–772, 1985.

30. Greenfield JC Jr, Reinbert JC, Tindall GT: Transient changes in cerebral vascular resistance during the valsalva maneuver in man. *Stroke* 15:76–79, 1984.

31. Barnet HJM: Platelet and coagulation function in relation to thromboembolic stroke. *Adv Neurol* 16:45–70, 1977.

32. Baker VV, Kort B, Cefalo RC: Effects of plasma on the platelet antiaggregatory action of prostacyclin in pregnancy. *Am J Obstet Gynecol* 156:974–977, 1987.

33. Fuchs A, Goeschen K, Husslein P, et al: Oxytocin and the initiation of human parturition. III. Plasma concentrations of oxytocin and 13,14-dihydro-15-keto-prostaglandin $F_2\alpha$ in spontaneous and oxytocin-induced labor at term. *Am J Obstet Gynecol* 147:497–502, 1983.

34. Sahmay S, Coke A, Hekim N, et al: Maternal, umbilical, uterine and amniotic prostaglandin E and $F_2\alpha$ levels in labour. *J Int M Res* 16:280–285, 1988.

35. Pennink M, White RP, Crockarell JR, et al: Role of prostaglandin $F_2\alpha$ in the genesis of experimental cerebral vasospasm. Angiographic study in dogs. *J Neurosurg* 37:398–406, 1972.

36. Moskowitz MA, Coughlin SR: Basic properties of the prostaglandins. *Stroke* 12:696–701, 1981.

37. Chyatte D: Prevention of chronic cerebral vasospasm in dogs with ibuprofen and high-dose methylprednisolone. *Stroke* 20:1021–1026, 1989.

38. Stern BJ, Kittner S, Sloan M, et al: Stoke in the young. *MD Med J* 40(7):453–462, 565–571, 1991.

39. Barno A, Freeman DW: Maternal deaths due to spontaneous subarachnoid hemorrhage. *Am J Obstet Gynecol* 125:384–392, 1976.

40. Biller J, Godersky JC, Adams HP Jr: Management of aneurysmal subarachnoid hemorrhage. *Stroke* 19:1300–1305, 1988.

40a. Dias MS, Sekhar LN: Intracranial hemorrhage from aneurysms and arteriovenous malformations during pregnancy and the puerperium. *Neurosurgery* 27:855–866, 1990.

41. Robinson JL, Hall CS, Sedzimir CB: Arteriovenous malformations, aneurysms, and pregnancy. *J Neurosurg* 41:63–70, 1974.

42. Giannotta SL, Daniels J, Golde SH, et al: Ruptured intracranial aneurysms during pregnancy. *J Reprod Med* 31:139–147, 1986.

43. Okawara S: Warning signs prior to rupture of an intracranial aneurysm. *J Neurosurg* 38:575–580, 1973.

44. Verweij RD, Wijdicks EFM, van Gijn J: Warning headache in aneurysmal subarachnoid hemorrhage. *Arch Neurol* 45:1019–1020, 1988.

45. Leblanc R: The minor leak preceding subarachnoid hemorrhage. *J Neurosurg* 66:35–39, 1987.
46. Eguchi K, Lin YT, Noda K, et al: Differentiation between eclampsia and cerebrovascular disorders by brain CT scan in pregnant patients with conclusive seizures. *Acta Med Okayama* 41:117–124, 1987.
47. Heros RC, Kistler JP: Intracranial arterial aneurysm: an update. *Stroke* 14:628–631, 1983.
48. Adams HP Jr, Kassell NF, Torner JC, et al: CT and clinical correlations in recent aneurysmal subarachnoid hemorrage: a preliminary report of the cooperative aneurysm study. *Neurology (Cleveland)* 33:981–988, 1983.
49. Solomon RA, Fink ME: Current strategies for the management of aneurysmal subarachnoid hemorrhage. *Arch Neurol* 44:769–774, 1987.
50. Wilkins RH: Attempts at prevention or treatment of intracranial arterial spasm: an update. *Neurosurgy* 18:808–825, 1986.
51. Nimotop (nimodipine). Miles Inc, Pharmaceutical Division, 1989 package insert.
52. Allen GS, Ahn HS, Preziosi TJ, et al: Cerebral arterial spasm—a controlled trial of nimodipine in patients with subarachnoid hemorrhage. *N Engl J Med* 308:619–624, 1983.
53. Huszar G, Naftolin F: The myometrium and uterine cervix in normal and preterm labor. *N Engl J Med* 311:571–581, 1984.
54. Tracy TS, Black CD: Calcium modulators: future agents, future uses. *Drug Intell Clin Pharm* 21:575–583, 1987.
55. Donchin Y, Amirav B, Sahar A, et al: Sodium nitroprusside for aneurysm surgery in pregnancy: report of a case. *Br J Anaesthesiol* 50:849–851, 1978.
56. Tuttleman RM, Gleicher N: Central nervous system hemorrhage complicating pregnancy. *Obstet Gynecol* 58:651–657, 1981.
57. Newman B, Lam AM: Induced hypotension for clipping of a cerebral aneurysm during pregnancy: a case report and brief review. *Anesth Analg* 65:675–678, 1986.
58. Willoughby JS: Sodium nitroprusside, pregnancy and multiple intracranial aneurysms. *Anaesth Intensive Care* 12:358–360, 1984.
59. Lennon RL, Sundt TM Jr, Gronert GA: Combined cesarean section and clipping of intracerebral aneurysm. *Anesthesiology* 60:240–242, 1984.
60. Conklin KA, Herr G, Fung D: Anaesthesia for caesarean section and cerebral aneurysm clipping. *Can Anaesthesiol Soc J* 31:451–454, 1984.
61. Buckland MR, Batjer HH, Giesecke AH: Anesthesia for cerebral aneurysm surgery: use of induced hypertension in patients with symptomatic vasospasm. *Anesthesiology* 69:116–119, 1988.
62. Kofke WA, Wuest HP, McGinnis LA: Cesarean section following ruptured cerebral aneurysm and neuroresuscitation. *Anesthesiology* 60:242–245, 1984.
63. Drake CG: Management of cerebral aneurysm. *Stroke* 12:273–283, 1981.
64. Acosta-Rua GJ: Familial incidence of ruptured intracranial aneurysms. *Arch Neurol* 35:675–677, 1978.
65. Miyasaka K, Wolpert SM, Prager RJ: The association of cerebral aneurysms, infundibula, and intracranial arteriovemous malformations. *Stroke* 13:196–203, 1982.

66. Wilkins RH: Natural history of intracranial vascular malformations: a review. *Neurosurgery* 16:421–430, 1985.
67. Suzuki J, Kodama N: Moyamoya disease: a review. *Stroke* 14:104–109, 1983.
68. de la Monte SM, Moore GW, Monk MA, et al: Risk factors for the development and rupture of intracranial berry aneurysms. *Am J Med* 78:957–964, 1985.
69. Levey AS, Pauker SG, Kassirer JP: Occult intracranial aneurysms in polycystic kidney disease. When is cerebral arteriography indicated? *N Engl J Med* 308:986–994, 1983.
70. Van Crevel H, Habbema JDF, Braakman R: Decision analysis of the management of incidental intracranial saccular aneurysms. *Neurology* 36:1335–1339, 1986.
71. Fleming C, Wong JB, Moskowitz AJ, et al: A peripartum neurologic event: shooting from the hip. *Med Decis Making* 8:55–71, 1988.
72. Ojemann RG: Management of the unruptured intracranial aneurysm. *N Engl J Med* 304:725–726, 1981.
73. Wiebers DO, Whisnant JP, O'Fallon WM: The natural history of unruptured intracranial aneurysms. *N Engl J Med* 304:696–698, 1981.
74. Ferguson GG, Peerless SJ, Drake CG: Natural history of intracranial aneurysms. *N Engl J Med* 305:99, 1981.
75. Borno RP, Kirkendall HL Jr, Stone BB, et al: Ruptured berry aneurysm in a pregnant patient at term. *Am J Obstet Gynecol* 121:573–574, 1973.
76. Meincke DL, Hurt WG, Young HF: Ruptured intracranial aneurysms in pregnancy. *Va Med* 103:878–881, 1976.
77. Hisley JC, Granados JL: Subarachnoid hemorrhage secondary to ruptured intracranial aneurysm during pregnancy. *South Med J* 68:1512, 1560, 1975.
78. Rish BL: Treatment of intracranial aneurysms associated with other entities. *South Med J* 71:553–557, 1978.
79. Young DC, Leveno MJ, Whalley PJ: Induced delivery prior to surgery for ruptured cerebral aneurysm. *Obstet Gynecol* 61:749–752, 1983.
80. Wiebers DO: Subarachnoid hemorrhage in pregnancy. *Semin Neurol* 8:226–229, 1988.
80a. Sadasivah B, Malik GM, Lee C, et al: Vascular malformations and pregnancy. *Surg Neurol* 33:305–313, 1990.
81. Stein BM, Wolpert SM: Arteriovenous malformations of the brain. II. Current concepts and treatment. *Arch Neurol* 37:69–75, 1980.
82. Leksell L: Stereotactic radiosurgery. *J Neurol Neurosurg Psychiatry* 46:797–803, 1983.
83. Lunsford LD, Flickinger JC, Steiner L: The gamma knife. *JAMA* 259:2544, 1988.
84. Kemeny AA, Dias PS, Forster DMC: Results of stereotactic radiosurgery of arteriovenous malformations: an analysis of 52 cases. *J Neurol Neurosurg Psychiatry* 52:554–558, 1989.
84a. Lunsford LD, Flickinger J, Coffey RJ: Stereotactic gamma knife radiosurgery. *Arch Neurol* 47:169–175, 1990.

84b. Heros RC, Korosue K: Radiation treatment of arteriovenous malformations. *N Engl J Med* 323:127–129, 1990.
85. Steinberg GK, Fabrikant JI, Marks MP, et al: Stereotactic heavy-charged-particle Bragg-peak radiation for intracranial arteriovenous malformations. *N Engl J Med* 323:96–101, 1990.
86. Caroscio JT, Brannan T, Budabin M, et al: Subarachnoid hemorrhage secondary to spinal arteriovenous malformation and aneurysm. *Arch Neurol* 37:101–103, 1980.
87. Collins JH Jr, Oser F Jr, Garcia CA, et al: Sudden paralysis in pregnancy due to spinal cord vascular accidents. *J LA State Med Soc* 138:44–48, 1986.
88. Aminoff MJ, Logue V: Clinical features of spinal vascular malformations. *Brain* 39:197–210, 1974.
89. Kulkarni MV, Burks DD, Price AC, et al: Diagnosis of spinal arteriovenous malformation in a pregnant patient by MR imaging. *J Comput Assist Tomogr* 9:171–173, 1985.
90. Laidler JA, Jackson IJ, Redfern N: The management of caesarean section in a patient with an intracranial arteriovenous malformation. *Anaesthesia* 44:490–491, 1989.
91. Bansal BC, Gupta RR, Prakash C: Stroke during pregnancy and puerperium in young females below the age of 40 years as a result of cerebral venous/venous sinus thrombosis. *Jpn Heart J* 21:171–183, 1980.
92. Estanol B, Rodriguez A, Conte G, et al: Intracranial venous thrombosis in young women. *Stroke* 10:680–684, 1979.
93. Srinivasan K: Cerebral venous and arterial thrombosis in pregnancy and puerperium: a study of 135 patients. *Angiology* 34:731–746, 1983.
94. Fehr PE: Sagittal sinus thrombosis in early pregnancy. *Obstet Gynecol* 59(Suppl):7S-9S, 1982.
95. Lavin PJM, Bone I, Lamb JT, et al: Intracranial venous thrombosis in the first trimester of pregnancy. *J Neurol Neurosurg Psychiatry* 41:726–729, 1978.
96. Monteiro MLR, Hoyt WF, Imes RK: Puerperal cerebral blindness. Transient bilateral occipital involvement from presumed cerebral venous thrombosis. *Arch Neurol* 41:1300–1301, 1984.
97. Bousser MG, Chiras J, Bories J, et al: Cerebral venous thrombosis: a review of 38 cases. *Stroke* 16:199–213, 1985.
97a. Einhaupl KM, Villringer A, Meister W, et al: Heparin treatment in sinus venous thrombosis. *Lancet* 338:597–600, 1991.
98. Averback P: Primary cerebral venous thrombosis in young adults: the diverse manifestations of an under-recognized disease. *Ann Neurol* 3:81–86, 1979.
98a. Hulcelle PJ, Dooms GC, Mathurin P, et al: MRI assessment of unsuspected dural sinus thrombosis. *Neuroradiology* 31:217–221, 1989.
99. Beal MF, Wechsler LR, Davis KR: Cerebral vein thrombosis and multiple intracranial hemorrhages by computed tomography. *Arch Neurol* 39:437–438, 1982.
100. Brant-Zawadzki M, Chang GY, McCarty GE: Computed tomography in dural sinus thrombosis. *Arch Neurol* 39:446–447, 1982.
101. Buonanno FS, Moody DM, Ball MR, et al: Computed cranial tomo-

graphic findings in cerebral sinovenous occlusion. *J Comput Assist Tomogr* 2:281–290, 1978.
102. Kingsley DPE, Kendall BE, Moseley IF: Superior sagittal sinus thrombosis: an evaluation of the changes demonstratad on computed tomography. *J Neurol Neurosurg Psychiatry* 41:1065–1068, 1978.
103. Gettelfinger DM, Kokmen E: Superior sagittal sinus thrombosis. *Arch Neurol* 34:2–6, 1977.
104. Younker D, Jones MM, Adenwala J, et al: Maternal cortical vein thrombosis and the obstetric anesthesioloqist. *Anaesth Analg* 65:1007–1012, 1986.
105. Haley EC, Brashear HR, Barth JT, et al: Deep cerebral venous thrombosis. *Arch Neurol* 46:337–340, 1989.
106. Hanley DF, Feldman E, Borel CO, et al: Treatment of sagittal sinus thrombosis associated with cerebral hemorrhage and intracranial hypertension. *Stroke* 19:903–909, 1988.
107. DiRocco C, Iannelli A, Leone G, et al: Heparin-urokinase treatment in aseptic dural sinus thrombosis. *Arch Neurol* 38:431–435, 1981.
108. Yatsu FM, Fisher M: Atherosclerosis: current concepts on pathogenesis and interventional therapies. *Ann Neurol* 26:3–12, 1989.
109. Mudd SH: Vascular disease and homocysteine metabolism. *N Engl J Med* 313:751–753, 1985.
110. Boers GHJ, Smals AGH, Trijbels FJM, et al: Heterozygosity for homocystinuria in premature peripheral and cerebral occlusive arterial disease. *N Engl J Med* 313:709–715, 1985.
111. Farine D, Andreyko J, Lysikiewicz A, et al: Isolated angitis of brain in pregnancy and puerperium. *Obstet Gynecol* 63:586–588, 1984.
112. Ishikawa K: Natural history and classification of occlusive thromboaortopathy (Takayasu's disease). *Circulation* 57:27–35, 1978.
113. Hall S, Barr W, Lie JT, et al: Takayasu arteritis. A study of 32 North American patients. *Medicine* 64:89–99, 1985.
114. Ishikawa K, Matsuura S: Occlusive thromboaortopathy (Takayasu's disease) and pregnancy: clinical course and management of 33 pregnancies and deliveries. *Am J Cardiol* 50:1293–1300, 1982.
115. Wong VCW, Wang RYC, Tse TF: Pregnancy and Takayasu's arteritis. *Am J Med* 75:597–601, 1983.
116. Winn HN, Setaro JF, Mazor M, et al: Severe Takayasu's arteritis in pregnancy: the role of central hemodynamic monitoring. *Am J Obstet Gynecol* 159:1135–1136, 1988.
117. Ishikawa K, Yonekawa Y: Regression of carotid stenoses after corticosteroid therapy in occlusive thromboaortopathy (Takayasu's disease). *Stroke* 18:677–679, 1987.
118. Gardner JD, Lee NR, Abdou NI: Takayasu's arteritis: reversal of pulse deficits after early treatment with corticosteroids. *J Rheumatol* 11:92–93, 1984.
119. Corrin LS, Sandok BA, Houser OW: Cerebral ischemic events in patients with carotid artery fibromuscular dysplasia. *Arch Neurol* 38:616–618, 1981.

120. Mettinger KL: Fibromuscular dysplasia and the brain. II. Current concept of the disease. *Stroke* 13:53–58, 1982.
121. Paulson GW, Boesel CP, Evans WE: Fibromuscular dysplasia. *Arch Neurol* 35:287–290, 1978.
122. Bellot J, Gherardi R, Poirier J, et al: Fibromuscular dysplasia of cervicocephalic arteries with multiple dissections and a carotid-cavernous fistula. A pathological study. *Stroke* 16:255–261, 1985.
123. Numaguchi Y, Higashida RT, Abernathy JM, et al: Balloon embolization in a carotid-cavernous fistula in fibromuscular dysplasia. *AJNR* 8:380–382, 1987.
124. Ezra Y, Kidron D, Beyth Y: Fibromuscular dysplasia of the carotid arteries complicating pregnancy. *Obstet Gynecol* 73:840–843, 1989.
125. Starr DS, Lawrie GM, Morris GC: Fibromuscular disease of carotid arteries: long-term results of graduated internal dilatation. *Stroke* 12:196–199, 1981.
126. Hart RG, Easton JD: Dissections. *Stroke* 16:925–927, 1985.
127. Mokri R, Sundt TM, Houser OW: Spontaneous internal carotid dissection, hemicrania, and Horner's syndrome. *Arch Neurol* 36:677–680, 1979.
128. Wiebers DO, Mokri B: Internal carotid artery dissection after childbirth. *Stroke* 16:956–959, 1985.
129. Rothrock JF, Lim V, Press G, et al: Serial magnetic resonance and carotid duplex examinations in the management of carotid dissection. *Neurology* 39:686–692, 1989.
130. McNeill DH, Dreisbach J, Marsden RJ: Spontaneous dissection of the internal carotid artery: its conservative management with heparin sodium. *Arch Neurol* 37:54–55, 1980.
131. Ehrenfeld WK, Wylie EJ: Spontaneous dissection of the internal carotid artery. *Arch Surg* 111:1294–1301, 1976.
132. Krajewski LP, Hertzer NR: Blunt carotid artery trauma: report of two cases and review of the literature. *Ann Surg* 191:341–346, 1980.
133. Bergquist BJ, Boone SC, Whaley RA: Traumatic dissection of the internal carotid artery treated by ECIC anastomosis. *Stroke* 12:73–76, 1981.
134. Stern WE: Carotid-cavernous fistula. In *Handbook of Clinical Neurology*. Edited by PJ Vinken and GW Bruyn. Amsterdam. North Holland Publishing Company, Inc., 1976, Volume 24, pp. 399–439.
135. Toya S, Shiobara R, Izumi J, et al: Spontaneous carotid-cavernous fistula during pregnancy or in the postpartum stage: report of two cases. *J Neurosurg* 54:252–256, 1981.
136. Hirata Y, Matsukado Y, Takeshima H, et al: Postpartum regression of a spontaneous carotid-cavernous fistula. *Neurol Med Chir (Tokyo)* 28:673–676, 1988.
137. Ahn HS, White RI Jr, Kumar AJ, et al: Carotid-cavernous fistula: intravascular treatment with a self-sealing detachable balloon. *Radiology* 149:583–584, 1983.
138. Raskind R, Johnson N, Hance D: Carotid cavernous fistula in pregnancy. *Angiology* 28:671–676, 1977.
139. Higashida RT, Halbach VV, Tsai FY, et al: Interventional neurovascular

treatment of traumatic carotid and vertebral artery lesions: results in 234 cases. *AJR* 153:577–582, 1989.

140. Debrun GM, Vinuela F, Fox AJ, et al: Indications for treatment and classification of 132 carotid-cavernous fistulas. *Neurosurgery* 22:285–289, 1988.

141. Gee W, Morrow RA, Stephens HW, et al: Ocular pneumoplethysmography in carotid-cavernous sinus fistulas. *J Neurosury* 59:40–45, 1983.

142. Bruno A, Adams HP Jr, Biller J, et al: Cerebral infarction due to moyamoya disease in young adults. *Stroke* 19:826–833, 1988.

143. Miyakawa I, Lee HC, Haruyama Y, et al: Occlusive disease of the internal carotid arteries with vascular collaterals (moyamoya disease) in pregnancy. *Arch Gynecol* 237:175–180, 1986.

144. Enomoto H, Goto H: Moyamoya disease presenting as intracerebral hemorrhage during pregnancy: case report and review of the literature. *Neurosurgery* 20:33–35, 1987.

145. Hashimoto W, Fujii K, Nishimura K, et al: Occlusive cerebrovascular disease with moyamoya vessels and intracranial hemorrhage during pregnancy. *Neurol Med Chir (Tokyo)* 28:588–593, 1988.

146. Brick JF: Vanishing cerebrovascular disease of pregnancy. *Neurology* 38:804–806, 1988.

147. Call GK, Fleming MC, Sealfon S, et al: Reversible cerebral segmental vasoconstriction. *Stroke* 19:1159–1170, 1988.

147a. Geraghty JJ, Hoch DB, Robert ME, et al: Fatal puerperal cerebral vasospasm and stroke in a young woman. *Neurology* 41:1145–1147, 1991.

148. Wickremasinghe HR, Peiris JB, Thenabadu PN, et al: Transient emboligenic aortoarteritis: noteworthy new entity in young stroke patients. *Arch Neurol* 35:416–422, 1978.

149. Asinger RW, Dyken ML, Fisher M, et al: Cardiogenic brain embolism: the second report of the cerebral embolism task force. *Arch Neurol* 46:727–743, 1989.

150. Shuiab A: Cerebral infarction and ventricular septal defect. *Stroke* 20:957–958, 1989.

151. Jones HR, Caplan LR, Come PC, et al: Cerebral emboli of paradoxical origin. *Ann Neurol* 13:314–319, 1983.

152. Lechat P, Mas JL, Lascault G, et al: Prevalence of patent foramen ovale in patients with stroke. *N Engl J Med* 318:1148–1152, 1988.

153. Rozier JC, Brown EH Jr, Berne FA: Diagnosis of puerperal ovarian vein thrombophlebitis by computed tomography. *Am J Obstet Gynecol* 159:737–740, 1988.

154. Savader SJ, Otero RR, Savader BL: Puerperal ovarian vein thrombosis: evaluation with CT, US, and MR imaging. *Radiology* 167:637–639, 1988.

155. Martin B, Mulopulos GP, Bryan PJ: MRI of puerperal ovarian-vein thrombosis (case report). *AJR* 147:291–292, 1986.

156. Homans DC: Peripartum cardiomyopathy. *N Engl J Med* 312:1432–1437, 1985.

157. Hodgman MT, Pessin MS, Homans DC: Cerebral embolism as tbe initial manifestation of peripartum cardiomyopathy. *Neurology* 32:668–671, 1982.

158. Lee W, Cotton DB: Peripartum cardiomyopathy: current concepts and clinical management. *Clin Obstet Gynecol* 32:54–67, 1989.
159. George J, Lamb JT, Harriman DGF: Cerebral embolism due to nonbacterial thrombotic endocarditis following pregnancy. *J Neurol Neurosurg Psychiatry* 47:79–80, 1984.
160. Jonas EG: Maternal death due to fat-embolism. *J Obstet Gynaecol Br Comm* 68:479–483, 1961.
161. Fyke FE III, Kazmier FJ, Harms RW: Venous air embolism. Life-threatening complication of orogenital sex during pregnancy. *Am J Med* 78:333–336, 1985.
162. Bernhardt TL, Goldmann RW, Thombs PA, et al: Hyperbaric oxygen treatment of cerebral air embolism from orogenital sex during pregnancy. *Crit Care Med* 16:729–730, 1988.
163. Younker D, Rodriguez V, Kavanagh J: Massive air embolism during cesarean section. *Anesthesiology* 65:77–79, 1986.
164. Aronson NE, Nelson PK: Fatal air embolism in pregnancy resulting from an unusual sexual act. *Obstet Gynecol* 30:127–130, 1967.
165. Bray P, Myers RAM, Cowley RA: Orogenital sex as a cause of nonfatal air embolism in pregnancy. *Obstet Gynecol* 61:653–657, 1983.
166. Hwang T, Fremaux R, Sears ES, et al: Confirmation of cerebral air embolism with computerized tomography. *Ann Neurol* 13:214–215, 1983.
167. Mader JT, Hulet WH: Delayed hyperbaric treatment of cerebral air embolism. *Arch Neurol* 36:504–505, 1979.
168. Barnett HJM, Boughner DR, Taylor DW, et al: Further evidence relating mitral-valve prolapse to cerebral ischemic events. *N Engl J Med* 302:139–144, 1980.
169. Devereux RB, Kramer-Fox R, Kligfield P: Mitral valve prolapse: causes, clinical manifestations, and management. *Ann Intern Med* 111:305–317, 1989.
170. Strasberg GD: Postpartum group B streptococcal endocarditis associated with mitral valve prolapse. *Obstet Gynecol* 70: 485–487, 1987.
171. Cheng TO: Transient ischemic attack: a complication of mitral valve prolapse in pregnancy. *Obstet Gynecol* 73:297, 1989.
172. Artal R, Greenspoon JS, Rutherford S: Transient ischemic attack: a complication of mitral valve prolapse in pregnancy. *Obstet Gynecol* 71:1022–1030, 1988.
173. Anzalone S, Landi G: Lacunar infarction in a puerpera with mitral valve prolapse. *Ital J Neurol Sci* 9:515–517, 1988.
174. Bergh PA, Hollander D, Gregori CA, et al: Mitral valve prolapse and thromboembolic disease in pregnancy: a case report. *Int J Gynecol Obstet* 27:133–137, 1988.
175. Jackson AC, Boughner DR, Barnett HJM: Mitral valve prolapse and cerebral ischemic events in young patients. *Neurology (Cleveland)* 34:784–787, 1984.
176. Marks AR, Choong CY, Sanfilippo AJ, et al: Identification of high-risk and low-risk subgroups of patients with mitral-valve prolapse. *N Engl J Med* 320:1031–1036, 1989.
177. Oakley C: Valve prostheses and pregnancy. *Br Heart J* 58:303–305, 1987.

178. Sareli E, England MJ, Berk MR, et al: Maternal and fetal sequelae of anticoagulation during pregnancy in patients with mechanical heart valve prostheses. *Am J Cardiol* 63:1462–1465, 1989.
179. Hall JG, Pauli RM, Wilson KM: Maternal and fetal sequelae of anticoagulation during pregnancy. *Am J Med* 68:122–140, 1980.
180. Oakley C, Doherty P: Pregnancy in patients after valve replacements. *Br Heart J* 38:1140–1148, 1976.
181. Ginsberg JS, Hirsh J: Anticoagulants during pregnancy. *Ann Rev Med* 40:79–86, 1989.
182. Hirsh J, Cade JF, O'Sullivan EF: Clinical experience with anticoagulant therapy during pregnancy. *Br Med J* 1:270–273, 1970.
183. Larrea JL, Nunez L, Reque JA, et al: Pregnancy and mechanical prostheses: a high-risk situation for the mother and the fetus. *Ann Thorac Surg* 36:459–463, 1983.
184. Hurwitz A, Milwidsky A, Medina A, et al: Failure of continuous intravenous heparinization to prevent stroke in a pregnant woman with a prosthetic valve and atrial fibrillation. *J Reprod Med* 30:618–620, 1985.
185. Brabeck MC: Ambulatory management of thromboembolic disease during pregnancy with continuous infusion of heparin. *JAMA* 257:1790–1791, 1987.
186. Barss VA, Schwartz PA, Greene MF, et al: Use of the subcutaneous heparin pump during pregnancy. *J Reprod Med* 30:899–901, 1985.
187. Iturbe-Alessio I, Fonseca MDC, Mutchinik O, et al: Risks of anticoagulant therapy in pregnant women with artificial heart valves. *N Engl J Med* 315:1390–1393, 1986.
188. Hughes LO, McFadyen IR, Raftery EB: Acute bacterial endocarditis on a normal aortic valve following vaginal delivery. *Int J Cardiol* 18:261–262, 1988.
189. Come PC, Riley MF, Bivas NK: Roles of echocardiography and arrhythmia monitoring in the evaluation of patients with suspected systemic embolism. *Ann Neurol* 13:527–531, 1983.
190. Knopman DS, Anderson DC, Asinger RW, et al: Indications for echocardiography in patients with ischemic stroke. *Neurology* 32:1005–1011, 1982.
191. Biller J, Johnson MR, Adams HP Jr, et al: Echocardiographic evaluation of young adults with nonhemorrhagic cerebral infarction. *Stroke* 17:608–612, 1986.
192. Zenker G, Erbel R, Kramer G, et al: Transesophageal two-dimensional echocardiography in young patients with cerebral ischemic events. *Stroke* 19:345–348, 1988.
193. Jonas S, Klein I, Dimant J: Importance of Holter monitoring in patients with periodic cerebral symptoms. *Ann Neurol* 1:470–474, 1977.
194. Easton JD, Sherman DG: Managenent of cerebral embolism of cardiac origin. *Stroke* 11:433–442, 1980.
195. Cerebral Embolism Study Group: Immediate anticoagulation of embolic stroke: brain hemorrhage and management options. *Stroke* 15:779–789, 1984.

196. Grotta JC, Manner C, Pettigrew LC, et al: Red blood cell disorders and stroke. *Stroke* 17:811–817, 1986.
197. Portnoy BA, Herion JC: Neurological manifestations in sickle cell disease: with a review of the literature and emphasis on the prevalence of hemiplegia. *Ann Intern Med* 76:643–652, 1972.
198. Wood DH: Cerebrovascular complications of sickle cell anemia. *Stroke* 9:73–75, 1978.
199. Russell MO, Goldberg HI, Hodson A: Effect of transfusion therapy on arteriographic abnormalities and on recurrence of stroke in sickle cell disease. *Blood* 63:162–169, 1984.
200. Fabian RH, Peters BH: Neurological complications of hemoglobin SC disease. *Arch Neurol* 41:289–292, 1984.
201. Boros L, Weiner WJ: Sickle cell anemia and other hemoglobinopathies. In *Handbook of Clinical Neurology.* Edited by PJ Vinken and GW Bruyn. Amsterdam, North Holland Publishing Co., Inc., Vol 38, 1979, pp. 33–51.
202. Chmel H, Bertles JF: Hemoglobin S/C disease in a pregnant woman with crises and fat embolization syndrome. *Am J Med* 58:563–566, 1975.
203. Shapiro MP, Hayes JA: Fat embolism in sickle cell disease: report of a case with brief review of the literature. *Arch Intern Med* 144:181–182, 1984.
204. Levine SR, Welch KMA: Antiphospholipid antibodies. *Ann Neurol* 26:386–389, 1989.
205. Young SM, Fisher M, Sigsbee A, et al: Cardiogenic brain embolism and lupus anticoagulant. *Ann Neurol* 26:390–392, 1989.
206. Wilson JJ, Zahn CA, Ross SD, et al: Association of embolic stroke in pregnancy with the lupus anticoagulant. A case report. *J Reprod Med* 31:725–728, 1986.
207. Levine SR, Welch KMA: The spectrum of neurologic disease associated with antiphospholipid antibodies. Lupus anticoagulants and anticardiolipin antibodies. *Arch Neurol* 44:876–883, 1987.
208. Briley DP, Coull BM, Goodnight SH Jr: Neurological disease associated with antiphospholipid antibodies. *Ann Neurol* 25:221–227, 1989.
209. Spencer JAD: Paroxysmal nocturnal haemoglobinuria in pregnancy: case report. *Br J Obstet Gynaecol* 87:246–248, 1980.
210. Wozniak AJ, Kitchens CS: Prospective hemostatic studies in a patient having paroxysmal nocturnal hemoglobinuria, pregnancy, and cerebral venous thrombosis. *Am J Obstet Gynecol* 142:591–593, 1982.
211. Vleymen BV, Dehaene I, Hoff AV, et al: Cerebral venous thrombosis in paroxysmal nocturnal haemoglobinuria. *Acta Neurol Belg* 87:80–87, 1987.
212. Jacobs P, Wood L: Paroxysmal nocturnal haemoglobinuria and pregnancy. *Lancet* 2:1099, 1986.
213. Beresford CH, Gudex DJ, Symmans WA: Paroxysmal nocturnal haemoglobinuria and pregnancy. *Lancet* 2:1396–1397, 1986.
214. Gramont AD, Krulik M, Debray J: Paroxysmal nocturnal haemoglobinuria and pregnancy. *Lancet* 1:868, 1987.
215. High KA: Antithrombin III, protein C, and protein S. *Arch Pathol Lab Med* 112:28–36, 1988.

216. Clouse LH, Comp PC: The regulation of hemostasis: the protein C system. *N Engl J Med* 314:1298–1304, 1986.
217. Schwartz ME, Harrington EB, Rand JH: Unusual venous thrombosis associated with protein C deficiency. *J Vasc Surg* 7:443–445, 1988.
218. Morrison AE, Walker ID, Black WP: Protein C deficiency presenting as deep venous thrombosis in pregnancy. Case report. *Br J Obstet Gynecol* 95:1077–1080, 1988.
219. Brenner B, Shapira A, Bahari C, et al: Hereditary protein C deficiency during pregnancy. *Am J Obstet Gynecol* 157:1160–1161, 1987.
220. Ueyama M, Hashimoto Y, Uchino M, et al: Progressing ischemic stroke in a homozygote with variant antithrombin III. *Stroke* 20:815–818, 1989.
220a. Camerlingo M, Finazzi G, Casto L, et al: Inherited protein C deficiency and nonhemorrhagic arterial stroke in young adults. *Neurology* 41:1371–1373, 1991.
221. Sacco RL, Owen J, Mohr JP, et al: Free protein S deficiency: a possible association with cerebrovascular occlusion. *Stroke* 20:1657–1661, 1989.
222. Kosik KS, Furie B: Thrombotic stroke associated with elevated plasma factor VIII. *Ann Neurol* 8:435–437, 1980.
222a. Hart RG, Kanter MC: Hematologic disorders and ischemic stroke: a selective review. *Stroke* 21:1111–1121, 1990.
223. Dorfman LJ, Marshall WH, Enzmann DR: Cerebral infarction and migraine: clinical and radiologic correlations. *Neurology* 29:317–322, 1979.
224. Cohen RJ, Taylor JR: Persistent neurologic sequelae of migraine: a caee report. *Neurology* 29:1175–1177, 1979.
225. Boguousslavsky JS, Regli F, Melle GV, et al: Migraine stroke. *Neurology* 38:223–227, 1988.
226. Rothrock JF, Walicke P, Swenson MR, et al: Migrainous stroke. *Arch Neurol* 45:63–67, 1988.
226a. Welch KMA, Levine SR: Migraine-related stroke in the context of the International Headache Society classification of head pain. *Arch Neurol* 47:458–462, 1990.
227. Bending JJ: Recurrent bilateral reversible migrainous hemiparesis during pregnancy. *CMA Journal* 127:508–509, 1982.
228. Titus F, Montalban J, Molins A, et al: Migraine-related stroke: brain infarction in superior cerebellar artery territory demonstrated by nuclear magnetic resonance. *Acta Neurol Scand* 79:357–360, 1989.
229. Mandel S: Hemiplegic migraine in pregnancy. *Headache* 28:414–416, 1988.
230. Stampfer MJ, Colditz GA, Willett WC, et al: A prospective study of moderate alcohol consumption and the risk of coronary disease and stroke in women. *N Engl J Med* 319:267–273, 1988.
231. Klatsky AL, Armstrong MA, Friedman GD: Alcohol use and subsequent cerebrovascular disease hospitalizations. *Stroke* 20:741–746, 1989.
232. Gorelick PB: The status of alcohol as a risk factor for stroke. *Stroke* 20:1607–1610, 1989.
233. Camargo CA Jr: Moderate alcohol consumption and stroke. The epidemiologic evidence. *Stroke* 20:1611–1626, 1989.
234. Gorelick PB. Alcohol and stroke. *Stroke* 18:268–271, 1987.

235. Hillbom M, Kaste M: Ethanol intoxication: a risk factor for ischemic brain infarction. *Stroke* 14:694–699, 1983.
236. Hillbom M, Kaste M: Ethanol intoxication: a risk factor for ischemic brain infarction in adolescents and young adults. *Stroke* 12:422–425, 1981.
237. Caplan LR, Hier DR, Banks G: Stroke and drug abuse. *Stroke* 13:869–872, 1982.
238. Levine SR, Welch KMA: Cocaine and stroke. *Stroke* 19:779–783, 1988.
239. Klonoff DC, Andrews BT, Obana WG: Stroke associated with cocaine use. *Arch Neurol* 46:989–993, 1989.
239a. Kaku DA, Lowenstein DH: Emergence of recreational drug abuse as a major risk factor for stroke in young adults. *Ann Intern Med* 113:821–827, 1990.
239b. Levine SR, Brust JCM, Futrell N, et al: Cerebrovascular complications of the use of the "crack" form of alkaloidal cocaine. *N Engl J Med* 323:699–704, 1990.
240. Henderson CE, Torbey M: Rupture of intracranial aneurysm associated with cocaine use during pregnancy. *Am J Perinatol* 5:142–143, 1988.
241. Mercado A, Johnson G Jr, Calver D, et al: Cocaine, pregnancy, and postpartum intracerebral hemorrhage. *Obstet Gynecol* 73:467–468, 1989.
242. Dagi TF, Maccabe JJ: Metastatic trophoblastic disease presenting as a subarachnoid hemorrhage: report of two cases and review of the literature. *Surg Neurol* 14:175–184, 1980.
243. Weir B, MacDonald N, Mielke R: Intracranial vascular complications of choriocarcinoma. *Neurosurgery* 2:138–142, 1978.
244. Pullar M, Blumbergs PC, Phillips GE, et al: Neoplastic cerebral aneurysm from metastatic gestational choriocarcinoma. *Neurosury* 63:644–647, 1985.
245. Seigle JM, Caputy AJ, Manz HJ, et al: Multiple oncotic intracranial aneurysms and cardiac metastasis from choriocarcinoma: case report and review of the literature. *Neurosurgery* 20:39–42, 1987.
246. Momma F, Beck H, Miyamoto T, et al: Intracranial aneurysm due to metastatic choriocarcinoma. *Surg Neurol* 25:74–76, 1986.
247. Watanabe AS, Smoker WRK: Computed tomography and angiographic findings in metastatic choriocarcinoma. *J Comput Assist Tomogr* 13:319–322, 1989.
248. Noterman J, Verhest A, Baleriaux D, et al: A ruptured cerebral aneurysm from choriocarcinomatous origin—a case report and a review. *Neurosurg Rev* 12:71–74, 1989.
249. Engstrom JW, Lowenstein DH, Bredesen DE: Cerebral infarctions and transient neurologic deficits associated with acquired immunodeficiency syndrome. *Am J Med* 86:528–532, 1989.
250. Yanker BA, Skolnik PR, Shoukimas GM, et al: Cerebral granulomatous angiitis associated with isolation of human T-lymphotropic virus type III from the central nervous system. *Ann Neurol* 20:362–364, 1986.
251. Katz DA, Berger JR: Neurosyphilis in acquired immunodeficiency syndrome. *Arch Neurol* 46:895–898, 1989.
252. Albers GW, Goldberg MP, Choi DW: N-methyl-D-aspartate antagonists: ready for clinical trial in brain ischemia? *Ann Neurol* 25:398–403, 1989.

253. Collins RC, Dobkin BH, Choi DW: Selective vulnerability of the brain: new insights into the pathophysiology of stroke. *Ann Intern Med* 110:992–1000, 1989.
254. Ritter JM, Farquhar C, Rodin A, et al: Low dose aspirin treatment in late pregnancy differentially inhibits cyclo-oxygenase in maternal platelets. *Prostaglandins* 34:717–722, 1987.
255. Caseby NG: Postpartum stroke successfully treated with high-dose pentobarbitone therapy: a case report. *Can Anaesthesiol Soc J* 30:77–83, 1983.
256. Miller JD: Barbiturates and raised intracranial pressure. *Ann Neurol* 6:189–193, 1979.
257. Ropper AH, Shafran B: Brain edema after stroke: clinical syndrome and intracranial pressure. *Arch Neurol* 41:26–29, 1984.
258. Ropper AH, King RB: Intracranial pressure monitoring in comatose patients with cerebral hemorrhage. *Arch Neurol* 41:725–728, 1984.
259. Battaglia F, Prystowsky H, Smisson C: Fetal blood studies. XIII. The effect of the administration of fluids intravenously to mothers upon the concentrations of water and electrolytes in plasma of human fetuses. *Pediatrics* 25:2–10, 1960.
260. Bruns PD, Linder RO, Drose VE, et al: The placental transfer of water from fetus to mother following the intravenous infusion of hypertonic mannitol to the maternal rabbit. *Am J Obstet Gynecol* 86:160–167, 1963.
261. Brott T, Reed RL: Intensive care for acute stroke in the community hospital setting. The first 24 hours. *Stroke* 20:694–697, 1989.

4

Brain Tumors in Pregnancy

Alessandro Olivi, M.D.
Rachel F. Brem, M.D.
Robert McPherson, M.D.
Henry Brem, M.D.

Introduction

The incidence of brain tumors during pregnancy does not appear to be different from that in the general population.[1,2] Nevertheless, since many intracranial tumors occur during the reproductive years and their clinical course may be influenced by pregnancy, it is important to be alert to the appearance of such tumors, and to consider both conditions in choosing strategies for treatment.

Several reports have suggested that physiological changes occurring during pregnancy influence the manifestations and progression of primary brain tumors.[3–6] Multiple mechanisms have been advocated, including an increase in blood volume, the accumulation of extra- and intracellular fluid with a consequent increased tendency to develop brain edema, and the direct effect of hormones on the tumor growth. The reported observations[3,7–9] that symptoms related to intracranial neoplasms often diminish or completely subside after parturition have corroborated the hypothesis of a direct hormonal influence. In the past, such observations have prompted clinicians to consider early termination of pregnancy as a therapeutic measure. As

From Goldstein PJ, Stern BJ, (eds): *Neurological Disorders of Pregnancy. Second Revised Edition.* Mount Kisco NY, Futura Publishing Co., Inc., © 1992.

a result of considerable advances in diagnostic modalities, anesthetic procedures, and surgical techniques, such "radical" measures can now be restricted to a very limited number of cases. Careful monitoring of the pregnancy, medications, or a surgical procedure with acceptable risks can be offered to the majority of patients. Furthermore, current information on the clinical behavior of different types of tumor allows the formulation of more comprehensive treatment plans.

This review describes the brain tumors that occur most frequently in women of childbearing age, their common presenting symptoms and signs, and an approach to the evaluation and treatment of patients affected by these tumors.

Pituitary Tumors

Pituitary adenomas are the most common intrasellar lesions, comprise 5% to 8% of all intracranial tumors, and have a peak incidence in women of childbearing age. Frequently, the hormonal changes associated with these tumors result in infertility, thus preventing their coexistence with pregnancy. Nevertheless, in those cases where the reproductive cycle is not affected, or when medical treatment (e.g., bromocriptine) has restored normal ovulatory function, this association can occur. In a recent study of 69 autopsy-obtained pituitaries from women who died during pregnancy, after abortion, or in the postpartum period, 8 (12%) noninvasive microadenomas were encountered.[10] This incidence is not significantly different from that observed in unselected adult autopsy series,[10,11] thus indicating that pregnancy does not have a pathogenic role in the development of pituitary adenomas.

Clinically, pituitary tumors manifest themselves with endocrinopathy and local mass effect. Functional adenomas produce excessive quantities of pituitary hormones, causing characteristic symptoms. For example, prolactin-secreting tumors, which are the most common, cause the amenorrhea-galactorrhea syndrome; growth hormone (GH)-secreting adenomas produce acromegaly; and ACTH-secreting tumors cause hypercortisolemia and Cushing's syndrome. As a consequence, functional adenomas often can be diagnosed when they are still small (microadenomas—less than 5 mm in diameter).

Nonfunctional adenomas usually manifest themselves by direct compression of the surrounding structures and therefore, as a general rule, are larger at the time of diagnosis.

The mass effect generated by any tumor in this area can result in compression of the following: the normal pituitary gland, producing pituitary insufficiency; the pituitary stalk, compromising the hypothalamic-hypophyseal axis (the so-called "stalk effect"); the optic pathways (most commonly the chiasm), causing visual deficits such as the typical bitemporal hemianopsia; and the cavernous sinuses causing oculomotor problems and, rarely, stroke. Headache, a symptom frequently associated with pituitary adenomas, is probably caused by stretching of the surrounding sensory innervated dura mater.

An important concern in a pregnant woman, whether she is diagnosed as having a pituitary adenoma before or during pregnancy, is the increase in size of the normal pituitary gland that occurs as a normal physiological consequence during pregnancy.[10,12] Complicating matters is the observation that pituitary adenomas may expand more rapidly in pregnant women. This effect is reported more frequently in patients with macroadenomas (5% to 20% of cases) than in those with microadenomas (1% of cases) and is usually more accentuated in the second and third trimester.[13] Patients should undergo frequent clinical evaluations (including ophthalmological testing) and laboratory and imaging studies to document progressive disease that would alter treatment.

Another fortunately rare event that can occur in any patient with a pituitary adenoma, and requires emergency treatment, is "pituitary apoplexy". This condition describes sudden hemorrhage or ischemic or hemorrhagic infarction of the pituitary adenoma that causes a rapid increase of the intrasellar pressure. A sudden and violent headache, often accompanied by vomiting, and rapid deterioration of vision or ocular motility are the most characteristic symptoms of this disorder. If this syndrome develops, an emergency decompressive surgical procedure should be performed to avoid progression of the deficit and possible death.

Diagnosis

When a pituitary tumor is suspected, a complete evaluation should include endocrinological testing, a neuro-ophthalmological evaluation including visual field assessment, and neuroimaging studies. As a general rule, the initial hormonal studies are directed toward a general baseline determination of the anterior and posterior pituitary functions. This evaluation commonly includes measurement of serum prolactin, an early morning cortisol, serum gonadotropins, urine volume, serum electrolytes and osmolarity, and a thyroid profile (T4, T3, and TSH levels). These tests can determine the presence of overproduction or lack of one or more of the trophic pituitary hormones. If a particular endocrinopathy is revealed by the clinical examination or initial laboratory testing, more specific endocrine tests are obtained. These tests include, for example, growth hormone and somatomedin-C levels and glucose suppression test for acromegaly; urinary free cortisol, dexamethasone suppression test, and ACTH levels for Cushing syndrome; and antidiuretic hormone serum level for diabetes insipidus.[14]

Imaging studies available to evaluate these patients have improved considerably in the last decade. Skull x-rays and polytomography, capable of detecting indirect signs of pituitary tumors in the form of bony erosion (sella and clinoids), have been replaced by high-resolution computed tomography (CT) and magnetic resonance imaging (MRI) (Fig. 1A). In most cases CT and MRI can outline even small tumors and their relationship with the surrounding neurovascular structures.[15–17] The use of intravenous contrast agents, iodine derivatives for CT and paramagnetic substances (e.g., gadolinium) for MRI, has also significantly improved the accuracy of these tests. Although allergic reactions to iodine agents are well known and caution should be taken when administered, there are no higher risks of side effects from these agents to the mother or the fetus.

Although CT utilizes ionizing radiation, each "slice" is highly collimated with minimal scatter. There are formulas for estimating the fetal radiation dose for any individual CT scanner at given distances from the fetus.[18] The dose of radiation to the fetus from a CT scan 30 cm or more away results in approximately 1/1000 of the maximum permissible dose of 0.5 rem.[19] Therefore, the resulting radiation to the fetus from a head CT represents little or no risk.[18,20] Magnetic resonance imaging does not utilize ionizing radiation and is currently believed to be harmless to the fetus.[21,22] Thus from a safety standpoint both imaging modalities are acceptable.

If available, however, MRI is the diagnostic procedure of choice

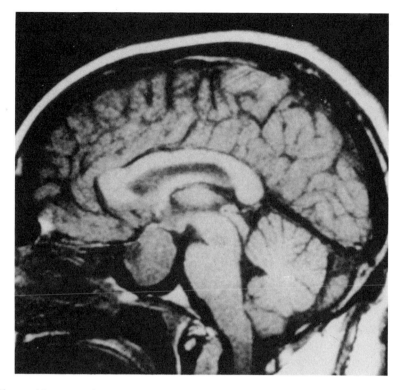

Figure 1A: Sagittal MRI (1.5 Tesla; T1 weighted image) of 39-year-old woman affected by a large nonfunctioning pituitary adenoma.

for pituitary adenomas. Magnetic resonance imaging enables visualization of details of the vascular structures and virtually eliminates the need for angiography in the evaluation of these patients. Furthermore, multiplanar views, important for a complete evaluation of pituitary tumors, can be obtained easily without changing the patient's position.

High-resolution CT scan provides detailed definition of the sella and surrounding bony structures. This information is particularly valuable in the preoperative evaluation of the sphenoidal bones when a transsphenoidal resection is planned.

Treatment

Bromocriptine has been used successfully to treat prolactin-secreting adenomas. The growth of the tumor is often significantly slowed or even arrested by this treatment and frequently normal endocrine function is restored, with reduction in size of the adenoma.[23] Patients with prolactinomas presenting with the classic amenorrhea-galactorrhea syndrome and placed on bromocriptine may resume regular ovulatory cycles and subsequently become pregnant. To minimize any possible effects of bromocriptine on the developing fetus, it is recommended that women discontinue taking this drug while trying to conceive.[24] Other medical therapies for hyperfunctional pituitary adenomas include cyproheptadine and ketoconazole for Cushing's disease and a somatostatin analog (SMS-201-995) for acromegaly, but no definitive information on the safety of these drugs in pregnancy is available.

Patients with tumors that do not respond to medical treatment, who show progression of the disease, either clinically or with imaging studies, or who develop pituitary apoplexy, require surgical treatment. Transsphenoidal resection of the lesion is generally the safest method for intrasellar tumors (Fig. 1B). Radiation therapy is often used as an adjunctive measure after surgery or as an initial form of treatment in selected cases.

In pregnant women who are clinically stable, show no changes on imaging studies, and have no visual deterioration, surgical intervention can be postponed until after delivery. Also, because radiation therapy for pituitary lesions is primarily used to prevent recurrences, it can generally be postponed until after delivery.

In summary, the majority of pregnant women affected by pituitary adenomas can be safely followed clinically with frequent ophthalmological evaluations and MRI or CT. Deterioration in the neuro-ophthalmic examination would indicate the need for imaging studies and possibly therapeutic interventions. Medical management may be quite effective. Only a small proportion require further surgical treatment before parturition.

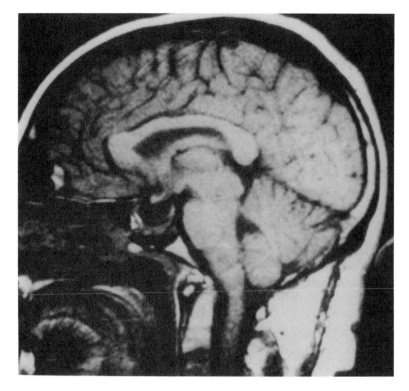

Figure 1B: Sagittal MRI (1.5 Tesla; T1 weighted image) of the same patient after transsphenoidal resection of the adenoma.

Glial Tumors

Glial tumors are the most common primary brain tumors of adults, comprising about half of all newly diagnosed brain tumors. They include different histological types (e.g., astrocytomas, oligodendrogliomas, ependymomas) and different grades of malignancy, from the rather quiescent pilocytic astrocytoma to the highly malignant glioblastoma multiforme. The presenting symptoms can be due to direct destructive or irritative involvement of the surrounding nervous tissue, or to increased intracranial pressure. While focal neurological deficits or seizures can be easily related to a new pathological process in the central nervous system (CNS), symptoms due to elevated intracranial pressure, such as headache, drowsiness, nausea, and vomiting are more difficult to distinguish from common disturbances of pregnancy. Accompanying signs such as papilledema, subtle changes in mental status, cranial nerve deficits, and motor or sensory dysfunction help in establishing the correct diagnosis.

A direct influence on tumor growth by the hormonal changes of pregnancy has been suggested, although no experimental evidence to support this has been demonstrated.[2]

The extent of brain edema surrounding glial tumors, which is a major factor in determining the severity of some neurological symptoms, may be influenced by the physiological changes occurring during pregnancy. The edema is thought to be the result of incompetent new neoplastic vessels that lack tight junctions between endothelial cells[25] and allow extracellular fluid to accumulate in the vicinity of the brain tumor. The tendency to retain extra- and intracellular fluid during pregnancy is considered a predisposing factor for the development of more extensive perineoplastic brain edema and, subsequently, more severe symptoms.[3,26] Fortunately, brain edema due to neoplasms has a significant (and at times dramatic) response to corticosteroid treatment. Corticosteroids can control the progression of symptoms and help in postponing, if necessary, surgical intervention. The hazards of the use of corticosteroids during pregnancy appear to be confined to the possible development of hypoadrenalism in the neonate, who therefore should be carefully observed after birth.[27]

Diagnosis

Once an intracranial neoplastic lesion is suspected from the clinical presentation, high-resolution CT scanning or MRI are the imaging tests of choice (Fig. 2A). As previously discussed, the choice of MRI or CT should be based on availability and clinical grounds because both modalities are safe for imaging brain lesions in pregnant women.[18] These diagnostic tests provide precise information on the configuration of the lesion, the relative vascularity, the presence of cystic components or concomitant obstructive hydrocephalus, and the extent of mass effect on the surrounding structures. The imaging studies may also provide clues about the histological type and grade of malignancy. Angiography, which utilizes significantly higher radiation doses,[17] is rarely needed. Electroencephalography is occasionally useful to optimally manage the patient's seizures.

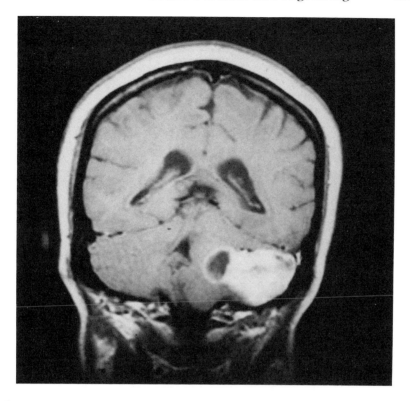

Figure 2A: Coronal MRI (1.5 Tesla; T1 weighted image) after injection of ga-dolinium-DTPA from a 37-year-old woman who was 7–months pregnant. An enhancing left cerebellar tumor exerting considerable mass effect on the fourth ventricle is evident.

Treatment

When the tumor is accessible, surgical resection is generally in-dicated (Fig. 2B). Radical excisions have been associated with longer survivals both in highly malignant and more quiescent glial tumors.[28] For deep-seated lesions, or tumors in direct proximity to eloquent portions of the cortex, limited diagnostic biopsies are performed. Re-cent technological advances have introduced precision stereotactic equipment that enables extremely accurate biopsies with a very low rate of morbidity. In a cooperative patient, a stereotactic biopsy can

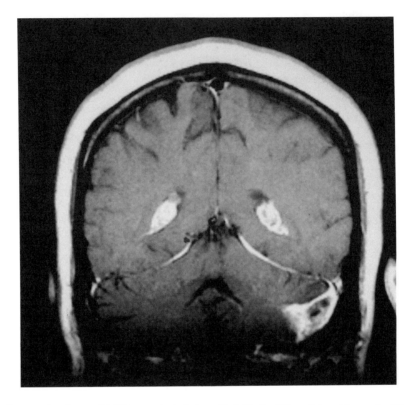

Figure 2B: Coronal MRI post-gadolinium (1.5 Tesla; T1 weighted image) of the same patient after an uncomplicated resection of a left cerebellar malignant astrocytoma. The patient subsequently delivered, at term, a healthy baby via cesarian section.

be performed with only local anesthesia. This approach is useful for particularly high-risk patients when a reliable tissue diagnosis is needed.

Conventional radiation therapy plays an important role in the treatment of glial tumors as an adjuvant measure after surgery. Stereotactic radiosurgery, utilizing precisely defined converging radiation beams (gamma knife and linear accelerators), provides a valid alternative to surgery for the radical treatment of small deep-seated lesions.[29–31] Such precise radiation therapy, which has minimal scatter to even the surrounding brain, has obvious advantages for the pregnant woman.

The treatment plan for a pregnant woman diagnosed with a glial tumor should be individualized. If the tumor is causing progressive symptoms, or if it is large or surrounded by edema causing considerable mass effect and/or increased intracranial pressure, a surgical resection and decompression are performed as soon as possible. If the increased intracranial pressure is the result of obstructive hydrocephalus, a shunting procedure should be performed. When the tumor is not producing much mass effect, the symptoms are not progressive, or the patient is clinically stable, the option of a diagnostic stereotactic biopsy or the postponement of any kind of invasive procedures until after delivery is available. In both cases, the patient should be followed with frequent neurological examinations, neuroimaging studies, and, when necessary, medical treatment throughout the pregnancy.

Two types of agents are commonly used to control the symptoms associated with glial tumors: synthetic corticosteroids (e.g., dexamethasone and methylprednisolone) to ameliorate the perineoplastic brain edema; and anticonvulsants for seizure control and prophylaxis. At present, it is not clear whether synthetic corticosteroids affect the development of the embryo or fetus. Prolonged use of these agents (as is frequently required in patients with malignant gliomas) can certainly inhibit the activity of the adrenal glands both in the mother and fetus. Consequent hypoadrenalism should be anticipated in infants born to mothers undergoing corticosteroid treatment during pregnancy. As with any other agent for which teratogenicity has not been determined, the use of corticosteroids is discouraged during the early phase of pregnancy unless the benefits of this treatment clearly outweigh the potential hazards to the mother and the fetus.

A different approach should be taken toward the use of anticonvulsants in pregnant women because of the association of these agents with teratogenicity. Although this controversial topic is discussed in detail in Chapter 2, a few recommendations can be made pertaining to pregnant women affected by brain tumors and seizures. Because no anticonvulsants are absolutely free of significant teratogenic effect, their use—even in patients with brain tumors—should be limited to those patients with generalized motor seizures or multiple seizures jeopardizing the health of the mother and fetus. When only a single focal seizure is reported, serious consideration should be given to deferring the initiation of anticonvulsant treatment. Likewise, pro-phylactic anticonvulsant treatment in women undergoing craniotomy and who have no history of seizures should be generally avoided. If anticonvulsant treatment is indicated, a single agent regimen is pref-erable. Phenobarbital or carbamazepine are often favored over other anticonvulsants, but good comparative data are lacking. Trimetha-dione and valproic acid should be avoided because of their well es-tablished teratogenic effect.[32,33]

Radiation Therapy and Chemotherapy

Both irradiation and chemotherapy are commonly used to treat patients with malignant gliomas. Although in most instances these therapies can be postponed until after delivery, if treatment is re-quired during gestation, it is important to take safety precautions for the best protection of the fetus. It is generally accepted that a fetus should not absorb more than 50 rad at any time during gestation.[34] Acute radiation during the 8th to 15th week of gestation with 100 rad (1 Gy) or more presents a substantial risk for abortion or mental re-tardation and congenital defects to the surviving embryo.[35] Consid-ering, however, the relatively long distance of the maternal brain from the abdomen, the limited scattering of the ionizing radiation through the body, and the use of appropriate lead shielding that reduces ra-diation diffusion through the air, the fetus can generally be ade-quately protected from dangerous radiation levels.

The use of chemotherapeutic agents should be avoided during the first trimester of pregnancy.[36] In particular, antimetabolites such as aminopterin and methotrexate have been associated with fetal ab-normalities when given during the first trimester.[37] Studies on ani-mals have indicated a teratogenic effect of carmustine (BCNU), the most widely used agent for malignant gliomas, when given early in pregnancy.[38] There is no evidence of an increased risk of teratogen-icity associated with the administration of cytotoxic drugs in the sec-ond and third trimester.[36,39,40] The possibility of reducing the sys-temic effects of chemotherapy by the interstitial implant of biocompatible polymers impregnated with chemotherapeutic agents has been recently investigated.[41] Conceivably, one of the important clinical applications of this novel method would be the adjuvant treatment of pregnant women affected by malignant brain tumors.

Meningiomas and Vascular Tumors

Meningiomas and vascular tumors have been frequently reported to present and progress during pregnancy.[42-45] Meningiomas originate from the meninges, are generally slow-growing, are more common in females than in males (3:1), and are usually surgically resectable. Among the vascular tumors, benign hemangioblastomas are the most common, characteristically occurring in the posterior fossa in young adults. Since the first observations by Cushing and Bailey,[46] these tumors have been reported to show rapid progression of symptoms during the course of pregnancy, followed by decrease and, at times, disappearance of the same symptoms after parturition.[44,45] The leading hypotheses on the mechanisms for an increase in size of the tumor during pregnancy are: (1) a rapid expansion of the vascular bed (vascular engorgement) as a result of the generalized increase of blood volume occurring during pregnancy;[44,47] and (2) a direct hormonal effect on the tumor's growth rate, mediated by progesterone and estrogen receptors that are frequently detected in meningioma cells.[48-50]

Treatment

Surgical resection is the only definitive treatment for these benign tumors. Pregnant women affected by these tumors should be followed very closely. Because these tumors are usually slow growing, it is generally safe to defer surgery until after pregnancy, unless progression of disease jeopardizes the health of the patient. In that event, surgical resection of the tumor can be done during pregnancy.

Other Tumors

Any other primary brain tumor of adulthood can occasionally become manifest in a pregnant woman. Acoustic neuromas,[51] ependymomas,[52] medulloblastomas,[1,5] and choroid plexus papillomas[5] have been reported to occur in pregnant women. Recently, with the increased prevalence of acquired immunodeficiency syndrome (AIDS), the incidence of primary brain lymphoma has increased.[53] This tumor is frequently associated with immunodeficient states and can also theoretically occur during pregnancy. Surgical intervention is oriented to establishing a tissue diagnosis usually by stereotactic biopsy, because the lymphoma is generally very radiation- and/or chemotherapy-sensitive.[53]

Metastatic tumors to the brain are more frequent in older patients but can also occur in women of childbearing age. The treatment is largely palliative and varies according to the nature of the primary tumor and the extent of the systemic and CNS dissemination.[54] In this disease too, establishing a definite tissue diagnosis is very important. In the case of solitary brain metastases that are surgically accessible, there is strong evidence that surgical resection followed by radiation treatment is the treatment that provides the longest survival.[55] Although lung cancer, breast cancer, and melanomas are statistically the most frequent primary tumors to metastasize to the brain, it is important to mention choriocarcinoma because of its possible occurrence during pregnancy and because it can metastasize to the brain.[56,57] This tumor, originating from the trophoblast that produces human chorionic gonadotropin, has a known tendency to spontaneous hemorrhage and can therefore cause acute CNS symptoms when an intratumoral bleed occurs. Irradiation and chemotherapy play a very important role in the treatment of this tumor,[58] with surgical treatment being reserved for selected cases.

Pseudotumor Cerebri

Pseudotumor cerebri, also known as benign intracranial hypertension, is a self-limited condition characterized by an abnormally elevated intracranial pressure with no apparent cause. It can occur in pregnant women, particularly during the first trimester, and some of its symptoms mimic the ones of a brain tumor.[59] Some of the most common presenting symptoms are headache, blurred vision, dizziness, vomiting, tinnitus, and paresthesias. Obtundation is never present. A small number of patients can experience progressive visual impairment, most likely as the result of chronic papilledema. The etiology is still unclear and several factors have been advocated to be related with the development of this condition including vascular obstructions of the draining sinuses, increased cerebral blood volume, endocrine dysfunction, and electrolyte imbalances. The diagnosis is usually one of exclusion. Imaging studies occasionally demonstrate small ventricles but are important in eliminating the occurrence of other structural diseases. Lumbar puncture, after a CT scan or MRI, rules out a mass lesion, has a role in confirming the diagnosis, eliminating the possibility of infectious or inflammatory states, and temporarily treating the symptoms. Patients affected by pseudotumor cerebri should be followed periodically with complete ophthalmological evaluations. Medical treatment with small doses of corticosteroids and acetazolamide or other diuretics is often successful in controlling the symptoms. Serial lumbar punctures or surgical insertion of a lumboperitoneal shunt should be reserved for the medically refractory patient with documented progression of tbe visual impairment. Optic nerve sheath decompression has recently been utilized for the rare patient with progressive visual loss. Pseudotumor cerebri is not a contraindication for vaginal delivery.[60]

Anesthetic Considerations

In dealing with pregnant patients affected by neurosurgical disorders, there are two anesthetic issues that should be addressed: the optimal anesthesia techniques for delivery in patients with intracranial lesions and the recommended anesthesia measures for the pregnant patients requiring craniotomy.

Delivery in Patients With Intracranial Lesions

The time of delivery is extremely important in infant viability. Traditionally, delivery was postponed until 36–38 weeks gestation to decrease the risk of the respiratory distress syndrome. Recent advances in the use of surfactant suggest that safe delivery at 32 weeks gestation may be an option.[61] The intracranial pathology greatly affects the anesthetic plan for delivery. If delivery is to be accomplished prior to neurosurgical treatment, the intracranial pathology must be carefully considered. If delivery and craniotomy are to be accomplished during the same anesthetic, the anesthetic management plan should be that required for craniotomy alone. Rapid initiation of general anesthesia with intravenous agents, endotracheal intubation and mild hyperventilation probably have little adverse effects on the fetus. The discussion will be divided into lesions with intracranial mass effect and those without mass effect. These two groups differ considerably in their potential response to regional anesthesia (subarachnoid block; epidural; caudal).

Patients ready for delivery harboring lesions causing mass effect are best anesthetized with general endotracheal anesthesia. The CNS effects of active labor in such patients are poorly understood but unlikely to be advantageous to the parturient. Cesarean section under general anesthesia is quick, safe and has only minor disadvantages to the fetus. The most likely problem would be respiratory depression in the newborn that can be treated quite easily. Regional anesthesia should be avoided because of the risk of loss of cerebrospinal fluid and herniation through the foramen magnum. Because accidental dural puncture is an accepted consequence of both epidural and caudal anesthesia, they are best avoided.

Patients with intracranial lesions not exerting mass effect, on the other hand, are excellent candidates for regional anesthesia, specifically epidural anesthesia. An instrumented delivery should be anticipated and, in fact, encouraged.

Anesthesia for Pregnant Women Requiring Craniotomy

Craniotomy in the pregnant patient may be required for both neoplastic and vascular processes. In the first trimester, the multiple drugs required might increase the risk of developmental abnormalities, whereas in the second and third trimesters drug-induced abnormalities would seem less likely. Coincidental surgery during pregnancy appears to increase the risk of first and second trimester spontaneous abortion but not the incidence of congenital abnormalities.[62]

The physiological changes of pregnancy require some special

consideration in surgery and anesthesia, particularly in drug doses and in surgical positioning. Pregnancy decreases anesthetic requirements by 30%,[63] increases plasma volume and total blood volume with a dilutional anemia, and increases cardiac output by 50%. The lung closing capacity is increased and the supine patient is at increased risk of atelectasis. Gastric morbidity is decreased and the patient is at increased risk of vomiting and aspiration upon induction of anesthesia.[64]

The pregnant patient should be positioned to prevent vena cava compression. In the supine patient a wedge (folded sheet) should be placed under the right hip to minimize caval compression. Positioning in either the sitting or park bench position should have little detrimental effect on uterine blood flow. However, the prone position should be avoided if possible because increased intrathoracic and intra-abdominal pressure may decrease uterine blood flow. Maintenance of normal uterine blood flow is important for the viability of the fetus. Potential causes of decreased uterine artery blood flow are vena cava compression by the uterus (supine hypotension syndrome), α-vasoconstrictors such as phenylephrine, and hyperventilation. A decrease in $PaCO_2$ from the normal for pregnancy ($PaCO_2$ = 32 mm Hg) to 25 mm Hg decreases uterine artery blood flow 25%, but the effect may be caused by mechanical ventilation rather than simple changes in $PaCO_2$.[65]

Controlled hypotension may be required and its effect on uterine blood and the fetus is important. There are several case reports of hypotension to a mean arterial blood pressure of 40–50 mm Hg for up to 40 minutes produced by either isoflurane or nitroprusside without injury to the fetus.[66–68]

Thus it appears that after the first trimester, a carefully controlled anesthetic offers little risk to the fetus. Hyperventilation probably should be used only sparingly, and vasoconstrictors avoided. Careful attention to positioning to avoid uterine effects on venous return is required. Monitoring of the fetus by Doppler will be a fair indication of the adequacy of oxygen delivery to the fetus.

Conclusions

Although it is clear that the physiological changes occurring during pregnancy can influence the severity and duration of symptoms associated with intracranial lesions, particularly for pituitary adenomas, glial tumors, meningiomas, and vascular tumors, there is no evidence that pregnancy predisposes women to develop primary or metastatic brain tumors. The incidence of CNS tumors during pregnancy is no greater than in the general population. Furthermore, the availability of sophisticated diagnostic tools allows early diagnosis and more precise patient evaluation. Both MRI and CT scans of the brain are considered safe during pregnancy and therefore the choice of imaging modality should be made on clinical grounds.

Careful monitoring of the patient during pregnancy, with frequent neurological examinations, neuroimaging studies, and medical treatment, usually permits postponement of invasive intervention until after delivery. If surgery is necessary, however, it can usually be performed with minimal risk to the patient and her fetus because of the improvement in surgical and anesthetic techniques. Even radiotherapy and chemotherapy can be administered with appropriate caution. Therefore, in the majority of cases, the clinical course of pregnant women with primary or metastatic brain tumors can be controlled without prematurely terminating gestation.

References

1. Smolik EA, Nash FP, Clawson JW: Neurological and neurosurgical complications associated with pregnancy and the puerperium. *South Med J* 50:561–572, 1957.
2. Roelvink NCA, Kamphorst W, Van Alpen HAM, et al: Pregnancy-related primary brain and spinal tumors. *Arch Neurol* 44:209–215, 1987.
3. Kemper MD: Management of pregnancy associated with brain tumors. *Am J Obstet Gynecol* 87:858–864, 1963.
4. Whitcher BR: Brain tumor complicating pregnancy. *J Med Soc NJ* 53:112–114, 1956.
5. Barnes JE, Abbott KH: Cerebral complications incurred during pregnancy and puerperium. *Am J Obstet Gynecol* 82:192–207, 1961.
6. Gregory JR, Watkins G: Eclamptic manifestations occurring in pregnancy complicated by brain tumor. *Am J Obstet Gynecol* 60:1263–1271, 1950.
7. Weyand RD: The effect of pregnancy on intracranial meningiomas occurring about the optic chiasm. *Surg Clin North Am* 31:1225–1233, 1925.
8. Bickerstaff ER, Small JM, Guest IA: The relapsing course of certain meningiomas in relation to pregnancy and menstruation. *J Neurol Neurosurg Psychiatry* 21:89–91, 1958.
9. Michelsen JJ, New PFJ: Brain tumour and pregnancy. *J Neurol Neurosurg Psychiatry* 32:305–307, 1969.

10. Scheithauer BW, Sano T, Kovacs KT, et al: The pituitary gland in pregnancy: a clinicopathologic and immunohistochemical study of 69 cases. *Mayo Clin Proc* 65:461–474, 1990.
11. Bergland RM, Ray BS, Torack RM: Anatomical variations in the pituitary gland and adjacent structures in 225 human autopsy cases. *J Neurosurg* 28:93–99, 1968.
12. Goluboff LG, Erzin C: Effect of pregnancy on the somatotroph and the prolactin cells of the human adenohypophysis. *J Clin Endocrinol Metab* 29:1533, 1969.
13. Gemzell C, Wang CF: Outcome of pregnancy in women with pituitary adenoma. *Fertil Steril* 31:363–372, 1979.
14. Tindall GT, Barrow DL: Current Management of pituitary tumors-Part I. *Contemp Neurosurg* Vol. 10, No. 2, 1988.
15. Creasy JL: CT and MRI compete in diagnosis of CNS disease. *Diagn Imaging* 12:96–101, 1990.
16. Kulkarni MV, Lee KF, McArdle CB, et al: 1.5 T MR imaging of pituitary microadenomas: technical considerations and CT correlation. *AJNR* 9:5–11, 1988.
17. Young SC, Grossman RI, Goldberg HI, et al: MR of vascular encasement in parasellar mass: comparison with angiography and CT. *AJNR* 9:35–38, 1988.
18. Felmlee JP, Gray JE, Leetzow ML, et al: Estimated fetal radiation dose from multislice CT studies. *AJR* 154:185–190, 1990.
19. Hall EJ: Effect of radiation on the embryo and fetus. In *Radiobiology for the Radiologist*. Philadelphia, PA. JB Lipincott Company, 1988, pp. 445–465.
20. Mole RH: Irradiation of the embryo and fetus. *Br J Radiol* 60:17–31, 1987.
21. Weinreb JC, Wolbarsht LB, Cohen JM, et al: Prevalence of lumbosacral intravertebral disk abnormalities on MR images in pregnant and asymptomatic nonpregnant women. *Radiology* 170:125–128, 1989.
22. Weinreb JC, Brown CE, Lowe TW, et al: Pelvic masses in pregnant patients: MR and US imaging. *Radiology* 159:717–724, 1986.
23. Thorner MO, Martin WH, Rogol AD, et al: Rapid regression of pituitary prolactinomas during bromocriptine treatment. *J Clin Endocrinol Metab* 51:438, 1980.
24. Evans WS, Thorner MO: Bromocriptine. In *Neurosurgery*. Edited by RN Wilkins and SS Rengachary. New York, NY. McGraw-Hill Book Co., 1985, pp. 873–878.
25. Brem H, Tamargo RJ, Guerin C, et al: Brain tumor angiogenesis. In *Advances in Neuro-Oncology*. Edited by PL Kornblith and MD Walker. Mount Kisco, NY. Futura Publishing Company, Inc., 1988, pp. 89–102.
26. O'Connell JEA: Neurosurgical problems in pregnancy. *Proc R Soc Med* 55:577–582, 1962.
27. Ohrander S, Gennser G, Nilsson KO, et al: ACTH test to neonates after administration of corticosteroids during gestation. *Obstet Gynecol* 49:691, 1985.
28. Laws ER Jr, Kern EB: Pituitary tumors treated by transnasal microsurgery: 7 years of clinical experience with 539 patients. In *Functioning Pituitary*

Adenoma: Proceeding of the First Workshop on Pituitary Adenomas. Edited by K Sano, K Takakura, T Fukushima. Tokyo, 1980, pp. 25–34.

29. Colombo F, Benedetti A, Pozza F, et al: : External stereotactic irradiation with linear accelerator. *Neurosurgery* 16:154–159, 1985.

30. Lundsford LD, Flickinger J, Linder G, et al: Stereotactic radiosurgery of the brain using the first United States 201 Cobalt-60 source gamma knife. *Neurosurgery* 24:151–159, 1989.

31. Lunsford LD, Flickinger J, Coffey RJ: Stereotactic gamma knife radiosurgery: initial North American experience in 207 patients. *Arch Neurol* 47:169–175, 1990.

32. Dalessio DJ: Seizure disorders and pregnancy. *N Engl J Med* 312:559, 1985.

33. Tein I, MacGregor DL: Possible valproate teratogenicity. *Arch Neurol* 42:291, 1985.

34. Brent RL: The effect of embryonic and fetal exposure to X-ray, microwaves, and ultrasound: counseling the pregnant and nonpregnant patient about these risks. *Semin Oncol* 16:347–368, 1989.

35. Otake M, Schull WJ: In utero exposure to A-bomb radiation and mental retardation: a reassessment. *Br J Radiol* 57:409–414, 1984.

36. Doll DC, Ringenberg QS, Yarbro JW: Antineoplastic agents and pregnancy. *Semin Oncol* 16:337–346, 1989.

37. Warkany J: Aminopterin and methotrexate: folic acid deficiency. *Teratology* 17:353–358, 1978.

38. Briggs, GG, Bodendorfer TW, Freeman RK, et al: *Drugs in Pregnancy and Lactation.* Baltimore, MD: Williams and Wilkins; 1983.

39. Lowenthal RM, Marsden KA, Newman NM: Normal infant after treatment of acute myeloid leukemia in pregnancy with daunorubicin. *Aust NZ J Med* 8:431–432,1978.

40. Nordlund JJ, De Vita VT, Carbone PP: Severe vinblastine-induced leukopenia during late pregnancy with delivery of a normal infant. *Ann Intern Med* 69:581–582, 1968.

41. Brem H, Mahaley SM, Vick NA, et al: Interstitial chemotherapy with drug polymer implants for the treatment of recurrent gliomas. *J Neurosurg* 74(3):441–446, 1991.

42. Scarcella G, Allen MB, Andy OJ: Vascular lesions of the posterior fossa during pregnancy. *Am J Obstet Gynecol* 82:836–840, 1961.

43. Ferrante L, Celli P, Fraioli B, et al: Hemangioblastomas of the posterior cranial fossa. *Acta Neurochir (Wien)* 71:283–294, 1984.

44. Robinson RG: Aspects of the natural history of cerebellar hemangioblastomas. *Acta Neurol Scand* 41:372–380, 1965.

45. Kasarkis EJ, Tibbs PA, Lee C: Cerebellar hemangioblastoma symptomatic during pregnancy. *Neurosurgery* 22:770–772, 1988.

46. Cushing H, Bailey P: *Tumours Arising from the Blood-Vessels of the Brain: Angiomatous Malformations and Hemangioblastomas.* Springfield IL, Charles C. Thomas, 1928.

47. Chesley L: Plasma and red cell volumes during pregnancy. *J Obstet Gynecol* 112:440–450, 1972.

48. Magdelenat H, Pertuiset BF, Poisson M: Progestin and oestrogen recep-

tors in meningiomas: biochemical characterization, clinical and pathological correlations in 42 cases. *Acta Neurochir* 64:199–213, 1982.
49. Martuza RL, MacLaughlin DT, Ojemann RG: Specific estradiol binding in schwannomas, meningiomas, and neurofibromas. *Neurosurgery* 9:665–671, 1981.
50. Vaquero J, Marcos ML, Martinez R: Estrogen- and progesterone-receptor proteins in intracranial tumors. *Surg Neurol* 19:11–13, 1983.
51. Allen J, Eldridge R, Koerbert P: Acoustic neuroma in the last month of pregnancy. Am J Obstet Gynecol 119:516–520, 1975.
52. Simon RH: Brain tumors in pregnancy. *Semin Neurol* 8(3):214–221, 1988.
53. O'Neill BP, Illig JJ: Primary central nervous system lymphoma. *Mayo Clin Proc* 64:1005–1020, 1989.
54. Galicich JH, Sundaresan N, Arbit E, et al: Surgical treatment of single brain metastasis: factors associated with survival. *Cancer* 45:381–386, 1980.
55. Patchell RA, Tibbs PA, Walsh JW, et al: A randomized trial of surgery in the treatment of single metastases to the brain. *N Engl J Med* 322:494–500, 1990.
56. Hammond C: Trophoblastic disease (symposium). *Obstet Gynecol Clin North Am* 15(3):1988.
57. Stilp TJ, Bucy PC, Brewer JI: Cure of metastatic choriocarcinoma of the brain. *JAMA* 221:276, 1972.
58. Hammond CB, Borchert LG, Tyrey L, et al: Treatment of metastatic trophoblastic disease: Good and poor prognosis. *Am J Obstet Gynecol* 115:451, 1973.
59. Greer M: Benign intracranial hypertension in pregnancy. *Neurology* 13:670, 1963.
60. Kassam SH, Hadi HA, Fadel HE, et al: Benign intracranial hypertension in pregnancy: current diagnostic and therapeutic approach. *Obstet Gynecol Surv* 38(6):314, 1983.
61. Davis JM, Veness-Meehan K, Notter RH, et al: Changes in pulmonary mechanics after the administration of surfactant to infants with respiratory distress syndrome. *N Engl J Med* 319:4476–4479, 1988.
62. Duncan PG, Pope WD, Cohen MM, et al: Fetal risk of anesthesia and surgery during pregnancy. *Anesthesiology* 64:790–794, 1986.
63. Palhniuk RJ, Shnider SM, Eger EI: Pregnancy decreases the requirement for inhaled anesthetic agents. *Anesthesiology* 41:82–83, 1974.
64. Pedersen H, Finster M: Anesthetic risk in the pregnant surgical patient. *Anesthesiology* 51:439–451, 1979.
65. Levinson G, Shnider SM, deLorimier AA, et al: Effects of maternal hyperventilation on uterine blood flow and fetal oxygenation and acid-base status. *Anesthesiology* 40:340–347, 1974.
66. Donchin Y, Amirav B, Sahar A, et al: Sodium nitroprusside for aneurysm surgery in pregnancy. *Br J Anaesth* 58:849–850, 1978.
67. Lam AM, Gelb AW: Cardiovascular effects of isoflurane-induced hypotension for cerebral aneurysm surgery. *Anesth Analg* 62:742–748, 1983.
68. Newman B, Lam AM: Induced hypotension for clipping of a cerebral aneurysm during pregnancy. *Anesth Analg* 65:675–678, 1986.

5

Headache

Ramesh Khurana, M.D.

Introduction

The National Health Examination survey found that 27.8% of women in the adult United States population suffered from headaches.[1] Therefore, it is not surprising that headache is a common complaint in pregnancy. Headache is a symptom originating from pain sensitive intracranial and extracranial structures.[2,3] The intracranial structures include the cranial sinuses and afferent veins, the dural arteries, parts of the dura mater in the vicinity of large vessels, the proximal portions of the large arteries forming the circle of Willis, and the pain-sensitive fibers of the 5th, 9th, 10th cranial nerves and 2nd and 3rd cervical nerves. The extracranial pain-sensitive structures include skin, scalp, fascia, periosteum, muscles, mucosa, and arteries. The insensitive portions of the cranium include the parenchyma of the brain, ependyma, choroid plexus, pia mater, arachnoid membrane, parts of the dura mater, and skull. In general, structures above the tentorium are supplied by the trigeminal afferents and those below the tentorium are innervated by the upper three cervical nerves and the 9th and 10th cranial nerves. The stimulation of structures in the territory of the trigeminal nerve causes pain in the anterior two thirds of the head, and pain from infratentorial structures is referred to the posterior third of the head. Because of this pattern of innervation and the resultant referred pain, pain arising from either intracranial structures or from extracranial tissues may be felt in the same regions of the head.

From Goldstein PJ, Stern BJ, (eds): *Neurological Disorders of Pregnancy. Second Revised Edition.* Mount Kisco NY, Futura Publishing Co., Inc., © 1992.

Based on the knowledge of pain pathways and clinical description, the Ad Hoc Committee on Classification of Headache described 15 different varieties of headache.[4] A modified classification recommended by Diamond and Dalessio[2] is as follows:

Headache Classification

1. *Vascular Headaches*
   A. Migraine: Classical, common, hemiplegic, and opthalmoplegic
   B. Cluster
   C. Toxic vascular
   D. Hypertensive
2. *Muscle-Contraction Headache*
   A. Cervical osteoarthritis
   B. Chronic myositis
   C. Depressive equivalents and conversion reactions
3. *Traction and Inflammatory Headaches*
   A. Mass lesions (tumors and hematomas, etc.)
   B. Diseases of the eye, ear, nose, throat, and teeth
   C. Arteritis, phlebitis and cranial neuralgias
   D. Occlusive vascular disease
   E. Atypical facial pain
   F. Temporomandibular joint disease

Unfortunately, for a number of reasons, no classification of headache is universally accepted. For example, recent studies with electromyography have demonstrated muscle tension with equal frequency in patients with migraine and those with muscle-contraction headaches.[5] On the other hand, regional cerebral blood flow studies have revealed spreading cerebral oligemia in classic migraine and normal blood flow in patients with common migraine, suggesting that these two varieties of migraine may not have as many similarities as previously believed.[6] In general, factors underlying the clinical signs and symptoms of headache are not well understood and knowledge about the pain of headache is insufficient to permit a definite taxonomy.

Recently, a classification committee chaired by Jes Olesen has proposed a hierarchically constructed classification, using up to four-digit levels.[7] Common migraine has been replaced by "migraine without aura". Migraine with aura includes classic migraine, hemiplegic migraine, complicated migraine, and migraine accompagne. Cluster headache syndrome is no longer classified under the vascular headache of migraine type. Muscle contraction headache has been labeled as tension-type headache that is subdivided into episodic and chronic varieties, with or without associated disorder of pericranial muscles.

This chapter will concentrate on those common headache varieties that are affected by pregnancy. The reader is referred to other monographs on the subject for aspects not discussed here[2,8,9]

Migraine

Migraine is one of the most common varieties of vascular headaches. According the the Ad Hoc Committee's definition,[4] vascular headaches of the migraine type consist of recurrent attacks of headache, widely varied in intensity, frequency and duration. Attacks are commonly unilateral in onset and are usually associated with anorexia and sometimes with nausea and vomiting. In some individuals, attacks are preceded by or associated with conspicuous sensory, motor, or mood disturbances. Migraine headaches tend to be familial. Patients with classic migraines have characteristic visual sensory or motor aura preceding the headache, but common migraine patients present without a striking prodrome.

Migraine without aura/common migraine, per International Headache Society Classification, has additional criteria of at least ten attacks of 4–72 hours duration (untreated or unsuccessfully treated). Patients with classic migraine (migraine with aura under I.H.S. Classification) should have had at least two attacks with fully reversible aura symptoms of focal hemispheric and/or brainstem dysfunction. Aura symptoms should develop gradually over more than 4 minutes and last no more than 60 minutes, and headache should follow with a free interval of less than 60 minutes.[7] The auras, in order of frequency, are: scotomata, teichopsia, photopsia, paresthesias, and visual and auditory hallucinations. The most common aura of hemianopic scintillating scotoma was well described by Sir William Gowers[10] during the latter half of the 19th century. In both types of migraines, organic disease should be excluded clinically or by neuroimaging studies.

There is no experimental animal model of migraine, and its benign nature in humans precludes in-depth study of its pathophysiology. Vascular involvement in migraine headaches is well known, but whether this is a primary or secondary event is debatable. Two theories, vascular and neurogenic, were proposed over a century ago. The vascular theory considers vasomotor disturbance as the primary event, with early symptoms being due to arterial spasm, and headache then being due to subsequent dilatation of vessels. In contrast, Living suggested the neurogenic hypothesis, which states that "nerve-storm" is a primary event and vasomotor disturbance is of secondary origin.[10] Gowers favored the latter view due to the localized involvement of the same region of the brain each time and due to simultaneous occurrence of symptoms attributable to excitation and inhibition. In the first half of the twentieth century, the vascular theory gained prominence because Wolff and associates[11] reported amelioration of the aura with inhalation of carbon dioxide or amyl nitrite, indicating the role of intracranial vasoconstriction in the production of aura. Further, ergotamine terminated the migraine headache by vasoconstricting the dilated extracranial vessels. Recently, Goadsby et al.[12] have demonstrated simultaneous occurrence of constriction in the cerebral vessels and dilatation in the extracranial vessels secondary to low frequency stimulation of the ipsilateral locus coeruleus. Furthermore, Lauritzen and colleagues[13] have observed that oligemia starts in the occipital region and moves anteriorly at a speed consistent with the slow march of migrainous symptoms. The cortical distribution of oligemia in this study did not relate to the distribution of major cerebral arteries and persisted throughout the headache phase. These studies have revived the neurogenic hypothesis.

Whether primary or secondary, cranial artery distention and dilatation are still implicated in the painful phase of migraine. Since vasodilatation in itself is usually insufficient to produce headache, sterile inflammation has been considered to be an important cofactor. Several vasoactive substances are known to be associated with neurogenic inflammation: serotonin, catecholamines, histamine, peptide kinins, prostaglandins, and slow-reacting substance of anaphylaxis.[2] Moskowitz[14] has suggested that the antidromic release of substance P from trigeminal nerve terminals may cause pain and vasodilation in the head.

Welch[15] has hypothesized a model of migraine based primarily on the functional changes within the central noradrenergic system.

Migraine, viewed as a biobehavioral disorder, has a threshold that when exceeded sets into motion the mechanism of an attack. Genetic makeup, age, sex, menstrual cycle, etc. are the potentiators acting on a neuronal circuit of orbito-frontal-brainstem projections to the intrinsic noradrenergic system. These prime the threshold so that activators of a migraine episode (glare, trauma, diet, radiological contrast media, etc.) can initiate event-related slow potential shifts in the cerebral cortex, thus precipitating a burst of neuronal activity followed by depression. Scintillating scotoma and spreading oligemia are possibly the respective clinical and physiological correlates of this neuronal dysfunction. This spreading depression depolarizes trigeminovascular fibers leading to release of substance P and other biochemical substances that cause sterile inflammation of the arteries and hence pain.

Women suffer from migraine headaches more often than men,[8] and statistics indicate that 70% of migraine sufferers are women of childbearing age.[16] The association of menses, oral contraceptives, and pregnancy with migraine suggests the relationship of migraine to steroid hormones.[17,18]

Headaches in pregnancy are of specific significance due to their effects on the pregnant mother as well as the fetus. Most authors report that pregnancy is associated with either complete cessation of symptoms or a decrease in frequency of migraine attacks. The improvement in headache begins gradually in the third or fourth month of pregnancy and is not related to social or emotional status.[19] Lance and Anthony[20] studied 120 migrainous women who had a total of 252 pregnancies and reported relief of migraine in 57.5% of pregnancies. In a retrospective study of 200 pregnant women, Somerville[21] reported 31 women with a history of migraines before pregnancy and 7 who developed migraines during pregnancy. Twenty-four of the 31 women (77%) showed improvement. Some experimental evidence supports these observations. Hardebo and colleagues[22] demonstrated reduced sensitivity of intracranial and extracranial vessels to α and β adrenergic agonists during late pregnancy in cats and rabbits. Sicuteri[23] found high levels of serum β endorphin-like immunoreactivity and held it responsible for the feeling of well being, euautonomia, and hyponociception in pregnant woman.

Recent studies have challenged the view that migraine attacks improve during pregnancy.[24–26] Graham[19] has observed aggravation of classic migraine, and other authors have described occurrence of common migraine during the second and third trimesters of pregnancy. Callaghan[27] reported the occurrence of migraine during pregnancy in 12.5% of multigravid as compared to 8% in primigravid women concluding that multiparity may be more stressful. Some authors report that migraine occurring in pregnancy may predispose the patients to eclampsia.[19,27]

Headaches may return in the first postpartum week or upon return of menstrual periods. Stein and associates[28] reported postpartum headaches in 39% of patients with migraine diathesis and ascribed it to the withdrawal of estrogen and progesterone. Sommerville[22] suggested that the prolonged elevated levels of estradiol may "prime" cranial vessels before withdrawal induces the migraine. Dooling and Sweeney[29] reported a 25-year-old woman with occurrence of familial hemiplegic migraine in relation to breast feeding and use of a breast pump, and postulated a complex effect of oxytocin on cerebral vessels in patients predisposed to vasospasm.

In a retrospective study, the incidence of congenital malformations in the children born to migrainous women was similar to those born to nonmigrainous women.[16] Similiarly, gender of the fetus does not affect the clinical course of headache.[20]

Muscle-Contraction Headache

Muscle-contraction headache (tension headache) is one of the common types of chronic recurring headaches in woman. Emotional lability, anxiety, and depression are also common in the first trimester.[30] Muscle-contraction headaches can occur during any trimester of pregnancy, and in contrast to migraine, women with these headaches are less likely to have relief during pregnancy.[31]

The clinical picture of muscle-contraction headache includes an ache or sensation of tightness, pressure, or constriction, which is widely variable in intensity and duration.[4] It is associated with sustained contraction of muscles and occurs without prodrome. The headache is usually bilateral and suboccipital and may cover the head like a tight cap. The duration of pain ranges from a few hours in an acute tension headache to days, weeks, or months in the chronic headache. Examination of these patients may reveal muscle contraction and tenderness of the scalp, particularly at the position of the insertion of muscles around the head. Within the aching muscles, one may palpate areas of local tenderness or nodules, which upon pressure, can cause spread and augmentation of pain and may even produce tinnitus, vertigo, and lacrimation.[32]

The mechanisms responsible for muscle-contraction headache are uncertain. Experimental work has focused primarily on two potential etiologies: electrical evidence of contraction in the head and neck muscles, and muscle blood flow. Earlier studies suggested that sustained contraction of skeletal muscle about the face, scalp, neck, and shoulders cause the headache. The pain and muscle potentials were eliminated by injection of procaine hydrochloride into muscles at the site of reported pain.[5] Diamond and Dalessio[2] state that reflex muscle contraction secondary to noxious stimulation from cervical osteoarthritis, chronic myositis, etc., is mediated by a multisynaptic withdrawal reflex and that a polysynaptic pathway transmits pain impulses cephalad. Furthermore, they believe that cortical influences via the reticulospinal tract activate the γ efferent neuron system perpetuating muscle contraction. Some authors have postulated that muscle contraction leads to accumulation of catabolic products such as potassium, prostaglandins, and kinins that sensitize muscle nociceptors and cause pain.[33,34] Others believe that direct mechanical stimulation of pain receptors via either contraction-induced pressure on muscle and nerve tissues or traction at the myofascial junction leads to pain. Recent studies demonstrate no significant differences in amplitude of electromyographic recordings from forehead and neck muscles in patients with muscle-contraction headaches and normal controls,[35] thus creating doubt about the role of excessive muscle activity in the etiology of these headaches.

Studies implicating vascular dysfunction in muscle-contraction headaches have been contradictory. Increased sensitivity of conjunctival vessels to dilute topical levarterenol, increase in headache intensity with administration of ergotamine or ipsilateral carotid artery compression, and improvement in 33 of the 42 patients with muscle-contraction headaches following intramuscular administration of nicotinic acid indicated relative ischemia of contraction muscles leading to build-up of vasoactive amines and lactic acid.[33,34,36,37] Conversely, radioactive sodium that was injected into the splenium capitis muscle cleared faster during headache than nonheadache phase, indicating increased capillary blood flow.[37] Likewise, there were reports of increase in severity of headache following inhalation of amyl nitrite or precipitation of headache following intravenous infusion of histamine in patients with muscle-contraction headache.[35,38] Whether muscular and vascular mechanism are acting independently or concurrently is not fully clear. Low levels of platelet serotonin have also been reported in patients with such headaches, suggesting defective serotonergic mechanisms.[39] Pain threshold to graded thermal stimuli, however, has been normal.[35] Other authors believe that psychological factors, for example depression, anxiety, and psychosomatic disorders, are of prime significance in the etiology of muscle-contraction headaches.[34] In any case, it is clear that muscle-contraction headache is a multifactorial problem.

Traction and Inflammatory Headache

Traction and inflammatory headache occurs infrequently but carries a serious prognosis. This type of headache is evoked by inflammation, displacement, and/or traction of pain-sensitive intracranial and extracranial structures. It is described as a deep and steady ache that may be intermittent at the onset but becomes continuous and progressively increases in severity. It can be precipitated or aggravated by coughing or straining. For example, headache is a prominent and usually an early feature of posterior fossa mass lesions. A 10-year study of maternal mortality during pregnancy and up to 6-months postpartum disclosed that 23% of all maternal deaths were due to central nervous system complications. Of these, the majority were caused by intracranial tumors, subarachnoid hemorrhage, intracranial hemorrhage, and arterial and venous occlusions.[40] Brain tumors, especially meningiomas and pituitary tumors, may grow rapidly in pregnancy, probably due to an increase in fluid content of tumor cells or hormonal stimulation.[41-44]

Traction headaches of particularly severe intensity occur in patients with intracranial hemorrhage. This is a condition characterized by severe explosive headache that demands definitive treatment to avoid high rates of recurrence and mortality. A retrospective study of 146 patients, 67 associated with pregnancy and 79 unassociated with pregnancy,[45] found the incidence of arteriovenous malformations to be four times greater in association with pregnancy. The arteriovenous malformations tended to bleed during the middle and end of pregnancy and fetal complications were common. Conversely, the incidence of hemorrhage from an aneurysm rose steadily during pregnancy with maximum tendency to bleed between the 30th and 40th weeks of pregnancy.

Strokes in pregnancy occur with an incidence of approximately 1:20,000 and carry a higher mortality. Major arterial occlusions are more common than venous occlusions[46,47] and most of them occur during the puerperium. The headache is intense, progressive, and resistant to simple analgesics in patients with venous thrombosis. Although primary venous thrombosis can occur in the first and second trimester, it usually occurs before, during, and after labor and is attributed to a hypercoagulable state. A more complete discussion of this subject is presented in Chapter 2.

Diagnosis

Headache may be a benign but disabling symptom or an extension of an underlying serious neurological disorder. An accurate diagnosis is essential to provide appropriate treatment. Diagnostic evaluation of headache patients should include history, physical examination, appropriate laboratory tests, evaluation of response to medications, and follow-up.[48]

A careful systematic history intended to elicit a headache profile is more important than the physical examination because the physical examination may not contribute to the diagnosis.[2,29] A headache profile consists of the temporal aspect of the symptom and features of a single attack from the onset to its termination. Age at the time of onset, frequency, periodicity, and progression of headache indicate the temporal relationship and provide a valuable clue to the differential diagnosis. To elicit a profile of an individual attack, a set of standard questions is utilized that includes: onset, premonitory symptoms, prodrome, location of pain, character and duration of pain, associated symptoms, precipitating factors, aggravating factors, and relieving factors. An accurate description of the onset of headache can be difficult to obtain because patients often confuse it with the time the headache becomes severe. An acute onset with neurological symptoms limits the differential diagnosis to condition such as subarachnoid hemorrhage, while subacute onset covers a wider spectrum of diagnoses. For the sake of brevity and simplicity, features of migraine, muscle-contraction headache, and traction and inflammatory headache are described in Table I.

A detailed physical examination is not only reassuring to patients with migraine and muscle-contraction headaches, but is essential in deciding the appropriate studies necessary to elucidate the diagnosis in patients with traction and inflammatory headaches.[2,29] Examination is usually normal in patients with migraine and muscle-contraction headaches. Patients with migraine may show various abnormalities of autonomic function: pale or flushed face, lacrimation, conjunctival injection, Horner syndrome, distended scalp vessels, and rhinorrhea. Observations of trigger spots, spasm of neck muscles, limitation of cervical movements, and temporomandibular joint dysfunction with spasms of muscles of mastication provide evidence for muscle-contraction headaches. Neurological abnormalities may be found in patients with traction and inflammatory headaches as may evidence of endocrinopathies or neurofibromata. In addition to the customary assessment of motor, sensory, and cerebellar function, the evaluation of such patients should include observations about disturbance of consciousness, anosmia, ocular abnormalities, sixth nerve paralysis, and auditory dysfunction.

Various laboratory tests may be utilized to rule out systemic causes of headache and to establish a database for pharmacotherapy. These include: complete blood cell count, erythrocyte sedimentation rate, blood sugar, urinalysis, and electrocardiogram. Noninvasive procedures include: psychological evaluation, electroencephalography, and thermography. Additional procedures to consider include x-rays of skull, cervical spine, chest and paranasal sinuses, lumbar puncture, computed tomography of the cranium, magnetic resonance imaging, and cerebral angiography. Visual evoked responses are occasionally used.

The electroencephalogram without administration of drugs is a harmless procedure of low diagnostic yield that may demonstrate abnormalities in patients with suspected focal lesions. Thermography is a procedure that pictorially records heat emission spectra over the forehead, temple, or back of the neck and shows focal hypothermia as the most common abnormality in patients with vascular headaches.[49] Lumbar puncture is without major complications in patients who do not have raised intracranial pressure from focal lesions but

Table I.
Features of Headache

	Migraine	Muscle Contraction Headache	Traction Inflammatory Headache
Family History	Usually present	May be present	Absent
Frequency	Periodic	Chronic, may be episodic	Intermittent at the onset
			Constant and progressive later
Duration of pain	Hours to days	Usually constant, hours to days in episodic type	Brief initially, prolonged later
Premonitory symptoms	Changes in mood, energy, or appetite	None	None
Prodromal symptoms	Visual or sensory	None	May occur in occipital or parietal lobe lesions
Location of pain diffuse	Unilateral or Bilateral	Bilateral and diffuse	Localized in early stages, with increase in intra-cranial
Character of pain	Throbbing	Band-like or vice-type sensation	Dull ache
			Pressure
Associated symptoms	Gastrointestinal e.g., nausea and vomiting	Tenderness of head and neck	Symptoms of CNS involvement depending upon the location of lesion
	Photophobia		
	Horner's syndrome		
	Lacrimation		
	Rhinorrhea		
	Sweating		
	Diarrhea		
	Fluid retention		
Precipitating factors	Alcohol, foods containing tyramine (e.g., wine, aged cheese), and emotional stress	Emotional stress	Valsalva maneuver, coughing and straining
Aggravating factors	Alcohol, stress, jolting	Emotional stress and anxiety	Coughing and staining
Relieving factors	Temporary relief by pressure on the distended scalp arteries, pregnancy, and sleep	Analgesics, relaxation	Decrease in intracranial pressure

can produce headache afterwards due to traction effects.[50] Lumbar puncture is definitely indicated in patients with suggested meningitis or encephalitis. Cranial computed tomography is probably the best tool to rule out intracranial pathology. Cerebral angiography is especially useful in patients with aneurysm, arteriovenous malformation, or tumor. When medically necessary, radiological studies should be performed with the abdomen appropriately shielded and field size as limited as possible.[51] Magnetic resonance imaging is a diagnostic tool devoid of radiation that seems to be safe in pregnancy.

In the majority of patients, laboratory and radiological investigations are not necessary. The tests are superfluous in patients with chronic, constant, nonprogressive headache, and in patients with chronic recurrent headache with clear-cut diagnosis. One can easily forego studies in patients who had tests prior to becoming pregnant and where the headache character has not changed. Neurological investigations are, of course, mandatory in acute cases of headache where organic disease is suspected.

Treatment

Management of headache in a pregnant patient is particularly challenging because of the potential complications of diagnosis and therapy to the mother and fetus. Accurate diagnosis and response to previous therapies are keys to proper treatment. Good rapport between the physician and patient is essential so as to tailor management to individual needs.[52] Pharmacotherapy has traditionally been the mainstay of treatment of migraine and muscle-contraction headaches. Any drug use during pregnancy needs to be carefully considered because of potential teratogenesis.[51,53,54] Drugs during pregnancy should therefore be used only when absolutely necessary and in minimal but effective doses. Whenever possible, nonpharmacological treatment should be used to help patients cope effectively with headaches.

Psychophysiological and psychological management is an extremely useful alternative to drug therapy in patients with migraine as well as muscle-contraction headaches.[2,29] Psychophysiological methods include biofeedback and relaxation techniques. Biofeedback is based upon the principle of operant conditioning and teaches a person to recognize internal cues and to control previously involuntary functions. Electromyographic and thermal feedback are usually effective in migraine patients, especially when combined with verbal relaxation techniques.[55] This therapy reduces headache intensity and frequency in a high proportion of patients. The psychological approach includes reassurance after detailed and sympathetic evaluation, explanation of mechanism of headache, encouragement to ventilate frustration and/or resentment (emotional decompression). Other strategies include adjustment of work patterns, modification of other stress factors, and teaching the patient how to cope with stress. Some patients may, however, need long-term psychotherapy.

Attention to physical factors can be of additional therapeutic benefit: for example, spectacles for refractive error, dental treatment for uneven bite, and physiotherapy to the cervical muscles. Injection with local anesthetic and steroids into trigger spots, use of a cervical collar, and traction for degenerative intervertebral cervical disc disease may alleviate muscle-contraction headache. Local use of ice packs for at least 12 minutes[56] and rest in dark and quiet surroundings will likewise provide comfort to patients with acute migraine attack.

Removal of trigger factors will diminish susceptibility to migraine attacks provided it is clear from the history that such factors are operational. These precipitating factors include emotional stress, bright sunlight, sun-on-snow glare, fatigue, heat, fasting for more than 5 hours during the day, or 13 hours overnight.[57] Additionally, foods that are allergic or that contain vasoactive substances such as tyramine, phenylethylamine, nitrites, and monosodium glutamate may be avoided. Red wine, chocolate, aged cheese, caffeine, alcohol, hot dogs, and Chinese food are all potential migraine triggers.

In general, pharmacotherapy for muscle-contraction headaches ranges from simple analgesics (acetaminophen and acetylsalicylic acid) to tranquilizers (diazepam) and serotonin uptake blockers (amitriptyline). The treatment of migraine headache in a nonpregnant patient is directed toward control of an acute attack and prophylaxis for recurrent attacks. For the acute attack, dihydroergotamine is the first-line drug. Other useful drugs for acute attacks include ergotamine, isometheptene mucate, naproxen sodium, and steroids. Recently, sumatriptan, a 5-HTl-like agonist has also be found to be useful.[58,59] Drugs recommended for prophylaxis include propranolol hydrochloride, amitriptyline, ergotamine, methysergide, cyproheptadine hydrochloride, and calcium channel blocking agents.[52,60]

Table II.
Commonly Used Drugs

Drug	Possible Effects on Fetus	Remarks
1. Acetaminophen	Kidney disease, liver damage, congenital dislocation of hip, club foot, oligohydromnios.	Benefit outweighs risk in first trimester.
2. Acetylsalicylic	Increased perinatal mortality, intrauterine growth retardation, congenital salicylate intoxication, depressed albumin binding capacity, hemorrhagic phenomenon in newborn, neonatal purpuric rash.	Occasional use not contraindicated. Avoid chronic use in amounts more than 3,250 mg/day. Avoid use close to term.
3. Meperidine	Possible maternal and neonatal addiction, respiratory depression, which is time- and dose-dependent.	Neonatal depression when given during labor in excess.
4. Prednisone	Immunosuppression and infection in newborn exposed to high dose throughout gestation.	None or small risk to the developing fetus.
5. Propranolol	Intrauterine growth retardation, hypoglycemia, bradycardia, respiratory depression at birth, small placenta.	Low fetal risks.
6. Amitriptyline	Limb reduction anomalies, Microngnathia, anomalous right mandible and pes equinovarus in one case. Swelling of hands and feet in one case, hypospadias in one case. Urinary retention due to its metabolite.	Limb reduction anomalies not confirmed in a study of 522,630. Benefit outweighs risk in the first trimester.
7. Cyproheptadine		Used to prevent habitual abortion in patients with increased serotonin production. Pregnancy normal. At 4 months of age, baby developed gastroenteritis and died.
8. Verapamil	Potential risk of hypotension, reduced intrauterine blood flow with fetal hypoxia and/or growth retardation.	Intrauterine growth retardation; possible stillbirths.

Pharmacotherapy in a pregnant patient should be used only when absolutely necessary and with full understanding of the risks and benefits, especially during the first trimester. Ergotamine, for example, is contraindicated in pregnant patients because of its oxytocic potential.[61] Table II enumerates some of the harmful effects of commonly used drugs on the fetus. Meperidine and acetaminophen can be used to treat acute migraine attacks. For prophylaxis, the β-adrenergic blocking agent propranolol and the tricylic antidepressant amitriptyline have been used. The teratogenic potential of these drugs has been substantiated in various studies.[53,62–64] Propranolol has been safely used during pregnancy to treat hypertension despite the possible risk of fetal growth retardation.[65,66] If necessary, for the prophylactic treatment of frequent refractory headaches, propranolol may be used, preferable in a low dose of 40–160 mg per day. These patients should be managed as "high-risk pregnancies". Use of multiple drugs in pregnancy should be discouraged[67] and prophylactic drugs should be discontinued 2 weeks before delivery.

References

1. Leviton A: Epidemiology of Headache. In *Advances in Neurology*. Volume 39. Edited by BS Schoenberg. New York, NY. Raven Press, 1978, pp. 341–353.
2. Diamond S, Dalesssio DJ: *The Practicing Physician's Approach to Headache*. Baltimore, MD. Williams & Wilkins, 1982.
3. Friedman AP: Nature of headache. *Headache* 19:163–167, 1979.
4. Ad Hoc Committee on classification of headache: Classification of headache. *JAMA* 179:717–718, 1962.
5. Pikoff H: Is the muscular model of headache still viable? A review of conflicting data. *Headache* 24:186–198, 1984.
6. Olesen J, Lauritzen M, Tfelt-Hansen P, et al: Spreading cerebral oligemia in classical and normal cerebral blood flow in common migraine. *Headache* 222:242–248, 1982.
7. Headache Classification Committee of The International Headache Society: Classification and diagnostic criteria for headache disorders, cranial neuralgias and facial pain. *Cephalgia* 8(Suppl 7):1–96, 1988.
8. Dalessio DJ: *Wolff's Headache and Other Head Pain*. New York, NY. Oxford University Press, 1980.
9. Lance JW: *Mechanisms and Management of Headache*. London, Butterworth Scientific, 1982.
10. Gowers WR: *A Manual of Diseases of the Nervous System*. Philadelphia, PA. P. Blakistan, Son and Co., 1888, pp. 1171–1189.

11. Dalessio DJ: *Wolff's Headache and Other Head Pain.* New York, NY, Oxford University Press, 1972, pp. 226–347.
12. Goadsby PJ, Lambert GA, Lance JW: Differential effects on the internal and external carotid circulation of the monkey evoked by locus coeruleus stimulation. *Brain Res* 249:247–254, 1982.
13. Lauritzen M, Olesen J: Regional cerebral blood flow during migraine attacks by xenox-133 inhalation and emission tomography. *Brain* 107:447–462, 1984.
14. Moskowitz MA: The neurobiology of vascular head and pain. *Ann Neurol* 16:157–168, 1984.
15. Welch KMA: Migraine: a biobehavioral disorder. *Arch Neurol* 44:323–327, 1987.
16. Wainscott G, Sullivan FM, Volans GN, et al: The outcome of pregnancy in women suffering from migraine. *Postgrad Med J* 54:98–102, 1978.
17. Rombert MH: *A Manual of the Nervous Disease of Man.* Volume I. Translated and edited by EM Sieverking. Printed for the Syndenham Society-London. 1853, pp. 176–178.
18. Grant ECG: Relation of arterioles in the endometrium to headache from oral contraceptives. *Lancet* 1:1143–1144, 1965.
19. Graham JR: Migraine: clinical aspects. In *Handbook of Clinical Neurology.* Volume 5. Edited by PJ Vinken, BW Bruyn. Amsterdam, North-Holland Publishing Company, 1968, pp. 45–48.
20. Lane JW, Anthony M: Some clinical aspects of migraine. *Arch Neurol* 15:356–361, 1966.
21. Somerville BW: A study of migraine in pregnancy. *Neurology* 22:824–828, 1972.
22. Hardebo JE, Edvinsson L: Reduced sensitivity to alpha and beta-adrenergic receptor agonists of intra and extracranial vessels during pregnancy: relevance to migraine. *Acta Neurol Scand* 56(Suppl):204–205, 1977.
23. Sicuteri F: Natural opiods in migraine. In *Advances in Neurology* Volume 33. Edited by M Critchley. New York, NY. Raven Press, 1982, pp. 65–74.
24. Massey EW: Migraine during pregnancy. *Obstet Gynecol Surv* 32:693–696, 1971.
25. Weinberger J, Lauersen NH: Vascular headache in pregnancy. *Am J Obstet Gynecol* 143:842–843, 1982.
26. Bending JJ: Recurrent bilateral reversible migrainous hemiparesis during pregnancy. *Can Med Assoc J* 127:508–509, 1982.
27. Callaghan N: The migraine syndrome in pregnancy. *Neurology* 18:197–201, 1968.
28. Stein G, Mortion J, Marsh A, et al: Headaches after childbirth. *Acta Neurol Scand* 69:74–79, 1984.
29. Dooling EC, Sweeney VP: Migrainous hemiplegia during breast-feeding. *Am J Obstet Gynecol* 118:568–570, 1974.
30. Nadelson C, Notman T, Ellis EA: Psychosomatic aspects of obstetrics and gynecology. *Psychosomatics* 24:871–884, 1983.
31. Blumenthal LS: Tension Headache. In *Handbook of Clinical Neurology.* Vol-

ume 5. Edited by PJ Vinken, GW Bruyn. Amsterdam, North-Holland Publishing Company, 1968, pp. 157–171.

32. Tunis MM, Wolff HG: Studies on headache, cranial artery vasoconstriction and muscle-contraction headache. *AMA Arch Neurol Psychiatry* 71:425–434, 1954.

33. Riley TL: Muscle-contraction headache. In *Neurologic Clinics*. Volume 1, Number 2. Edited by RC Packard. Philadelphia, PA. WB Saunders Company, 1983, pp. 489–500.

34. Brazil P, Friedman AP: Craniovascular studies in headache. A report and analysis of pulse volume tracings. *Neurology* 6:96–102, 1956.

35. Martin PR, Mathews AM: Tension headache: psychophysiological investigation and treatment. *J Psychosomatic Res* 22:389–399, 1978.

36. Ostfeld AM, Reis DJ, Wolff HG: Studies of headache: bulbar conjectival ischemia and muscle-contraction headahce. *Arch Neurol Psychiatry* 77:113–119, 1957.

37. Onel Y, Friedman AP, Grossman J: Muscle blood flow studies in muscle-contraction headaches. *Neurology* 11:935–939, 1961.

38. Krabbe AA, Olesen J: Headache provocation by continuous intravenous infusion of histamine: clinical results and receptor mechanisms. *Pain* 8:253–265, 1980.

39. Lance JW: Headache. *Ann Neurol* 10:1–10, 1981.

40. Barnes JE, Abbott KH: Cerebral complications incurred during pregnancy and the puerperium. *Am J Obstet Gynecol* 82:192–206, 1961.

41. Michelson JJ, New PFJ: Brain tumor and pregnancy. *J Neurol Neurosurg Psychiatry* 32:305–307, 1969.

42. Bickerstaff ER, Small JM, Guest IA: The relapsing course of certain meningiomas in relation to pregnancy and menstruation. *J Neurol Neurosurg Psychiatry* 21:89–91, 1958.

43. Child DF, Gordon H, Mashiter K, et al: Pregnancy, prolactin and pituitary tumors. *Br Med J* 4:87–89, 1975.

44. Powell JJ: Pseudotumor cerebri and pregnancy. *Obstet Gynecol* 40:713–718, 1972.

45. Robinson JL, Christopher SH, Sedzimir CG: Arteriovenous malformations, aneurysms and pregnancy. *J Neurosurg* 41:63–70, 1974.

46. Cross JN, Castro PO, Jennett WB: Cerebral strokes associated with pregnancy and puerperium. *Br Med J* 3:214–218, 1968.

47. Carroll JD, Leak D, Lee HA: Cerebral thrombophlebitis in pregnancy and the puerperium. *Q J Med* 139:347–368, 1966.

48. Kunkel RS: Evaluating the headache patient: history and work-up. *Headache* 19:122–126, 1979.

49. Matthew NT, Alvarex L: The usefulness of thermography in headache. In *Progress in Migraine Research 2*. Edited by CF Rose. Great Britain, The Pittman Press, 1984, pp. 232–245.

50. Spielman FJ: Post-lumbar puncture headache. *Headache* 22:280–283, 1982.

51. Howard FM, Hill JM: Drugs in pregnancy. *Obstet Gynecol Surv* 34:643–653, 1979.

52. Saper JR: Migraine treatment. *JAMA* 293:2480–2484, 1978.

53. Cefalo RC: Drugs in pregnancy: which to use and which to avoid. *Drug Therapy* 13:167–175, 1983.
54. Stirrat GM: Prescribing problems in the second half of pregnancy and during lactation. *Obstet Gynecol Surv* 31:1–7, 1976.
55. Diamond S: Biofeedback and headache. In *Neurologic Clinics.* Volume 1, Number 2. Edited by RC Packard. Philadelphia, PA. WB Saunders Company, 1983, pp. 479–488.
56. Robbins LD: Cryotherapy for headache. *Headache* 29: 598–600, 1989.
57. Olesen J: The significance of trigger factors in migraine. In *Progress in Migraine Research, 2.* Edited by FC Rose. London, The Pittman Press, 1984, pp. 18–29.
58. Glover V, Littlewood J, Sandler M, et al: Dietary migraine: looking beyond tyramine. In *Progress in Migraine Research, 2.* Edited by FC Rose. London, The Pittman Press, 1984, pp. 113–119.
59. Median JL, Diamond S: The role of diet in migraine. *Headache* 18:31–34, 1978.
60. Matthew NT: Abortive versus prophylatic treatment of migraine reappraisal. *Headache* 30:238–239, 1990.
61. Davis ME, Adair FL, Rogers G, et al: A new active principle in ergot and its effects on uterine motility. *Am J Obstet Gynecol* 29:155–167, 1935.
62. Briggs GG, Bodendorfer TW, Freeman RK, et al: *Drugs in Pregnancy and Lactation: A Reference Guide to Fetal and Neonatal Risk.* Baltimore, MD. Williams and Wilkins, 1983.
63. Donaldson JO: *Neurology of Pregnancy.* Philadelphia, PA. W.B. Saunders Company, 1989, pp. 217–227.
64. Louis R Jr: Headaches in pregnancy. *Semin Neurol* 8:187–192, 1988.
65. Rubin PC: Current concepts: beta-blockers in pregnancy. *N Engl J Med* 305:1323–1326, 1981.
66. Redmond GP: Propranolol and fetal growth retardation. *Semin Perinatol* 6:142–147, 1982.
67. Hughes HE, Goldstein DA: Birth defects following maternal exposure to ergotamine, beta blockers, and caffeine. *J Med Genetics* 25:396–399, 1988.

6

Infections of the Nervous System During Pregnancy

Michael L. Levin, M.D.
Janet Horn, M.D.
Lois Eldred, M.P.H.
John Meyerhoff, M.D.

Introduction

All agents that infect the nonpregnant patient are capable of infecting the pregnant patient.[1] The morbidity and mortality resulting from such infections depend on the number and virulence of the infecting organism and the immunological health of the patient.

Pregnancy is a state of immunosuppression that is necessary for fetal growth and survival.[2] Immune system changes may be most pronounced in the third trimester of pregnancy and include: (1) decreased neutrophil chemotaxis, myeloperoxidase levels,[3] and cell-mediated immunological function;[2] (2) alterations in the hexosemonophosphate shunt, decreasing the ability of the white blood cell to attack effectively and eradicate microbes; and (3) increased levels of humoral immunosuppressants such as corticosteroids, prostaglandins, α-fetoprotein and blocking antibodies. Additionally, cell-mediated immunity is suppressed as evidenced by a decreased T helper/suppressor cell ratio that returns to normal 3 months postpartum.[2] The T-cell suppression plays an important role in preventing rejection of the fetal-placental unit from the maternal uterus.[2] Clinically, these

From Goldstein PJ, Stern BJ, (eds): *Neurological Disorders of Pregnancy. Second Revised Edition.* Mount Kisco NY, Futura Publishing Co., Inc., © 1992.

immunological changes are associated with an increased susceptibility to viral infections during pregnancy.

The Collaborative Perinatal Project documented the frequencies of clinically recognized viral infections during pregnancy (per 10,000 pregnancies): rubella, 8; rubeola, 0.6; mumps, 10; and varicella-zoster virus, 5. Of the 30,000 pregnancies surveyed, 4.8% were complicated by one infection and 0.4% by two infections. Common infections were influenza or flu-like illnesses followed by cold sores/herpes simplex, viral gastroenteritis, and viral laryngopharyngitis/tonsillitis. The more specific infections (e.g., infectious mononucleosis, pneumonia) occurred at rates varying from 1 to 15 per 10,000 pregnancies.[4]

Because of the altered immune system in pregnancy, viruses may persist as chronic infections that then predispose the host to secondary bacterial infection. The virus may disseminate from the respiratory system to the central nervous system (CNS).[5] In 1977, Zinserling[6] described the CNS lesions that result from respiratory viruses such as influenza A and predispose to severe secondary bacterial infections (e.g., *Neisseria meningitidis*) at the same anatomical site.

Bacterial infections can also cause severe problems for the pregnant patient. Streptococcal puerperal infection may present without clinical evidence of extragenital involvement, but can spread rapidly from the genital tract to cause an acute purulent meningitis.[7] Disease resulting from obligate intracellular bacteria such as mycobacterium, salmonella, listeria, and brucella may cause infections in the pregnant patient just as in the nonpregnant patient.

Bacterial Infections

Meningitis

Bacterial infections in pregnancy can cause either a primary or secondary invasion of the CNS. Primary bacterial meningitis during pregnancy most frequently is caused by *S. pneumoniae* and *N. meningitidis*, and less commonly by *H. influenza* and *Listeria monocytogenes*. These infections have been treated successfully with neither resultant premature labor nor sequelae to mother or fetus.[8,9] Early in bacterial meningitis, the cerebrospinal fluid (CSF) may reveal a paucity of white blood cells and no visible bacteria on Gram's stain. The same CSF findings may be seen in partially treated meningitis. In these cases, the use of CSF counterimmunoelectropheresis may assist in rapid identification of the causative bacteria. Bacterial meningitis is an infectious disease emergency necessitating prompt parenteral antimicrobial therapy, even when the exact etiologic agent is not known. A reasonable empiric regimen for acute bacterial meningitis during pregnancy includes high-dose ampicillin for Listeria and a third generation cephalosporin (e.g., ceftriaxone) for other aforementioned microbes. If there are focal neurological signs or a depressed sensorium, a computed tomographic (CT) scan or magnetic resonance imaging (MRI) of the brain should be done prior to lumbar puncture, to exclude the possibility of a mass lesion producing increased intracranial pressure. Antibiotic therapy should not be withheld from the patient if there is an undue delay in obtaining an imaging study.

Although it is an uncommon infection, *Listeria monocytogones* presents a risk of infection during pregnancy. The largest outbreak of listeriosis in North America during the past decade occurred in 1985 in California and was associated with consumption of Mexican soft cheese. Of 145 cases, 48 (34%) occurred in pregnant women.[10] Listerial infections of the CNS may present in several ways: (1) fulminant meningitis; (2) meningoencephalitis; (3) an indolent chronic meningitis with low-grade fever and mental status changes; and (4) rhinoencephalitis. Because Gram's stain of the CSF is negative in 50% of cases of *Listeria meningitis*, delay of appropriate treatment is common if the diagnosis is not considered. Ampicillin is the drug of choice.

Secondary bacterial meningitis in pregnancy most commonly arises from an endovascular source. These infrequent CNS infections have an incidence of 1:8,000 deliveries and are associated with both increased maternal and fetal mortality.[4] Infective endocarditis may present with metastatic CNS abscesses, with or without focal neurological deficits.[11] Rarely has meningitis associated with endocarditis been reported in pregnancy.[12] Pregnant women with any form of meningitis are best delivered without using regional analgesia or anesthesia, in order to avoid contaminated CSF.

Tuberculosis

The effect of the immunosuppressed state of pregnancy on untreated pulmonary tuberculosis, a chronic granulomatous disease, is evidenced by an increased mortality of infected women in their reproductive years.[13,14] The highest morbidity occurs in the first trimester and postpartum period, when reactivation or worsening of active lesions occurs in 5% to 15% of these patients.[15] Pregnancy does not provide increased risk for reactivation of pulmonary tuberculosis in those patients who have received adequate chemotherapy. There is no need to offer isoniazid chemotherapy solely because of pregnancy in patients with only a positive purified protein derivative (PPD), but inactive tuberculosis.[16]

Pregnancy has little effect on adequately treated tuberculosis. Similarly, treated tuberculosis has little deleterious effect on pregnancy.[17–21] However, if tuberculosis remains unrecognized and untreated, both mother and fetus are at risk for complications. Unrecognized tuberculosis is not uncommon, especially in southeast Asians, where the incidence of isoniazid-resistant mycobacteria is higher. In addition, *Mycobacterium tuberculosis* infections are also more common in the HIV-infected individual. Congenital tuberculosis, though very uncommon, does occur. Placental tubercles are evident and organisms migrate transplacentally to the fetus. Indeed, extensive transplacental infection can occur without evidence of fetal infection.[22]

Breast feeding is contraindicated for women with active uncontrolled pulmonary tuberculosis—not because of the fear that mycobacteria will disseminate through lactation—but rather because of aerosolization of tubercle bacillus droplet nuclei from the nursing mother's respiratory tree to her child during breast feeding.

Tuberculosis of the CNS in pregnancy presents most commonly during the fifth through seventh months of gestation or the first few weeks postpartum.[23] Involvement of the CNS most frequently presents as meningitis. Untreated, tuberculous meningitis is uniformly fatal, usually within 2 months. Live births can occur in term mothers with tuberculous meningitis.[24] Tuberculoma accounts for only 0.15% of intracranial masses, except in developing countries where the incidence still remains high.[25]

Miliary tuberculosis may present with meningeal disease. In such cases, sputum examination rarely reveals acid-fast bacilli, as miliary tuberculosis results from hematogenous dissemination of myobacteria. Centrifugation of more than 5 cc of CSF, with examination and culture of the pellicle from the bottom of the test tube, may provide a greater diagnostic yield. Tuberculosis of the CNS may also present as multiple small mass lesions, or tuberculomas, on CT or MRI scans of the brain.

Currently, triple antituberculous therapy is advocated for CNS mycobacterial infection. All medications may be offered together once daily to increase compliance. The regimen approved for pregnancy is oral isoniazid (5 mg/kg), rifampin (600 mg), and ethambutol (15–20 mg/kg). Pyrazinamide may be selected as an alternate antituberculous agent in the seriously ill patient because of its excellent penetration into the CSF. There are, however, minimal data regarding its potential toxic effects to the fetus.

Untreated women infected with *Mycobacterium tuberculosis* may deliver either vaginally or by cesarean section. The majority of infants born to such women initially demonstrate no stigmata of tuberculosis, though 20% may demonstrate tuberculosis within the first month of life. If untreated, the majority of these infants die.[26] Thus, therapy should be provided for the actively infected pregnant woman once a diagnosis is made, and not delayed until the postpartum period.[27]

Spirochetes

Syphilis (Treponema pallidum)

Although adequate chemotherapy for syphilis has been available for more than four decades, this infection persists, and indeed its incidence is increasing, especially among intravenous drug users. More than 18,000 cases of primary and secondary syphilis were reported among women in the United States in 1989, During this same period, the Center for Disease Control (CDC) reported 700 cases of congenital syphilis, the largest number since the 1950s.[28]

Although secondary syphilis is generally a systemic infection without involvement of the CNS, it may present as acute aseptic meningitis with a predominantly mononuclear CSF pleocytosis. The CSF Venereal Disease Research Laboratory test (VDRL), being diagnostic, should always be obtained.[28,29] This form of syphilis is difficult to distinguish clinically from other forms of aseptic meningitis. Effective treatment can be achieved with 2,400,000 units benzathine penicillin intramuscularly (IM) or 600,000 units procaine penicillin IM daily for 5 days.[30] More frequently, neurosyphilis occurs in the latent asymptomatic stage, or presents with the classic neurological symptoms of dementia or tabes dorsalis with its associated loss of position and vibratory sensation.

Appropriate serological tests are helpful in establishing a diagnosis. Pregnancy does not alter the results of the serological test for syphilis.[31] However, during pregnancy, biological false-positive serum nontreponemal tests (e.g., rapid plasma reagin test [RPR]) for syphilis can occur. The use of a treponemal specific test, such as the fluorescent treponemal antibody absorption test (FTA-ABS) may differentiate true syphilis from a biological false-positive result. It should be noted, however, that even the FTA-ABS test is not 100% specific. The same conditions that result in a false-positive nontreponemal reaginic test (RPR or VDRL) may also rarely give a positive FTA-ABS reaction. If entertaining the diagnosis, to exclude a "prozone" phenomenon, one should request the laboratory to obtain serological testing with serial dilutions rather than accepting an undiluted "nonreactive" result as excluding the diagnosis.

Pregnancy does not necessitate a change in either the dosage or the schedule of therapy for syphilis. In the event that penicillin is contraindicated in an allergic patient, erythromycin is effective therapy for maternal syphilis. Erythromycin does not prevent congenital syphilis because of its limited transplacental transfer.[32,33] Thus, infants born to mothers previously treated with erythromycin should be treated with penicillin at birth. If the neonatal CSF examination is abnormal, treatment should include intravenous penicillin. If the CSF is normal, a single dose of penicillin G benzathine is sufficient for the neonate. Tetracycline should be avoided during pregnancy, despite its antisyphilitic potential, because of adverse fetal effects.

Appropriate follow-up care for the pregnant patient with syphilis includes quantitative serological testing 1, 2, 3, 6, 9, and 12 months after treatment to ensure efficacy of therapy. A failure for the titer to fall fourfold within 6 months, or a rise in titer, demands retreatment. Present therapy for neurosyphilis includes aqueous penicillin 2,400,000 units intravenously (IV), every 4 hours or penicillin G benzathane 3,000,000 units IM weekly for 3 weeks. If treatment precipitates a Jarisch-Herxheimer reaction in the second half of pregnancy, women are at risk for premature labor or fetal distress. Thus, careful monitoring for several hours postantimicrobic therapy is warranted.

Lyme Disease (Borrelia Burgdorferi)

Lyme disease is a multisystem disease that affects, in order of frequency, the skin, joints, central and peripheral nervous systems, and the heart. *B. burgdorferi*, the etiologic spirochete of Lyme disease, is carried by the small arthropod, *Ixodes damini*. The most common presenting manifestation of Lyme disease is the pathognomonic rash, erythema chronicum migrans (ECM). The rash is usually erythematous and enlarges from an initially small (several millimeters in diameter) lesion to 10 cm of more in size with clearing of the central portion of the lesion. These lesions usually last about 3 weeks, if not treated, and may recur for long periods of time. With careful staining technique, borrelia can be demonstrated in as many as 40% of Lyme skin lesions.[34] It is not clear how many of the lesions represent a direct response to the organism in the skin and how many are due to immune complex or serum sickness-like rashes.

Articular manifestations are the next most common manifestations and a similar uncertainty exists as to the cause of the synovial inflammation. Cultures of joint fluid are usually negative. Untreated, the average case of Lyme arthritis consists of three episodes of an inflammatory arthritis lasting a week or so each, usually involving at least the knee. About 10% of untreated patients develop a chronic arthritis, almost always involving the knee.

Lyme disease causes cardiac conduction abnormalities resulting in rapid fluctuations in rhythm. Patients may have transient first-, second-, and third-degree heart block. Rare patients may develop pericardial and myocardial inflammation.

The most worrisome and difficult complications are neurological.[35-38] Many patients have an aseptic meningitis with headache, stiff neck and malaise shortly after the initial tick bite. This usually clears without complication. Patients begin to develop central and peripheral nervous system signs and symptoms days to months later.

As evident from its European name, lymphocytic meningoradiculitis, involvement of the meninges and peripheral nervous system (PNS) is the most common manifestation in Europe, while in the United States, encephalitic manifestations are as common as PNS findings. In the first series from this country, of 18 patients, 78% had meningitis, 72% had encephalitis, 56% had cranial neuritis, 44% had a radiculoneuritis, and 5% had a myelitis.[35] In contrast, in a Swedish study of 46 patients, 72% had meningitis, 67% had PNS findings, and only 15% had CNS findings.[36] Simultaneous involvement of different parts of the nervous system is characteristic of Lyme disease.

The initial symptom is either a peripheral facial nerve palsy or a particularly painful radiculitis. The radicular involvement may be sensory or motor and often involves multiple roots asymmetrically. Meningeal symptoms follow and often are chronic but fluctuating in intensity. Cerebrospinal fluid analysis usually reveals approximately 100 white blood cells (WBC) (mostly mononuclear), but cell counts may range up to 500 and rarely into the thousands.[39] Cerebrospinal fluid protein levels are variable, with levels up to 325 mg/dL reported.[38] The encelphalitic symptoms may be subtle but debilitating, with memory loss, cognitive difficulty, and emotional lability. Other reported findings are chorea, paraparesis, ischemic strokes, somnolence, and hemianopsia. Magnetic resonance images have shown periventricular small bright signals on T2 weighted scans in patients with encephalopathic symptoms and multiple sclerosis-like symptoms.[40]

Other neurological complications include myositis and neuropathy. In one study, 60 of 82 patients had significant neurophysiological abnormalities.[41] Sensory nerve conduction was abnormal in 43 patients, motor nerve conductions in 34, and F responses in 34. Slowing of median nerve conduction at the carpal tunnel was noted in 21 patients. Sural nerve biopsies demonstrated changes consistent with a mild axonal neuropathy. Neurological involvement appears not to resolve without treatment as often as do the skin and joint manifestations. Some patients may therefore develop significant disability due to neurological disease.

The diagnosis of acute Lyme disease is not difficult when patients present with ECM or an intermittent arthritis, particularly when they live in an endemic area. Because of the difficulty culturing borrelia, testing for antibody to borrelia is necessary to confirm infection. A positive IgM antibody will document the acute nature of the infection. If a patient has a negative IgM, but a positive IgG antibody test, then the symptoms might be due to an infection that occurred months to years earlier. There is an unknown number of people who have positive antibody tests, who are not ill, and who have no history of Lyme disease symptoms. When such individuals present with rheumatologic or neurological symptoms, it may be difficult to know if these symptoms represent late sequelae of Lyme disease or some other disease.

There are patients who have neurological symptoms consistent with Lyme disease who do not have elevated levels of serum antibodies to *B. burgdorferi*, but do have elevated levels of specific antiborrelia antibody by enzyme-linked immunosorbent assay (ELISA) in the CSF and may have Wastern blot tests showing bands directed against borrelia antigens.[36] This has been reported from Europe, but in the United States it has been seen only in patients whose initial oral antibiotic regimens were of lower dose or shorter duration.

Treatment of acute Lyme disease (ECM lesions) with 14–21 days of amoxicillin or erythromycin will usually result in faster resolution of ECM and seems to reduce the frequency of rheumatologic, neurological, and cardiologic complications. The doses and duration of recommended antibiotic regimens have increased, since the initial lower doses have not always prevented further disease manifestations.[42]

Lyme disease and pregnancy, of course, do occur together. Maternal-fetal transmission of borrelia has been reported, but the effect of this transplacental infection is not clear.[43] There have been a number of reports of congenital malformations and fetal deaths in association with Lyme disease.[44] However, a prospective study in New York, from endemic and nonendemic areas, found no difference in congenital malformations between the two regions.[45] There was also no association between the presence of antibody to borellia and congenital malformations. There are no reports of worsening of Lyme disease, including the neurological symptoms, during pregnancy. Certainly, any pregnant woman who is discovered to have Lyme disease should be treated with appropriate antibiotics, erythromycin or penicillin. For late disease, ceftriaxone 2 gm IV daily for 21 days is recommended. Tetracyclines, effective for early Lyme disease, are contraindicated in pregnancy. While most patients do respond to this regimen, some continue to have symptoms.

Tetanus

The incidence of reported cases of tetanus in the United States remains 0.03/100,000 population.[46] Initial symptoms of tetanus include weakness, either localized or generalized stiffness, cramping, or difficulty swallowing or chewing. Increasing muscle rigidity ensues, leading to reflex spasms within 1–4 days of exposure. In its generalized form, tonic contractions of any muscle group may produce findings such as abdominal rigidity, opisthotonos, or laryngospasm.[46]

Maternal tetanus does not result in toxic effects on the fetus.[47,48] In some underdeveloped countries, umbilical tetanus results from the use of fecally contaminated materials to cover the severed cord. Unfortunately, umbillically contracted tetanus, as well as that associated with parenteral drug use, has a very poor prognosis.

Routine laboratory studies are of little use in the diagnosis of tetanus. The CSF of the patient with tetanus is normal, and Gram's stain and anaerobic culture of the wound may not reveal typical organisms. The diagnosis is based on a history of tissue injury followed by the development of the characteristic neurological signs and symptoms. The treatment modalities include: (1) human hyperimmune globulin (when the human preparation is not available, horse serum antitoxin can be used, if sensitivity to horse serum has been excluded by intradermal tests); (2) removal of injured tissue, if possible; (3) administration of procaine penicillin once daily, or intravenous aqueous penicillin every 6 hours for 10 days; and (4) intensive medical care provided in a quiet environment.

Severe tetanus does not confer immunity. Active immunization should be started with the absorbed tetanus toxoid; a three-dose course is required. This may be done during pregnancy. Maternal immunization protects the infant from neonatal tetanus unless the amount of toxin produced by umbilical tetanus exceeds the infant's complement of maternal antibody. Antitoxin and toxoid should not be administered simultaneously at the same anatomic site.

Epidural Abscess

Mild-to-moderate back pain is not uncommon with pregnancy, but severe back pain may be a harbinger of a more serious underlying problem.[49] It is not uncommon for spinal disc prolapse to begin in pregnancy. The presence of an epidural abscess, however, is exceedingly rare. This infectious disease emergency usually arises from hematogenous dissemination (usually genitourinary) or secondary to a contiguous spread from an osseous focus. It does have a disastrous outcome for mother and fetus if not rapidly diagnosed and treated. Diagnosis is best made with MRI of the spine. Emergency neurosurgical intervention is mandated, with appropriate drainage. Broad spectrum antimicrobials are administered; the specific agents used depend on the site of the origin of the infection but must provide adequate CSF antimicrobic levels to cover possible contiguous microbial spread.

Fungal Infection

Cryptococcus neoformans is the mycosis most commonly associated with CNS infection. Experimental animal work has failed to reveal transplacental passage of *C. neoformans*, a not unexpected finding considering the relatively large size of the fungus. The perinatal outcome depends both on the infection per se, as well as on the adverse effects of the chemotherapy used to treat the infections. Cryptococcal disease most commonly presents as a subacute or chronic meningitis in patients with a chronic underlying disease that alters the immune system. It also, however, occurs in patients who are immunosuppressed by virtue of corticosteroid therapy or human immunodeficiency virus (HIV) infection. Occasionally, there are multiple small mass lesions, cryptococcomas, that may present with focal neurological signs.

Diagnosis is based on a CSF evaluation showing a predominantly mononuclear pleocytosis, occasional hypoglycorrachia and elevated protein. The India ink preparation is positive in only 50% of cases of *Cryptococcal meningitis*; titered cryptococcal antigen is far more sensitive (positive in > 90% cases). In addition, fungal culture is confirmatory for diagnosis, but not immediately. A complete discussion of the therapy for cryptococcal meningitis is included in the sections discussing HIV-infected patients.

Though still unusual, there have been reports of deep mycotic CNS infections, such as blastomycosis, nocardiosis, and coccidioidomycosis during pregnancy.[50–52] Coccidioidomycosis, a noncontagious respiratory mycotic infection, is the only deep mycosis predisposed to dissemination because of the pregnant state. This is especially true if the infection occurs during the last half of pregnancy.[53] Therefore, though the infection is usually a self-limited pulmonary process, dissemination can occur hematogenously with spread to meninges, skin, bone, or joint. One third to one half of coccidioidomycotic patients present with CNS disease as the only organ involved. During pregnancy, disseminated coccidioidomycosis involves the meninges in one-third of reported cases. In these infections, *C. immitis* has been reported to infect the placenta by the hematogenous route.

The combination treatment of intravenous amphotericin B and oral 5-flucytosine (class C) is recommended for antifungal therapy because of its additive and synergistic effects. Both of these agents cross the placenta in therapeutic concentrations, though they cross the meninges poorly.[54,55] The major side effects of amphotericin B are potassium-losing nephropathy, bone marrow suppression, fevers, chills, and vomiting. They appear to be no worse in the pregnant patient than in the nonpregnant one.[56] High-dose amphotericin B (0.4–0.6 mg/kg/day) is the treatment of choice for fungal meningitis. However, embryotoxic and teratogenic effects in animals are reported with this agent.

Parasitic Infection

Toxoplasmosis

Toxoplasma gondii is the most common parasite infecting pregnant women in the United States today. In one study, the sera from 23,000 pregnant women revealed that 38% of the women had toxoplasma antibody titers equal to or greater than 1:256, suggesting active or recent infection. In New York City, toxoplasmosis infection is present in 1:1300 deliveries; in Birmingham, Alabama in 1:500 deliveries.[62–64] In the United States, 3,000 of the three million babies born each year are believed to have congenital toxoplasmosis.[65] Though many of these infants appear normal at delivery, over 90% will be symptomatic by the age of 10 years.[66]

Toxoplasmosis may present as one of four syndromes. Acute toxoplasmosis usually presents as a "mononucleosis-like syndrome". Symptoms include sore throat, fatigue, malaise, atypical lymphocytosis and lymphadenopathy and heterophile-negative serologies. The infection is usually self-limited, requiring no treatment. Acute toxoplasmosis may be asymptomatic, which is particularly dangerous in pregnancy because acute infection may be overlooked. Rarely, acute toxoplasmosis may present as an aseptic meningitis or myocarditis. The only way to establish the diagnosis of acute toxoplasma infection is by serological conversion from IgM negative to IgM positive, or by a fourfold rise in IgM titers.

The second and third forms of presentations of toxoplasmosis, which occur in the neonate and infant, are congenital toxoplasmosis and chorioretinitis, respectively. The fourth form of toxoplasmosis occurs in the immunocompromised host and is generally a severe infection that presents as either an encephalitis or cerebral abscess. This syndrome is very common in the HIV-infected individual, and will be discussed in the section concerning HIV infection.

Malaria

Malaria results from the bite of an infected female Anopheles mosquito, with resultant parasitemia of the erythrocyte by the protozoa, plasmodium. Infrequently, transfusion-associated malaria is reported. The density of parasite burden determines the severity of illness. Plasmodium falciparum infection results in the illness with the highest degree of morbidity, mortality, and is the most common plasmodia to involve the CNS.

Nonspecific presenting symptoms of fever, chills, headaches and sweats occur in the illness, though nausea, vomiting, and myalgias are not uncommon. Heavy (> 5% to 10% RBC) parasitemia associated with *P. falciparum* results in an acute hemolysis of red blood cells. Severe dehydration, adult respiratory distress syndrome, acute pulmonary edema, acute renal failure, (blackwater fever), and acute cerebral edema are life-threatening sequelae of falciparum malaria.

Malaria associated with pregnancy is thought to be hazardous. Falciparum malaria is particularly dangerous for both the pregnant woman and her fetus, and in tropical climates is a major cause of maternal death, abortion, stillbirth, premature delivery, and low birth weight. A grossly abnormal placenta reveals sinusoids packed with parasitized erythrocytes. Recent studies support the hypothesis that malaria per se, rather than the therapeutic agent, quinine, is responsible for the mortality and morbidity associated with falciparum malaria. Painless uterine contractions and fetal distress have been found in a significant number of women beyond the 30th week of gestation with acute falciparum malaria. Signs of fetal distress disappeared as associated fever abated.

More than 80% of fetal cases of *P. falciparum* malaria have clinical features of cerebral malaria with concomitant histopathological features. Cerebral malaria is a diffuse encephalopathy associated with irreversible coma, extensor plantar responses, conjugate gaze disturbances, tone alterations, and absent abdominal reflexes. The coma develops abruptly followed by generalized seizures. Only 50% of survivors have persistent neurological deficits after 2–3 days of unconsciousness. Mortality, despite appropriate antimalaria therapy and supportive measures, approaches 15% to 50%.[57–59] Hypoglycemia may occur in pregnancy as a result of quinine-induced insulin secretion.[60]

Mefloquine, a newer agent prescribed for *P. falciparum* prophylaxis, especially for those traveling in chloroquine-resistant areas, is contraindicated during pregnancy.

Bilharzia (Schistosomiasis)

Bilharzia is a parasitic infestation of schistosoma. One species of this parasite lays eggs in the urinary bladder after gaining entry percutaneously. The most frequent site for CNS infestation is spinal cord involvement in the lower thoracic and upper lumbar segments because of the associated vascular communication between the pelvic organs via Batson's venous plexes anastomoses and the vertebral circulation.

Placental involvement with schistosoma has been reported, though congenital bilharzia has not. A solitary report documents transverse myelitis during pregnancy attributed to *Schistosoma hematobium* infestations. One dose of praziquantel provides effective therapy (Pregnancy Category B).[61]

Viral Infections

An association between congenital CNS developmental anomalies and viral infections in pregnancy has been documented with rubella and cytomegalovirus (CMV).[67] When evaluating retrospective studies that relate fetal malformation to maternal infection, it should be appreciated that a considerable number of mothers with normal babies also have serological evidence of viral infection during pregnancy.

Uncomplicated viral meningitis in the pregnant patient has not been shown to increase fetal or maternal morbidity or mortality. The majority of these patients are not toxic, though vomiting, fever, anorexia, and nuchal rigidity may require short-term hospitalization for symptomatic treatment. Mumps and picornaviruses are the most frequent etiologic agents of viral meningitis in both pregnant and non-pregnant women. Currently, there is no available antimicrobial therapy for these infections.

DNA Viruses

Herpes Encephalitis

The few cases of life threatening maternal CNS herpetic infections in pregnancy have followed two patterns: encephalitis per se or hepatitis with or without CNS involvement. Viremic spread from mother to fetus occurs with resulting widespread dissemination in the fetus. The question of whether offspring in successive pregnancies of women previously infected with herpes encephalitis are normal remains unanswered.[68]

Although definitive diagnosis of herpetic encephalitis can be established only through utilization of brain biopsy, the diagnosis may be strongly suspected on the basis of the classic clinical presentation with fever, headache, and focal cerebral signs and the exclusion of other types of encephalitis and meningitis. Neuroradiologic imaging using MRI may be normal in herpes encephalitis, or may show focal cerebritis, particularly in the temporal lobe. Lumber puncture may reveal normal CSF but more commonly reveals a nonspecific inflammatory pattern. As there currently exists excellent therapy, which is both safe and effective for herpes encephalitis, it is especially important in the pregnant woman to consider herpes simplex infection and begin empiric treatment. Acyclovir therapy for herpes encephalitis during the third trimester of pregnancy has resulted in a good outcome for mother and child.[69] Because there is a wide therapeutic to toxic ratio with this drug, no adverse effects of acyclovir have been apparent to either the fetus or mother. To date, there has been no documentation of fetal mutagenicity.[70]

Cytomegalovirus

Cytomegalovirus represents the most common cause of intra-uterine infection. In one study of women with CMV antibodies present before conception, 1.9% delivered congenitally infected offspring. Three and one-half percent of women excreted the virus during pregnancy, and 0.5% to 1.0% of newborns in the United States were infected with CMV at birth. Maternal viremia and secondary transplacental spread provide the pathway for fetal involvement.[71–74] Urine, saliva, and blood are also capable of chronic transmission of the virus. Recent studies confirm that CMV may not only be present in newborns, but may also be acquired by healthy infants within 6 weeks of delivery. A recent report showed that congenital CMV infections are asymptomatic in almost 90% of neonates.[75]

Though not common, CMV infection may present as an aseptic meningitis or encephalitis. The encephalitis typically presents in the immunocompromised patient, particularly the HIV-infected individual. Unlike rubella, CMV infections are more difficult to prevent and are capable of infecting the fetus during the entire gestational period. Also, unlike rubella, which is a self-limited disease because of protective antibody production, CMV produces a subclinical latent infection that, despite antibody production, is capable of future activation and subsequent active infection. Therefore, pre-existing maternal infection, unlike that occurring with toxoplasma or rubella, does not prevent subsequent intrauterine infection, even in the absence of an immunosuppressed state.

Although gancyclovir can suppress CMV infection, it has not been approved for use during pregnancy.

RNA Viruses

Rabies

The recent reported incidence of animal rabies in the United States peaked in 1981, with more than 7,118 cases. Only 14 human rabies cases have been reported during the 10 years between 1979 and 1989.[76] A dramatic increase in the reporting of rabid animals in the eastern United States between 1983 and 1985 reinforces the need for an adequate postexposure immunization program despite the 1989 prevalence of less than 0.01/100,000 cases.[77]

Human infection with rabies, a neurotropic virus, is almost universally fatal without immunization. Evidence in animals indicates that both rabies virus and antibody cross the placenta. Aggressive postexposure antirabies prophylaxis during the third trimester of pregnancy can lead to an apparently normal child. The current recommendations from the CDC utilize both human rabies immunoglobulin (HRIG) for passive immunization and human diploid cell rabies (HDCR) for active immunization. These newer agents are associated with a significantly lower incidence of postimmunization side effects. They are both safe and effective postexposure antirabies prophylaxis during pregnancy.[76]

Picornavirus

Enterovirus

Enteroviral infections during pregnancy are capable of spreading transplacentally to the neonate and causing neonatal meningitis, myocarditis, hepatitis, and death.

Equine Encephalitis

The 1989 cumulative reported incidence of arborviral encephalitis in the United States is 0.04/100,000 population.[46] Venezuelan equine encephalitis (VEE), a togavirus, is distributed in northern South America, Central America, and Texas. Mosquitos act as the vector with the horse as the primary host. Human disease does occur, albeit less frequently. Recent data suggest VEE may have both toxic and teratogenic capabilities for both embryo and fetus. Infection during pregnancy has resulted in fetal wastage. Postmortem examination of fetuses delivered from VEE-infected pregnant women revealed major pathological CNS changes incompatible with fetal life.[78]

Subacute Sclerosing Panencephalitis

Subacute sclerosing panencephalitis (SSPE) is a CNS infection caused by measles virus, or a virus similar to the measles virus. It usually affects children and young adults and is fatal within 12–24 months after onset of symptoms. High titers of measles antibodies in both the serum and CSF or amniotic fluid are characteristic. Oligoclonal immunoglobulin in the CSF may also assist in confirming the diagnosis. Currently, there is no effective antiviral therapy. The state of natural immunosuppression during pregnancy may be a factor in activating and permitting presentation of fulminant SSPE.[79,80]

Human Immunodeficiency Virus

Human immunodeficiency virus, a RNA virus exhibiting reverse transcriptase activity, selectively infects CD4 lymphocytes, creating cellular immunodeficiency. Human immunodeficiency virus also infects monocytes, multinucleated giant cells, and other cells that express CD4 antigen. It is neurotropic for glial cells and has been cultured from CSF and neuronal tissue.[81]

Acquired immunodeficiency syndrome (AIDS), initially reported in homosexual men in 1981, is increasingly infecting women. They accounted for 7.4% of the total cases reported to the CDC through 1986. In 1989 alone, women accounted for 11.2% of the reported AIDS cases.[82,83] The percentage increase in cases continues to be greatest for women and infants infected through perinatal transmission. Over two thirds of the female AIDS cases occur in women of childbearing age.

The risk behaviors associated with acquisition of HIV may further complicate care of the HIV-infected pregnant woman. Of the female AIDS cases in the United States, 52% occur in women with a history of intravenous drug use.[84]

In the female who has not used intravenous drugs, the risk profile for acquiring HIV infection is similar to the profile for women at increased risk of acquiring any sexually transmitted disease. Risk factors include early age of first intercourse, multiple sexual partners, and multiple sexually transmitted diseases. In one study, genitourinary tract infections and sexually transmitted disease were more common in HIV-infected pregnant women than in noninfected pregnant controls.[85] Risk assessment questionnaires designed to detect pregnant women at high risk for HIV infection have failed to detect the majority of HIV-infected patients.[86–88] Women may be unaware of HIV exposure from a sexual partner, or be unwilling to admit high-risk behaviors. Human immunodeficiency virus infection should be considered in any pregnant patient with clinical evidence of cellular immunodeficiency, whether or not the patient has a high-risk profile.

Maternal-Infant Transmission of HIV

Infants born to HIV seropositive mothers passively acquire maternal HIV antibodies. By 15 months of age, most infants will lose maternal antibody; if truly infected, they will produce their own antibodies to HIV at this time. Because HIV infection cannot be detected serologically in the neonate and newborns are usually asymptomatic, HIV maternal-infant transmission rates are difficult to determine.

Among larger cohort studies, approximately one third (24% to 39%) of infants born to HIV-infected women developed laboratory or clinical evidence of HIV infection.[89–91] Neonatal infection rates appear to be higher in infants of mothers who have previously delivered an HIV-infected baby.[92] It is postulated that women bearing a second HIV-infected child may have an increased viremic load; whether this is related to length of maternal infection and therefore more advanced disease is not known. There are preliminary data to suggest that perinatal transmission rates are higher in HIV positive mothers with a low CD4 count, p24 antigenemia, and high HIV viral replication.[93]

Human immunodefiency virus may be transmitted to the fetus throughout pregnancy. The virus has been isolated from a fetus as early as 15 weeks gestation[95] and directly isolated from the placenta at 39 weeks.[94] While the potential for maternal-infant transmission exists at the time of delivery, the mode of delivery—cesarean section versus vaginal delivery—appears to be unrelated to the risk of neonatal infection.[90,96] There have been several case reports of postpartum maternal-infant transmission of HIV through breast milk.[97,98] Free virus has been isolated from breast milk.[99] It is recommended that women who are HIV infected abstain from breast feeding.[100]

Fetal Outcome

Studies vary regarding adverse fetal outcome in infants born to HIV-infected mothers. In a study comparing HIV-infected and non-infected infants born to mothers in all stages of HIV infection, infants did not differ with respect to weight, height, head circumference, or rate of malformations. The infected infants did have higher IgM concentrations at birth and significantly lower CD4 counts.[101] Another study examining infants of mothers with AIDS found a significant increase in low birth weight, low gestational age at birth, low ratio of head circumference to height, and chorioamnionitis.[89] In a third study, more than one third (34.6%) of pregnancies in HIV-infected women were complicated by preterm labor.[85] Prematurity, low birth weight, and premature rupture of membranes have been noted in another study,[96] although intravenous drug use may be a confounding variable in some reports. Craniofacial dysmorphism in infants HIV-infected in utero was reported in 1986.[101] A subsequent controlled study could not substantiate the existence of an HIV embryopathy.[102]

Maternal Outcome

The suppression of cellular immunity normally seen in the last trimester of pregnancy is similar to that associated with HIV infection; both conditions produce decreased CD4 cells and CD4:CD8 ratio. Although pregnancy was originally thought to hasten progression of HIV disease,[101] subsequent controlled studies have shown only minor effects of pregnancy on HIV disease progression.[103] Decreases in CD4 cell counts have been 10% to 20% greater in HIV-infected pregnant patients than in their noninfected pregnant controls.[104]

Use of Zidovudine (AZT) in Pregnancy

Zidovudine (AZT) has not been used in pregnant women, in other than early investigations. In vitro, it crosses the human placenta in a manner consistent with simple diffusion.[105] This drug is extensively metabolized by the placenta into as yet unidentified metabolites. It is unknown if the placental accumulation of these metabolites will exert an antiviral action on the fetus. While AZT's safety in pregnancy has not been established, in vitro and animal studies have not revealed mutagenicity or malformation at this time. It is unknown if maternal use of AZT will affect the placental transmission of HIV or prove beneficial to an HIV-infected fetus.

Neurological Disease and HIV Infection

Approximately 10% of AIDS patients present with neurological illness; nearly 40% of all AIDS patients experience neurological symptoms during the course of their disease.[81,82] The majority of CNS diseases associated with AIDS are of an infectious etiology.

Diffuse Encephalopathy

Brain parenchymal diseases are easily divided into those that are accompanied by diffuse dysfunction and those that cause predominantly focal symptoms. Although these disorders do overlap, this division is clinically useful. For instance, herpes simplex encephalitis usually presents with a diffuse encephalopathy in the HIV-infected population, but may also present with focal brain disease. Likewise, cerebral toxoplasmosis usually presents with focal symptoms, but may also manifest as a diffuse encephalitis.

Metabolic encephalopathy may develop as sequelae of systemic diseases in AIDS patients just as in non-AIDS patients (e.g., hypoxia associated with pneumonia). Very commonly, these metabolic encephalopathies may have an unmasking effect on an underlying HIV dementia. In addition to the metabolic encephalopathies, infectious causes resulting in diffuse brain disease include cytomegalovirus, herpes simplex virus types I and II, *Toxoplasma gondii* and *Varicella zoster* virus (VZV). In addition, acute HIV infection may present as an acute encephalitis as well as an aseptic meningitis.

AIDS Dementia Complex/HIV Encephalopathy

Unique to AIDS, HIV encephalopathy, also known as the AIDS dementia complex or subacute encephalitis, is the most common neurological illness in this patient population. This disorder occurs in the later stages of HIV infection and is characterized by cognitive, motor, and behavioral dysfunction.[106–108] The demential complex usually appears initially as a confusional state. Characteristically manifesting after patients develop opportunistic infections or neoplasia, the AIDS dementia complex may also be the presenting syndrome in some patients, prior to the development of other systemic complications. The early presentation of the AIDS dementia complex has recently resulted in this being a diagnostic criteria for AIDS.

Initially, symptoms usually include poor concentration, intellectual slowing, forgetfulness, apathy, and social withdrawal. Occasionally, there are motor symptoms such as leg weakness and loss of balance. Other manifestations include mutism, psychosis, or psychomotor slowing. At the end stage of the disease, patients may become vegetative.

It is extremely important that other treatable etiologies be considered before attributing the cognitive changes to the AIDS dementia complex. All patients should undergo neuroimaging procedures and CSF examination. The neuroimaging findings in the AIDS dementia complex include cerebral and cerebellar atrophy and enlarged ventricles. The CSF reveals a mildly elevated protein and a mild mononuclear pleocytosis. Because intravenous drug use is the most common risk factor for HIV infection in women, drug toxicity or withdrawal must also be excluded.

Currently, the only available treatment for this devastating syndrome is zidovudine (AZT). In one study, the neurological symptoms have demonstrated a rapid improvement with this drug.[109] This is problematic, because zidovudine is not approved for use during pregnancy. As yet, there are no data to suggest that the course of HIV encephalopathy differs in the pregnant patient.

Focal Brain Disease

In the patient with cellular immunodeficiency, any diseases can present with discrete findings. Central nervous system toxoplasmosis is the most common cause of focal lesions in AIDS patients, followed by CNS lymphoma. Tuberculoma, cryptococcoma and other fungal diseases, and Kaposi's sarcoma may all present with a similar clinical and radiographic picture. Cytomegalovirus and herpes simplex virus types 1 and 2 may occasionally present as a mass lesion though typically they produce a diffuse encephalitis. Progressive multifocal leukoencephalopathy (PML) is a demyelinating disease caused by a papovavirus, Jacob-Crutzfeld (JC) virus. The white matter lesions characteristically demonstrated on CT and MRI may be difficult to distinguish from toxoplasmosis or lymphoma. Intravenous drug users are predisposed to septic emboli that can lead to intracranial abscess. In addition, patients may be susceptible to bacterial abscesses from posterior extension of chronic sinusitis, an infection commonly seen in AIDs patients.

While infection with *Toxoplasma gondii* in the immune competent host is often asymptomatic or mild and self-limiting, in the immunodeficient host it is frequently severe and often fatal if untreated. Most immunodeficient HIV-infected patients present with focal neurological deficits; fewer patients present with fever, headache, and seizures. Because serological titers for toxoplasmosis in AIDS patients are similar to titers in healthy patients with inactive infections, serology is rarely helpful except when negative. However, there have been case reports of AIDS patients with pathologically proven toxoplasmosis and undetectable titers of specific IgG.[110]

Magnetic resonance imaging is the preferred procedure for the HIV-infected immunocompromised pregnant patient with findings suggestive of an intracranial mass. The MRI contrast agent gadolinium is designated by the FDA as a Pregnancy Category C drug. If MRI reveals single or multifocal lesions, the patient should be treated empirically for toxoplasmosis. If the patient fails to show clinical or imaging improvement within 7 to 10 days, stereotactic needle biopsy should be performed to establish a diagnosis.

The most effective therapy for toxoplasmosis encephalitis, a combination of pyrimethamine and sulfadiazine, provides a sequential blockade of folic acid metabolism. Concomitant use of folinic acid (calcium leucovorin) with pyrimethamine should not be used in the first 14–16 weeks of pregnancy because of its teratogenic effects. The efficacy of sulfonamides without pyrimethamine in the treatment of CNS toxoplasmosis is not known.

Meningitis

Meningitis in the HIV-infected patient may be caused by a variety of opportunistic pathogens or by direct HIV invasion of the CNS. Aseptic meningitis presenting with headache, fever, cranial neuropathies, and meningismus may be the first manifestation of HIV disease, occurring at the time of initial HIV seroconversion. A mononuclear pleocytosis with low CD4 and elevated CD8 counts may be found in the CSF. Acute symptoms are usually self-limited with resolution in 1 to 4 weeks. Human immunodeficiency virus disease should be considered in any pregnant woman with unexplained aseptic meningitis. Most patients seroconvert within 3 months of exposure to HIV; however, more frequent testing may be warranted in the pregnant woman because she may choose to terminate the pregnancy based on HIV seropositivity.

Cryptococcus neoformans is the most common organism found in AIDS-associated meningitis. It occurs in 11% of patients with progressive HIV infection.[110] Cryptococcal meningitis typically presents with headache, meningismus, altered mentation, and nausea. India ink smears detect cryptococci in 50% of patients with cryptococcal meningitis. The presence of cryptococcal antigen in CSF and serum are extremely reliable indicators of infection; fungal cultures of CSF are specific but insensitive.

An initial 6-week course of amphotericin B is followed by long-term antifungal treatment to prevent relapse of cryptococcal meningitis in the immunodeficient patient. Maintenance amphotericin B therapy is administered weekly or biweekly, and may be given in an outpatient setting. A new imidazole, oral fluconazole, (200–400 mg daily) is available as maintenance therapy for cryptococcal meningitis. It may not be as effective as amphotericin B as initial therapy in the AIDS patient.

Syphilis in HIV-Infected Patients

In the HIV-infected host, the clinical manifestations, efficacy of antimicrobial therapies, serological responses, and frequency of syphilitic complications may be altered. While most HIV-infected patients demonstrate a normal serological response to *Treponema palli-*

dum, case studies have reported negative nontreponemal and treponemal tests in the face of biopsy-confirmed secondary syphilis.[111]

The CDC developed new recommendations for the diagnosis and treatment of syphilis in HIV-infected patients:[112]

(1) Persons with HIV infection acquired through intravenous drug use or sexual contact should be tested for syphilis. Likewise, persons with syphilis should be tested for HIV, with the informed consent of the patient.

(2) In cases of congenital syphilis, the mother should be offered counseling and testing for HIV, with appropriate medical follow-up of mother and infant if the mother is HIV seropositive.

(3) When the clinical examination suggests syphilis, and serological tests are negative, darkfield microscopy and direct fluorescent antibody staining for *T. pallidum* (DFA-TP) of the lesion and its exudate should be pursued.

(4) Neurosyphilis should be considered in the differential diagnosis of neurological disease in all HIV-infected persons.

Case reports suggest the more frequent occurrence of treatment failures of syphilis in HIV-infected patients, including progression to neurosyphilis. In one study, 3 of 4 patients who failed standard treatment for secondary syphilis (single injection of 2.4 million units of benzathine penicillin) were HIV infected.[113] While current CDC recommendations involve no change in the therapy for early syphilis for HIV-coinfected patients, there is considerable debate on this issue. Some authorities advise CSF examination in all HIV-coinfected patients, and treatment with a therapeutic regimen appropriate for neurosyphilis in these patients regardless of the clinical stage of syphilis.

HIV-infected pregnant women who report a history of penicillin allergy should be carefully questioned regarding the details of their reaction and, if necessary, receive skin testing with both major and minor determinants to confirm penicillin allergy. Truly allergic patients should be referred for desensitization.

Peripheral Nervous System Complications Related to HIV Infection

The peripheral nervous system complications related to HIV infection can be divided into four distinct syndromes: distal symmetric peripheral neuropathy, inflammatory demyelinating polyradiculo-neuropathy, mononeuropathy multiplex, and progressive polyradi-culopathy.[114]

The most common syndrome involving the peripheral nervous system in HIV-infected patients is a distal symmetric peripheral poly-neuropathy. The symptoms and signs are initially mild and yet chron-ically progressive, and include paresthesias, hypesthesia, weakness, and hypoactive muscle stretch reflexes. Affecting sensory function more than motor function, this syndrome may or may not be painful. Dysautonomia may rarely occur. The CSF is generally normal unless there are other coexisting processes. Zidovudine has shown promise in the treatment of this entity. Symptomatic treatments include ami-triptyline and nonsteroidal anti-inflammatory drugs. There is no spe-cific data to suggest a difference in the progression of symptoms dur-ing pregnancy. Because zidovudine is not approved in pregnancy, treatment for this disorder must be symptomatic.

Inflammatory demyelinating polyradiculoneuropathy can pres-ent as an acute, subacute, or chronic process in HIV-infected patients. This syndrome usually presents with prominent distal weakness, but there may be proximal weakness as well as sensory loss. The CSF has an elevation of protein and a mild pleocytosis. Electromyography and nerve conduction velocity tests suggest a demyelinating poly-radiculopathy. Treatment with plasmapheresis has been very suc-cessful when demyelination predominates over axonal loss. Predni-sone is ineffective. Spontaneous improvement occasionally occurs.

Mononeuropathy multiplex is less common than inflammatory demyelinating polyradiculoneuropathy. It mostly occurs in HIV-in-fected patients who have not yet developed AIDS. This condition is characterized by the rapid development of sensory and motor loss in the distribution of one or more nerve trunks or cranial nerves. The presentation is very similar to the mononeuropathy multiplex caused by diabetes mellitus or polyarteritis nodosa. The CSF reflects inflam-mation. Electromyography and nerve conduction studies show changes suggesting combined axonal loss and demyelination. Treat-ment with plasmapheresis is sometimes successful.

Progressive polyradiculopathy is a distinct syndrome that can present either as a radiculopathy or radiculomyelopathy occurring in patients with "full-blown" AIDS. It begins with asymmetric leg weak-ness which progresses cephalad over several weeks. Sensory loss is also prominent. Urinary retention is typical. The CSF characteristically shows hypoglycorrhachia in addition to elevated protein and a mononuclear cell pleocytosis. Nerve conduction studies are usually normal, and the electromyogram shows a reduced recruitment pattern. Prognosis for this particular neurological complication is very poor, even when it is caused by herpes simplex virus or cytomegalovirus, which are treatable with specific antiviral agents. Herpes zoster virus may also cause polyradiculopathies as can meningeal lymphomatosis.

Again, as with the diffuse encephalopathies seen in HIV-infected patients, there are no data to suggest a difference in presentation or progression of these neurological complications in the pregnant HIV-infected patient.

Vacuolar Myelopathy

Patients with advanced HIV disease may also develop a myelopathy often associated with AIDS-related dementia. A noninflammatory vacuolar myelopathy manifests as a spastic paraparesis and sensory ataxia. Spastic paraparesis may also be caused by HTLV-1. Another cause of myelopathy is vitamin B_{12} deficiency.

Myopathies

Myopathies are less well characterized and less common than the neuropathies. These may also occur at several stages of HIV-1 infection with a wide range of possible presentations, from an asymptomatic elevation of creatine kinase to progressive proximal muscle weakness.[115,116] Zidovudine may also cause a necrotizing myopathy.

Antimicrobial Therapy

Genetic differences in the fetus can influence the likelihood of drug-induced developmental toxicity. Even if a prospective study uncovers no increase in neonatal malformations compared with untreated populations, it does not exclude the possibility that the drug in question may act as a teratogen in a small number of patients.

Details regarding safety in pregnancy are incomplete for many of the newer antimicrobial agents. Therefore, use in pregnancy is advocated only if the potential benefits justify the potential risk to the fetus.

The number of women receiving antimicrobial therapy during pregnancy has been reported variously at 21% to 37%.[117,118] The standard regimen for antimicrobial dosage may be inadequate when applied to the pregnant patient. In part, this is due to increased intravascular volume and circulation to the maternal kidney, which results in more rapid renal clearance and more transfer of drug to the fetus. Increased blood flow to the uterus also contributes to a variable fetal exposure to antimicrobial agents.

During pregnancy, there is an associated decrease in albumin binding of many antibiotics. Therefore, the increased unbound antibiotic fraction maintains effective serum and tissue levels despite a decrease in the total serum antimicrobial level. It is beyond the scope of this chapter to discuss the individual antibiotics and their use during pregnancy.

Risk Assessment for Drugs Used During Pregnancy

The Food and Drug Administration has defined categories to determine the level of risk a drug poses to the fetus.[119] Briggs et al.[118] use these definitions to assign risk factor categories to drugs according to available data. Because there have been few controlled trials of drugs in pregnant women, data is based primarily on animal studies and incident reports, or lack thereof. The definitions used for risk factors are as follow:

Category A: Controlled studies in women fail to demonstrate a risk to the fetus in the first trimester (and there is no evidence of a risk in later trimesters), and the possibility of fetal harm appears remote.

Category B: Either animal-reproduction studies have not demonstrated a fetal risk but there are no controlled studies in pregnant women, or animal-reproduction studies have shown an adverse effect (other than a decrease in fertility) but this was not confirmed in controlled studies in women in the first trimester (and there is no evidence of a risk in later trimesters).

Category C: Either studies in animals have revealed adverse effects on the fetus (teratogenic or embryocidal or other) and there are no controlled studies in women or studies in women and animals are not available. Drugs should be given only if the potential benefit justifies the potential risk to the fetus.

Category D: There is positive evidence of human fetal risk, but the benefits from use in pregnant women may be acceptable despite the risk (e.g., if the drug is needed in a life-threatening situation or for a serious disease for which safer drugs cannot be used or are ineffective).

Category X: Studies in animals or human beings have demonstrated fetal abnormalities or there is evidence of fetal risk based on human experience or both, and the risk of the use of the drug in pregnant women clearly outweighs any possible benefit. The drug is contraindicated in women who are or may become pregnant.

See Table I for appropriate use of antibiotics in pregnancy.

Immunizations

Immunizations during pregnancy should not include live viral vaccines because of potential fetal risk. However, they may be administered as part of postpartum care for women at risk. This includes single dose measles (rubeola), rubella, and yellow fever immunization. If possible, postponement of travel is preferable to yellow fever immunization during pregnancy.[126] Its risk to fetus or neonate is unknown. Evidence now exists of deleterious fetal effects with the live altered strain of Venezuelan equine encephalitis (VEE) administered during pregnancy.[127]

Inactivated vaccines do not appear to present increased risk to the pregnant patient or her fetus. Inactivated, enhanced-potency poliomyelitis vaccines have become available and provide greater efficacy. No data are available on adverse effects of the product administered during pregnancy although unintentional inoculated polio vaccine appears safe. With this inactivated enhanced polio vaccine available, it is no longer necessary to administer a live polio vaccine to pregnant patients with recent exposure. The CDC suggests that for pregnant women requiring immediate immunization against po-

Table I.
Antimicrobic Agents in Pregnancy

Name	Safety in Pregnancy	Class	Concentration in CSF	Comments
Aminoglycosides				VIII nerve damage
Streptomycin	0	D		
Gentamicin	+	D	+/0	
Tobramycin		D		
Amikacin		D		
Netillmycin		D		
Kanamycin		D	0	
Cephalosporins				
1st Generation	+ + +		0	
(Ancef, Kefzol, etc.)				
2nd Generation	+ + +	B	0	
Cefmandole	+ + +	B	0	
Cefuroxime	+ + +	B	0	
Cefoxitin	+ + +	B	0	
Cefotetan	+ + +	B	0	
3rd Generation	+ + +	B		
Ceftriaxone	+ + +	B	+ +	
Cefotaxime	+ + +	B	+ +	
Ceftazidime	+ + +	B	+ +	
Cefoperazone	+ + +	B	0	
Ceftizoxime	+ + +	B	+ +	
Chloromycetin	+/0	C	+ +	"Gray-baby" syndrome at term
Glycopeptides				
Vancomycin	+	C	+/0	
Macrolides				
Erythromycin	+ + +	B	0	Not estolate-hepatotoxicity
Clindamycin	+		0	
Metronidazole	+ +	B	+/0	Carcinogenic in animals

Monobactams				
Aztreonam	+++	B	+/0	
Penicillins				
Penicillin	+++	A	++	
Ampicillin	+++	A	++	
Ticarcillin		B	0	
Nafcillin; Oxacillin; Methicillin		B		
Ureidopenicillins				
Mezlocillin	+++	B	0	
Piperacillin	+++	B	0	
Azlocillin	+++	B	0	
Penems				
Imepenem-Cilastin	+	C	+/0	High-dose lead to seizures
Quinolones				
Ciprofloxacin	0	C	+/0	associated cartilagenous lesions
Norfloxacin	0	C	0	
Ofloxacin	0	C		
Temafloxacin	0	C		
Sulfonamides				
Sulfamethozasole	+	C	++	Hyperbilirubinemia[122-25] at term/
Trimethoprim	+	C	++	Combined with sulfamethozasole
Tetracyclines				
Tetracycline HCL	0	D	+	Dental staining;
Vibramycin	0	D	+	Bone growth decreased;
Minocycline	0	D	+	+/– hepatic failure post 28th week gestation
Antifungals				
Amphotoricin B	++	B	+	
Ketoconazole	+	C	0	
Fluconazole	0	C	++	
Itraconazole (investigational)		—	0	carcinogenic
Pentamadine	+	C	0	
5-Fluorocytosine		C	0	

(continued)

Table I. Antimicrobic Agents in Pregnancy (Continued)

Name	Safety in Pregnancy	Class	Concentration in CSF	Comments
Antimalarials				
Chloroquin Phosphate	+ + +	C		VIII nerve damage; decreased platelets;
Quinine	+	X		deafness; malformations and abortions;
Emetine	0	X	0	fetotoxic
Mefloquin	0	X	0	
Antiparasitic				
Praziquantel	+ + +	B	0	
Mebendazole	+	C		
Thiabendazole	+	C		
Quinacrine HCl	+	C		
Niclosamide	+ + +	B		
Pyrimethamine	+	C		malformation
Antituberculars				
Isoniazid	+	C	+	some intrautero abnormalities benefit may
Ethambutol	+	C	0	outweigh risks
Rifampin	+	C	+ +	
Pyrazinamide	+	C	+ +	
Antivirals				
Zovirax	+	C	+ +	
Gancyclovir	0	X	+ +	
Zidovudine	+	C	+ +	
Vidarabine	+	C	+ +	
Didanosine	unknown	B	unknown	

liomyelitis, either oral polio vaccine (OPV) or inactivated (IPV) polio vaccine may be used.[128]

A mass oral trivalent polio vaccine (OPV) immunization program, started in February of 1985 in Finland following a poliomyelitis outbreak, occurred with no significant variations from baseline in the prevalence of all fetal malformations[129] during the months after vaccinations. This suggests OPV had no harmful effects on fetal development.

If circumstances necessitate such administration, vaccines may be offered including influenza and rabies immunization. No fetal abnormalities have been associated with rabies immunization during pregnancy, and pregnancy is not a contraindication for postexposure prophylaxis.

Administration of dead vaccines to pregnant women poses no increased risk. The U.S. National 1976 Swine Flu Influenza Immunization Program was the only such undertaking to be associated with an increase in postimmunization Guillain-Barré syndrome. Subsequent annual influenza immunization program studies failed to establish such a relationship.

Immunizations derived from portions of whole viruses or bacteria have proven to be effective immunogens and are safe to administer during pregnancy. These include meningococcal vaccine and genetically engineered recombinant hepatitis B vaccine, (though the latter is listed as Pregnancy Category C).

References

1. Brabin BJ: Epidemiology of infection in pregnancy. *Rev Infect Dis* 7:579–603, 1985.
2. Gall, SA: Maternal adjustments in the immune system in normal pregnancy. *Clin Ob-Gyn* 26:521–536, 1983.
3. El-Maliem H, Fletcher J: Impaired neutrophil function and myeloperoxidase deficiency in pregnancy. *Br J Haematol* 44:375–381, 1980.
4. Sever JL: Infections in pregnancy: highlights from the collaborative perinatal project. *Teratology* 25:227, 1982.
5. Harris JW: Influenza occurring in pregnant women: a statistical study of thirteen hundred and fifty cases. *JAMA* 72:978–980, 1919.
6. Zinserling AV, Aksenov OA, Melnikova VF: Extrapulmonary lesions in influenza. *Tohoku J Exp Med* 140:259–272, 1983.
7. Hutchinson PT, Kinney A, Eykyn S: Neonatal death due to pneumococcal infection. *Obstet Gynecol* 31:130, 1984.

8. Lucas AO: Pneumococcal meningitis in pregnancy and the puerperium. *Br Med J* 1:92–95, 1969.
9. Sandberg T: Meningitis and septicemia due to H, influenzal Type B in pregnancy. *Br Med J* 282:946, 1981.
10. Linnan MJ, Mascola L, Lou XD: Epidemic Listeriosis associated with Mexican style cheese. *N Engl J Med* 319:823–828, 1988.
11. Payne DG, et al: Bacterial endocarditis in pregnancy. *Obstet Gynceol* 2:247, 1960.
12. McComb JM, McNamee PT, Sinnamon GD, et al: Staphylococcal endocarditis presenting as meningitis in pregnancy. *Int J Cardiol* 1:325, 1982.
13. Stephanopoulos C: The development of tuberculous meningitis during pregnancy. *Am Rev Tuber* 76:1079, 1956.
14. Mehta BR: Pregnancy and tuberculosis. *Dis Chest* 39:505, 1961.
15. Petrini B, Gentz J, Winbladh B, et al: Perinatal transmission of tuberculosis, meningitis in mother, disseminated in child. *Scand J Infect Dis* 15:403, 1983.
16. Joint Statement of the ATS, National TBC and Respiratory Disease Association and CDC. *Am Rev Dis* 104:460, 1973.
17. D'Cruz IA, Dandekar AC: Tuberculosis meningitis in pregnant and puerperal women. *Obstet Gynecol* 31(6):775–778, 1968.
18. Weinstein L, Murphy T: The management of tuberculosis during pregnancy. *J Perinatol* 1:395, 1974.
19. Brandstetter RD, Murray HW, Mellow E: Tuberculous meningitis in a puerperal woman. *JAMA* 224:2440, 1980.
20. Garrioch DB: Puerperal tuberculosis. *Br J Clin Pract* 29:280, 1975.
21. deMarch P: Tuberculosis and pregnancy. *Chest* 6:800, 1975.
22. Ramos AD, Hibbard LT, Craig JR, et al: Congenital tuberculosis. *Obstet Gynecol* 43:61, 1974.
23. Centeno RS, Winter J, Bentson J: Central nervous system tuberculosis related to pregnancy. *J Comput Tomogr* 6:141–145, 1982.
24. Golditch I: Tuberculosis meningitis and pregnancy. *Am J Obstet Gynecol* 110:1144, 1971.
25. Adams RD, Victor M, (eds): *Principles of Neurology, Part IV*. New York, NY. McGraw Hill, 1981, p. 492.
26. Wilson EA: Tuberculosis complicated by pregnancy. *Am J Obstet Gynecol* 115:526, 1973.
27. National ACCP Consensus Conference on Tuberculosis. *Chest* 2:87, 1985.
28. Harter CA, Benirschice K: Fetal syphilis in the first trimester. *Am J Obstet Gynecol* 124:705, 1976.
28a. Morbidity and Mortality Weekly Report. Centers for Disease Control Annual Summary of Notifiable Diseases, United States, 1989.
29. Mascola L, Pelosi R, Blount JH, et al: Congenital syphilis: why is it still occurring? *JAMA* 252:1715, 1984.
30. Thompson SE: Treatment of syphilis in pregnancy. *J Am Vener Dis Assoc* 3:159, 1976.

31. Jones JE, Harris RE: Diagnostic evaluation of syphilis during pregnancy. *Obstet Gynecol* 5:611, 1979.
32. Hashisaki P, Wertzberger GG, Conrad GL, et al: Erythromycin failure in a treatment of syphilis in a pregnant woman. *Sex Transm Dis* Jan-Mar 10(1):36–38, 1983.
33. Fenton LF, Light J: Congenital syphilis after maternal Lyme treatment with erythromycin. *Obstet Gynecol* 47:492, 1976.
34. Berger BW. Dermatologic manifestations of Lyme Disease. *Rev Inf Dis* 11(Suppl 6):S1475-S1481, 1989.
35. Reik L, Steere AC, Barenhagen NH, et al: Neurologic abnormalities of Lyme Disease. *Medicine* 58:281–294, 1979.
36. Stiernstedt G, Skoldenberg B, Garde A, et al. Clinical manifestation of *Borrelia* infections of the nervous system. *Zbl Bakt Hyg A* 263:289–296, 1986.
37. Bateman DE, Lawton NF, White JE, et al. The neurological complications of *Borrelia burgdorferi* in the New Forest area of Hampshire. *J Neurol Neurosurg Psych* 51:699–703, 1988.
38. Sindic CJM, Depre A, Bigaignon G, et al: Lymphocytic meningoradiculitis and encephalomyelitis due to *Borrelia burgdorferi*: a clinical and seriological study of 18 cases. *J Neurol Neurosurg Psychiatry* 50:1565–1571, 1987.
39. Reik L, Burgdorfer W, Donaldson JO. Neurological abnormalities in Lyme disease without erythema chronicum migrans. *Am J Med* 81:73–78, 1986.
40. Halperin JJ, Luft BJ, Anand AK, et al: Lyme neuroborreliosis: central nervous system manifestations. *Neurology* 39:753–759, 1989.
41. Halperin JJ, Pass HL, Anand AK, et al: Nervous system abnormalities in Lyme disease. *Ann NY Acad Sci* 539:24–34, 1988.
42. Dattwyler RJ, Halperin JJ. Failure of tetracycline therapy in early Lyme disease. *Arthritis Rheum* 30:448–50, 1987.
43. Schlesinger PA, Duray PH, Burke BA, et al: Maternal-fetal transmission of Lyme disease spirochete, *Borrelia burgdorferi*. *Ann Intern Med* 103:67–68, 1985.
44. Markowitz LE, Steere AC, Benach JL, et al: Lyme disease during pregnancy. *JAMA* 255:3394–3396, 1986.
45. Williams CL, Benach JL, et al: Lyme disease during pregnancy. A cord blood serosurvey. *Ann NY Acad Sci* 539:504–506, 1988.
46. Morbidity and Mortality. CDC Annual SUmmary of Notifiable Diseases, United States, 1989: Vol. 38; 54; 41 & 54.
47. Januszkiewicz J, Galazka A, Adamczyk J, et al: Severe tetanus in late pregnancy. *Scand J Infect Dis* 5:233, 1973.
48. Adams VB, Curtis DR, et al: Puerperal tetanus. *Am J Obstet Gynecol* 69:169, 1955.
49. Chunter JR, Ryan MD: Spinal epidural abscess in pregnancy. *Aust NZ J Surg* 47:672, 1977.
50. Neiberg AD, Mavromatis F, Dyke J, et al: Blastomycoses dermatitidis treated during pregnancy: report of a case. *Am J Obstet Gynecol* 128:911–912, 1977.

51. Ismail MA, Lerner SA: Disseminated blastomyocosis in a pregnant woman. *Am Rev Respir Dis* 126:350–351, 1982.
52. Opsahl MS, O'Brien W: Systemic Nocardiosis in pregnancy. *J Reprod Med* 28:621, 1983.
53. Smale LE: Dissemination of Coccidioidomycosis in pregnancy. *Trans Pac Coast Obstet Gynecol Soc* 37:24–29.
54. Mahmaud I, Lerner S: Amphotericin B usage during pregnancy. *Am Rev Resp Dis* 126:350, 1982.
55. Aitken GWE, Symonos EM: Cryptococcal meningitis in pregnancy treated with amphotericin B. *J Obstet Gynecol Br Comm* 69:6779, 1962.
56. Ismail MA, Lerner SA: Disseminated blastomycosis in a pregnant woman: review of amphotericin B usage during pregnancy. *Am Rev Resp Dis* 126:350–353, 1982.
57. Aropa RC, Garg RK, Jap, I: *Cerebral Malaria Caused by Plasmodium vivax.* 36(9):564, 1983. 58. Warrell DA: Pathophysiology of severe falciparum malaria in man. *Parasitology* 94(Suppl):S53-S76, 1987.
59. Looareensuwan S, Phillips RE, White NJ, et al: Quinine and severe falciparum malaria in late pregnancy. *Lancet* VV:4–8, 1985.
60. White NJ, Warrell DA, Chanthavinich P, et al: Severe hypoglycemia and hyperinsulinemia in falciparum malaria. *N Engl J Med* 309:61–66, 1983.
61. Bittencourt AL, Cardoso de Almeida MA, Iunes MA, et al: Placental involvement in *Shistosoma mansoni. Am J Trop Med Hyg* 29:571–575, 1980.
62. Sever JL: Infections in pregnancy. *Teratology* 25:227, 1982.
63. Kimball AC, Kean BH, Fuchs F, et al: Toxoplasmosis. Risk variations in New York City obstetric patients. *Am J Obstet Gynecol* 119:208, 1974.
64. Desmonts G, et al: Congenital toxoplasmosis. *Br J Obstet Gynaecol* 19:417, 1984.
65. Congenital toxoplasmosis (editorial). *Lancet* 2:578–579, 1980.
66. Bettie CP: Congenital toxoplasmosis (editorial). *Br J Obstet Gynaecol* 19:417–418, 1984.
67. Grillner L, Forsgren M, Barr B, et al: Outcome of rubella during pregnancy with special reference to the 17th–24th weeks of gestation. *Scand J Infect Dis* 15:321–325, 1983.
68. Lynn E: Letter to the editor. *JAMA* 239:1960, 1978.
69. Hankey GJ, Bucens MR, Chambers JS: Herpes simplex encephalitis in third trimester of pregnancy: successful outcome for mother and child. *Neurology* 37:1534–1537, 1987.
70. Beser R: Successful treatment of HSV encephalitis during pregnancy. *Neurology* 39(5):748, 1989.
71. Diosi P, Babusceac L, Nevinglovschi O, et al: Cytomegalovirus infection associated with pregnancy. *Lancet* 2:1063–1066, 1967.
72. Hildebrandt R, Sever JL, Margileth AM, et al: Cytomegalovirus in the normal pregnant woman. *Am J Obstet Gynecol* 98:1125–1128, 1967.
73. Reynolds DW, Stagno S, Hosty TS, et al: Cytomegalovirus excretion and perinatal infection. *N Engl J Med* 289:1–5, 1973.
74. Nankervis G: Prospective study of maternal cytomegalovirus infection and its effects on the fetus. *Am J Obstet Gynecol* 149:435, 1984.
75. Peckham CS, Chin KS, Coleman JC, et al: Cytomegalovirus infection in

pregnancy: preliminary findings from a prospective study. *Lancet* 1:1352–1355, 1983.

76. Cates W: Treatment of rabies exposure during pregnancy. *Obstet Gynecol* 44:894, 1974.
77. Rabies: CDC surveillance summaries. *MMWR* 34, No ISS, 15SS, 1989.
78. London WT, Levitt NH, Kent SG, et al: Congenital cerebral and ocular malformations induced in rhesus monkeys by Venezuelan equine encephalitis virus. *Teratology* 16:285–290, 1977.
79. Wirguin I, Steiner I, Kidron D, et al: Fulminant subacute sclerosing panencephalitis in associated pregnancy. *Arch Neurol* 45:1324–1325, 1988.
80. Risk WS, Hadpad FS. The variable natural history of SSPE. *Arch Neurol* 36:610–614, 1979.
81. Levy RM, Bredesen DE, Rosenblum NL: Neurological manifestation of the acquired immunodeficiency syndrome (AIDS): experience at UCSF and review of the literature. *J Neurosurg* 62:475–495, 1985.
82. Center for Disease Control, AIDS Weekly Surveillance Report. Jan 5, 1987.
83. Centers for Disease Control, Morbidity and Mortality Weekly Report Update: Acquired Immunodeficiency Syndrome—United States 1989. Feb. 9, 1990, Vol. 39, No. S, p 82.
84. Centers for Disease Control, AIDS Weekly Surveillance Report. Dec. 12, 1988.
85. Gloeb DJ, O'Sullivan MJ, Efantis J, et al: The effects of human immunodeficiency virus on pregnancy. *Am J Obstet Gynecol* 159(3):756–761, 1988.
86. Barbacci M, Chaisson R: Routine versus targeted prenatal testing for human immunodeficiency virus. Sixth International Conference on AIDS. San Francisco, Abstract #Th.C.41. 1990.
87. Krasinski K, Borkowsky W, Bebenroth D, et al: Failure of voluntary testing for human immunodeficiency virus to identify infected parturient women in a high-risk population (letter). *N Engl J Med* 318(3):185, 1988.
88. Landesman S, Minkoff H, Holman S, et al: Serosurvey of human imunodeficiency virus in parturients: implication for human immunodeficiency virus testing programs of pregnant women. *JAMA* 258 2701–2703, 1987.
89. Ryder WR, Nsa W, Hassig SE, et al: Perinatal transmission of the human immunodeficiency virus type 1 to infants of seropositive woman in Zaire. *N Engl J Med* 320(25):1637–1642, 1989.
90. Mother-to-child transmission of HIV infection. The European Collaborative Study. *Lancet* 2(8619):1039–1046, 1988.
91. Blanche S, Rouzioux C, Moscato ML, et al: A prospective study in infants born to women serospositive for human immunodeficiency virus type 1. *N Engl J Med* 320(25):1643–1648, 1989.
92. Scott GB, Fischl MA, Klimas N, et al: Mothers of infants with the acquired immune deficiency syndrome. Evidence for symptomatic and asympomatic carriers. *JAMA* 253:263–236, 1985.
93. Boue F, Pons JC, et al: Risk for HIV-1 perinatal transmissions vary with

the mother's stage of HIV infection. Sixth International Conference on AIDS. San Francisco, Abstract #Th.C.44, 1990.

94. Sprecher S, Soumenkoff G, Puissant F, et al: Vertical transmission of HIV in 15 week fetus [letter]. *Lancet* 2:288–289, 1986.
95. Hill WC, Bolton V, Carlson JR, et al: Isolation of acquired immune deficiency syndrome virus from the placenta. *Am J Obstet Gynecol* 157:10–11, 1987.
96. Minkoff H, Nanda D, Menez R, et al: Pregnancies resulting in infants with acquired immunodeficiency syndrome or AIDS-related complex, *Obstet Gynecol* 69:285–287, 1987.
97. Lepage P, Van De Perre P, Carael M, et al: Postnatal transmission of HIV from mother to child [letter]. *Lancet* 2:400, 1987.
98. Ziegler JB, Cooper DA, Johnson RO, et al: Postnatal transmission of AIDS associated retrovirus from mother to infant. *Lancet* 1:896–898, 1985.
99. Thiry L, Sprecher-Goldberger S, Jonckheer T, et al: Isolation of AIDS virus from cell free breast milk of three healthy virus carriers. *Lancet* 2:891–892, 1985.
100. Centers for Disease Control. Recommendations for assisting in the prevention of perinatal transmission of human T lymphotrophic virus type III/lymphadenopathy associated virus and acquired immunodeficiency syndrome. *MMWR* 34:721, 1985.
101. Marion RW, Wiznia AA, Hutcheon G, et al: Human t cell lymphotrophic virus type embryopathy. A new dysmorphia syndrome. *Am J Dis Child* 140:638–640, 1986.
102. Qazi QH, Sheikh TN, Fikrig S, et al: Lack of evidence for craniofacial dysmorphism in perinatal HIV infection. *J Pediatr* 112:7, 1988.
103. Schaefer A, Grosch-Woerner I, et al: The effects of pregnancy on the natural course of HIV disease. Fourth International Conference of AIDS, Stockholm, 1988, Abstract #4039.
104. Biggar RJ, Pahwa S, et al: Helper and suppressor lymphocyte change in HIV-infected mothres and their infants. Fourth International Conference on AIDS. Stockholm, 1988. Abstract #4031.
105. Liebes L, Mendoza S, Wilson D, et al: Transfer of zidovudine (AZT) by human placenta. *J Infect Dis* 161:203–207, 1990.
106. Sidtis JJ, Price RW: Early HIV-1 infection and the AIDS dementia complex. *Neurology* 40:323–326, 1990.
107. Navia BA, Jordan BD, Price RW, et al: The AIDS dementia complex. I Clinical features. *Ann Neurol* 19:517–524, 1986.
108. Price RW, Brew BJ: The AIDS dementia complex. *J Infect Dis* 158:1079–1083, 1988.
109. Schmitt FA, Bigley JW, McKinnis R, et al: Neuropsychological outcome of azidothymidine (AZT) in the treatment of AIDS and AIDS-related complex: a double blind placebo-controlled trial. *N Engl J Med* 319:1573–1578, 1988.
110. McArthur JC. Neurologic manifestation of AIDS. *Medicine* 66(6):407–437, 1987.
111. Hicks CB, Benson PM, Lupton GP, et al: Seronegative secondary syphilis

in a patient infected with the human immunodeficiency virus (HIV) and Kaposi's sarcoma. *Ann Int Med* 107:492–495, 1987.

112. Centers for Disease Control. Sexuallly transmitted diseases treatment guidelines. *MMWR* 38(S-8):13, 1989.

113. Lukehart SA, Hook EW, Baker-Zander SA, et al: Invasion of the central nervous system by treponema pallidum: implications for diagnosis and treatment. *Ann Int Med* 109:855–862, 1988.

114. Janssen RS, Cornblath DR, Epstein LG, et al: Human immunodeficiency virus (HIV) infection and the nervous system: report from the American Academy of Neurology AIDS Task Force. *Neurology* 39:119, 1989.

115. Dalakas MC, Pezeshpour GH, Gravell M, et al: Polymyositis associated with AIDS retrovirus. *JAMA* 256:2381–2383, 1986.

116. Simpson DM, Bender AN: Human immunodeficiency virus associated myopathy: analysis of 11 patients. *Ann Neurol* 24:79–84, 1988.

117. Stewart K: Bacterial infection. *Clin Obstet Gynecol* 8:315, 1981.

118. Doering PL, Stewart RB: The extent and character of drug consumption during pregnancy. *JAMA* 239(9):843–846, 1978.

119. Federal Register 44:3734–3767, 1980.

120. Briggs GG, Bodendorfer TW, Yaffe SJ, et al: *Drugs in Pregnancy and Lactation: A Reference Guide to Fetal and Neonatal Risk*. Baltimore, MD. Williams and Wilkins, 1986, xxi.

121. Safety of antimicrobial drugs in pregnancy. *Med Lett Drugs Ther* 27(700): 93–95, 1985.

122. Lucey JF, Dirscoll TJ Jr: Hazard to newborn infants of administration of long-acting sulfonamides to pregnant women. *Pediatrics* 24:498–499, 1959.

123. Kantor HI, Sutherland DA, et al: Effects of bilirubin metabolism in the newborn of sulfisoxazole administration to the mother. *Obstet Gynecol* 17:494–500, 1961.

124. Dynn PM: The possible relationship between the maternal administration of sulfamethoxypyridazine and hyperbilirubinemia in the newborn. *J Obstet Gynaecol Br Commonw* 71:128–131, 1964.

125. Baskin CG, Law S, et al: Sulfadiazine rheumatic fever prophylaxis during pregnancy: does it increase the risk of hernicterus in the newborn? *Cardiology* 222–225, 1965.

126. Barry M, Frank BA: Pregnancy and Travel. *JAMA* 261(5):728–731,1989.

127. Casamassima AC, Hess LW, Marty A, et al: TC-83 Venezuelan equine encephalitis vaccine exposure during pregnancy. *Teratology* 36:287–289, 1987.

128. Immunization practices advisory committee: Polio. *MMWR* 36:795–798, 1987.

129. Harjulehto T, Aro T, Hovi T, et al: Congenital malformation and oral poliovirus vaccination during pregnancy. Preventive medicine. *Lancet* 1(8641):771–772, 1989.

7

Multiple Sclerosis and Pregnancy

Richard A. Rudick, M.D.
Kathy A. Birk, M.D.

Introduction

Multiple sclerosis (MS) is the most common crippling neurological disease affecting young adults. Nearly 250,000 Americans are
thought to have MS. Characterized by episodic inflammation and
demyelination in the brain, optic nerves, and spinal cord, MS causes
symptoms and signs of neurological dysfunction that wax and wane
in an unpredictable pattern over years or decades. Physical impairment gradually accumulates in a significant proportion of patients.
Motor and visual impairment are cardinal clinical features of MS, but
patients may also experience emotional or cognitive impairment, family and vocational problems, and economic distress caused indirectly
by the illness.

The onset of MS is greatest between the ages 20 and 35 and
women are affected twice as often as men. Consequently, the interaction between MS and pregnancy is of great concern to many women
and their physicians. The purpose of this chapter is to review the
relationship between MS and pregnancy and to propose management
strategies on a number of issues raised by women with MS.

From Goldstein PJ, Stern BJ, (eds): *Neurological Disorders of Pregnancy. Second
Revised Edition.* Mount Kisco NY, Futura Publishing Co., Inc., © 1992.

Overview of Multiple Sclerosis

Common initial symptoms of MS include blurring of vision, double vision, weakness, numbness, imbalance, or clumsiness. Symptoms typically worsen for several days, stabilize, and then improve during the course of 4–8 weeks. New symptoms occur months or years later. Some combination of motor, sensory, visual, and cerebellar dysfunction may accumulate with time as patients experience episodic exacerbations with incomplete recovery between attacks. Progression of symptoms is more gradual in about one third of patients and continues over months or years. This is particularly common in patients experiencing disease onset after the age of 35, and commonly presents as a progressive gait impairment. Approximately 30% of patients have benign MS, characterized by intermittent symptoms but without progressive impairment.

The diagnosis of MS is based primarily on clinical features, although laboratory testing is often used to substantiate a clinical diagnosis. To satisfy diagnostic criteria for MS,[1] there must be evidence for more than one area of central nervous system involvement spread over time. The history and neurological examination are of primary importance in determining that there have been multiple attacks of neurological dysfunction. Alternative diagnoses that can mimic MS must be excluded (Table I).

Magnetic resonance imaging (MRI) is very sensitive for signal changes in the periventricular white matter and is used to document disseminated white matter lesions. Lesions visualized by MRI are nonspecific, however, because similar changes are seen with vascular disease such as hypertensive cerebrovascular disease, multicentric inflammatory diseases like sarcoidosis, and with normal aging. Incorrect diagnoses of MS based largely on MRI findings are made with alarming frequency. Sensory evoked potential testing of visual, auditory, or somatosensory systems will demonstrate abnormalities in the majority of patients with clinically definite MS.[2] Cerebrospinal fluid (CSF) changes consist of a slightly increased number of mononuclear cells, normal glucose, and normal or slightly elevated total protein, but increased concentration of IgG. The latter abnormality can be measured in a number of ways. Cerebrospinal fluid gamma globulins form discrete bands—called oligoclonal bands—when the CSF proteins are separated by electrophoretic methods.[3] The amount

Table I.
**Conditions Incorrectly Diagnosed as
Multiple Sclerosis**

Vascular Diseases
Hypertensive cerebrovascular disease
Vasculitis
Structural Lesions
Cranial cervical junction
Posterior fossa
Spinal cord
Degenerative Diseases
Motor system disease
Spinocerebellar degeneration
Other
Cobalamin deficiency
Sjögren's syndrome
Sarcoidosis
HTLV-1 infection
Nonspecific MRI abnormalities

of CSF IgG synthesized within the nervous system each day can be estimated by measuring CSF and serum IgG and albumin and applying a formula developed for that purpose.[4] Free κ light chains, similar to Bence-Jones proteins, have been detected in CSF of MS patients and the finding appears to be more specific for MS than nonspecific IgG tests.[5] As with MRI and evoked potential abnormalities, CSF changes are not specific. Abnormalities support a clinical diagnosis of MS, but a diagnosis based mostly on the CSF test results should be held with skepticism.

The cause of MS is currently unknown, but accumulating evidence suggests that an environmental trigger, possibly a viral infection, triggers an autoimmune attack on CNS myelin in a genetically-susceptible individual (see below). The disease is common in certain high-prevalence geographic regions but uncommon in other areas. Migration studies[6] have suggested that exposure prior to the age of 13 determines whether a person from a high-prevalence zone carries the high risk with him when he migrates to a low-prevalence zone. Much attention has focused on viruses as a causative environmental factor, although no virus has been reproducibly isolated from the brain tissue of MS patients. In any event, given the proper environmental trigger, a genetically susceptible individual develops immune-mediated demyelination. Cells from the immune system, particularly lymphocytes and macrophages, leave the circulation and invade the perivascular space, infiltrate parenchyma, and cause myelin destruction.

Medical treatment include symptoms pharmacotherapy, disease treatments, and experimental therapies. Comprehensive reviews of this subject have been published recently.[7] Management issues of particular interest to the obstetrician will be considered here.

Multiple Sclerosis and Pregnancy

Multiple Sclerosis Does Not Affect Pregnancy: Multiple sclerosis does not affect pregnancy, does not change a woman's fertility and has little impact, if any, on the course and outcome of pregnancy. In a large review, Tillman[8] found that the number of pregnancies per woman was similar to a control group of healthy women. He concluded that infertility was not a feature of MS. Shapira[9] found fertility diminished by 13% but attributed that to physical disability and a prevailing view by physicians that women with MS should not have children, a view also shared by other investigators.[10]

Similarly, MS has little if any effect on the course of pregnancy, labor, or delivery. Tillman[8] followed 70 pregnant MS patients and found that MS did not change the course of pregnancy, labor, or delivery. Although there was an increased rate of elective surgical abortions, Tillman was unable to identify evidence for a "fetal lethal factor" associated with MS. In 36 pregnant MS patients reviewed by Sweeney,[11] the only obstetric complications were two cases of mild vomiting. Subsequent studies similarly found no increase in spontaneous abortions, complications of pregnancy or delivery, malformations, or stillbirths.[12] Thus, MS does not appear to be associated with increased spontaneous abortions, fetal malformations, or labor complications.

Pregnancy Does Not Cause Multiple Sclerosis: There is no current evidence to support the hypothesis that pregnancy causes MS, although some authors have suggested that pregnancy could "precipitate" the onset of MS.[13] Tillman reviewed prevailing views in 1950[8] and cast doubt on the view that pregnancy can cause MS. Data presented by Thompson et al.[14] would seem to establish that the pregnancy months themselves are not associated with an increased risk of MS onset. Thompson et al.[14] found that of 178 women, only 10 (6%) had MS onset during pregnancy. Data presented on the number of pregnancies in the group suggest that pregnancy months accounted for approximately 10% to 15% of the total months represented in the sample. Thus, pregnancy months may have been associated with a slight decrease in MS onset compared with nonpregnancy months.

Pregnancy Transiently Suppresses Multiple Sclerosis Disease Activity: While pregnancy does not appear to precipitate MS, there is little doubt that pregnancy alters the course of MS in a predictable way. The nine gestational months, particularly the second and third trimesters, are characterized by decreased disease activity as reflected by the rate of clinical exacerbation; the rate of exacerbation in the first six months postpartum, however, is dramatically increased.[9–11,15–18] These studies (reviewed by Birk[19]) suggest that pregnancy is relatively protective for women with MS, but that the postpartum period is one of high risk for relapses or worsening disease. There is general agreement among these studies on the magnitude of the postpartum risk. Between 20% and 40% of MS patients will experience a clinical relapse or worsening of the disease during the 3 months following delivery.

Why does pregnancy reduce MS disease activity? Tissue damage in MS is thought to be caused at least in part by autoreactive antibodies and cells that gain access to the central nervous system. This is the rationale for the various immunosuppressive strategies that have been used in an attempt to treat the disease. The apparent benefit from intensive immune suppression with cyclophosphamide[20] or total lymphoid irradiation[21] and the deleterious effect of gamma interferon[22] support the hypothesis that MS is caused by an autoimmune attack on CNS myelin.

The suppressive effect of pregnancy on MS disease activity further supports our concept of MS as an autoimmune disease. Pregnancy apparently is a state of immunosuppression [23–26] that presumably allows the fetus to survive as an allograft, despite paternal histocompatibility antigens immunologically foreign to the mother. Probably as a consequence of pregnancy-associated immunosuppression, pregnant women have increased susceptibility to viral illnesses, decreased responses to intradermal purified protein derivative (PPD) injection, and increased survival time of skin grafts. Several putative autoimmune diseases in addition to MS improve during gestation and worsen postpartum, including rheumatoid arthritis, autoimmune thyroiditis, and systemic lupus erythematosus.

The mechanisms of immunosuppression of pregnancy have received considerable attention. Cellular immune responses are diminished,[27,28] while humoral immune responses to exogenous antigens and to fetal proteins remain intact.[29] Plasma and amniotic fluid from pregnant women suppress lymphocyte and antibody responses to mitogens and antigens.[30] The placenta and fetus produce pregnancy-specific proteins that have immunosuppressive activity, including fetal α-fetoprotein (AFP), human chorionic gonadotropin (HCG), human placental lactogen (HPL), progesterone, and estrogen. Maternal factors include increased synthesis of adrenal corticosteroids and a number of pregnancy-associated plasma proteins, including pregnancy-associated plasma protein A (PAPP A) and pregnancy-associated α-glycoprotein (PAG), both large molecular weight substances with potent immunosuppressive properties. The specific effects of these soluble factors as they relate to MS have been reviewed.[19]

Pregnancy also clearly ameliorates the severity of experimental allergic encephalomyelitis (EAE), an animal model of multiple sclerosis. Autoimmune inflammatory demyelination can be induced by inoculating animals with brain or spinal cord or with encephalitogenic regions of myelin basic protein or proteolipid protein, the major protein constituents of myelin. The severity and course of EAE are clearly influenced by pregnancy or certain hormones. Experimental allergic encephalomyelitis was more difficult to induce and was less severe in animals that were pregnant at the time of immunization with encephalitogenic protein.[31,32] Abramsky et al.[33] demonstrated a beneficial effect of AFP on the course of EAE in guinea pigs, possibly due to an immunosuppressive effect of AFP. Arnason and Richman[34] found that oral contraceptives, particularly those high in estrogens, inhibited EAE in rats. Greig[35] found that melengestrol acetate, a progestational agent with some glucocorticoid activity, prevented EAE in rats when given after sensitization and was capable of reversing established disease. Melengestrol acetate was accompanied by fewer side effects and had a better therapeutic ratio than did hydrocortisone acetate. Thus, both pregnancy and exogenous pregnancy-associated hormones can prevent or ameliorate autoimmune encephalomyelitis.

<u>Does Pregnancy Alter the Ultimate Disability of a Woman with</u>

MS? Studies to date do not definitively clarify the effect of pregnancy on the ultimate course or extent of disability in MS, although there appears to be no obvious substantial deleterious effect associated with one or more pregnancies. The lack of definitive information on this question should not be surprising. It is notoriously difficult to determine the effect of a therapeutic intervention on the course of MS. For that purpose, one must select a large and homogeneous group of MS patients, randomize them to two or more interventions, and follow their course without knowledge of the intervention. Such a design to determine the effect of pregnancy on MS is obviously not possible or desirable.

Consequently there are only three studies with any significant data beyond anecdotes and opinion that bear on the question. Poser[10] reviewed gestational histories on 512 women with MS, reporting that pregnancy was not apparently associated with an increased rate of disease progression. Similarly, Thompson et al.[14] found no relationship between the number of pregnancies and the subsequent level of disability. Both Poser[10] and Thompson et al.[14] suggested that pregnancy or the number of pregnancies had no effect on subsequent disability. The data in these studies do not permit a definitive conclusion, however, because there may have been selection biases unavoidable in the sample. For example, women with more severe disability may have elected fewer pregnancies. Birk et al.[18] presented data suggesting that the pregnancy year may be associated with increasing disability. Eight women with MS were followed prospectively through pregnancy. Each was systematically examined twice during pregnancy and twice during the 6 months postpartum. Six of the eight women experienced postpartum relapses, mostly consisting of mild symptom flares; disability status scores increased between 35 weeks gestation and 6-months postpartum in 6 of the 8 women. Mean Kurtzke expanded disability scores[36] (EDSS) increased from 2.4 at 35-weeks gestation to 3.4 at 6-months postpartum. The number of patients was small and the duration of follow-up too short to draw definite conclusions related to the effect of pregnancy on disability, but the average increase EDSS noted would seem unlikely to have occurred due to the natural history of MS.[37,38] Thus, while pregnancy or the number of pregnancies does not appear to have a dramatic or predictable effect on worsening disease, the exact effect of pregnancy on the ultimate course of MS remains unclear.

Susceptibility to Multiple Sclerosis is Inherited But the Risk of

Transmission is Low: There is clearly a genetically determined susceptibility to MS. Multiple sclerosis is not transmitted by a single gene. The susceptibility to develop MS is probably determined by multiple genes. In most temperate zones, an individual's lifetime risk for developing MS is about 0.1% (1 in 1,000). The importance of genetic factors is evident when one considers that the lifetime risk increases 400-fold to 40% if an identical twin has MS. The lifetime risk of developing MS for a child of an MS patient has been estimated as approximately 3%,[39] a 30-fold increase over the baseline risk. The risk of transmission from father to offspring appears to be considerably lower than the risk from mother to offspring.[40] The nature of MS susceptibility genes is currently under investigation; there are no gene markers that can be used at present for genetic counseling or prenatal diagnosis.

Reproductive Counseling (Table II)

Women with MS bring many issues related to pregnancy to their neurologist, obstetrician, internist, or family physician. In many cases

---

Table II.
Major Issues Raised by Women With Multiple Sclerosis
Contemplating Pregnancy (See text for discussion)

Issues Related to Whether to Have a Baby
Will pregnancy make my MS symptoms worse?
Can I decrease the risk of postpartum relapse?
Will my ultimate disability be worse as a result of pregnancy?
Will I pass MS on to my children?
Should I have a baby?
Issues Related to Pregnancy
Will MS affect the management of my pregnancy?
Will termination of pregnancy affect my disease?
Will MS affect my delivery?
What anesthetics are safe during labor or cesarean section?
Can I breastfeed with MS?
Which drugs are safe during pregnancy or during breastfeeding?
Should my MS treatments be altered?

---

the answers are clearly supported based on the studies reviewed above. In other instances, there are incomplete data to allow a definite recommendation. The following positions represent the authors'approach to many of these questions and have been published previously.[19,41]

Will Pregnancy Make My MS Symptoms Worse? Retrospective work reviewed above suggests increased risk of a flare in disease activity for 6-months postpartum. The risk of such a flare appears to be about two to three times the expected relapse rate. In the individual patient, the risk for a postpartum exacerbation is probably 20% to 40%. Pregnant women with MS need to know about the increased risk so that they plan their postpartum period appropriately. There should be a plan for adequate help in the home to assist with infant care and nighttime feedings. Women with MS should plan to take 3-months maternity leave from work if possible.

Can I Decrease the Risk of Postpartum Relapse? There are no measures that have been shown to decrease the risk of postpartum relapse. However, adequate rest and alleviation of stress in the post-partum period seems prudent and may diminish the frequency or severity of attacks.

Will My Ultimate Disability be Worse as a Result of Pregnancy? Current knowledge supports the notion that pregnancy does not alter the overall course of MS, including long-term disability. One must exercise caution in rendering this opinion, however, since prior studies are inconclusive on this point. Most investigators have found no difference in overall disability related to the number of pregnancies, but there may be important selection factors that bias these studies.

Will I Pass MS on to My Children? There does seem to be some increased risk of MS in offspring of mothers or fathers with MS. For example, Sadovnick[28] found a 3% lifetime risk of developing MS for a child born to a parent with MS, compared to a 0.1% risk for the general population in British Columbia. Genetic counseling on this issue may be useful for couples. It is important to inform the patient about the increased risk of MS in offspring, but equally important to stress that the actual risk of transmission is small.

Should I Have A Baby? This is often the ultimate question faced by women with MS contemplating a family. In general, the decision to have a baby should be based on a range of personal, family, and economic issues, among which is the presence of MS. Rarely should the decision be based exclusively on the presence of MS. We recommend that physicians support a couple's decision to have a baby in the face of MS, particularly if physical impairment is minimal or moderate and the couple is committed to the plan. The couple needs information about the effect of pregnancy on the course of MS and needs information about the genetic susceptibility to MS. Individuals vary, however, in how they respond to the same information. The physician should take an educational, supportive, and optimistic role in helping a couple with the decision to have a baby.

Pregnancy Counseling (Table II)

Will MS Affect the Managment of My Pregnancy? Once pregnant, a woman with MS should have routine prenatal care. Prenatal iron should be taken to avoid anemia. A high index of suspicion for and prompt treatment of urinary tract infections is vital. Multiple sclerosis and pregnancy are both associated with increased urinary tract infections and pyelonephritis is an extremely serious complication during pregnancy. Therefore, prophylaxis with nitrofurantoin or ampicillin should be considered for the patient with a history of recurrent urinary tract infections or if intermittent catheterization is required. Nitrofurantoin has a broader spectrum of activity than ampicillin, but has been associated with peripheral neuropathy. It should be discontinued postpartum if used during pregnancy.

Multiple sclerosis is not associated with increased complications of pregnancy. Complications, should they arise, should be treated routinely, including the use of sympathomimetics for preterm labor or magnesium sulfate for pregnancy-induced hypertension. Multiple sclerosis is not associated with increased congenital malformations or with poor fetal outcome.

Gynecologic care for women with MS does not differ significantly from routine practice with a few exceptions relating to drugs commonly used in the MS population. A proper decision about an appropriate method for contraception should consider concurrent medications. Many antibiotics decrease the effectiveness of oral contraceptives by changing the enterohepatic circulation. Birth control pills are also less effective when used with medications that induce hepatic enzymes, including phenytoin, barbiturates, and hypnotics. Immunosuppression may increase the risk of pelvic infection related to an intrauterine device. Given these problems, barrier contraception should be considered as an alternative for women with MS when antibiotic or immunosuppressive medication is used. For women with occasional antibiotics use, an oral contraceptive with 50 μm of estrogen rather than the lower dose pills may be prescribed. During the time of antibiotic or immunosuppressant drug use, another method of birth control should supplement the pill.

A second concern is the relationship of cervical dysplasia and neoplasia to any immunosuppressive drug[42,43] including azathioprine. Any women being treated with immunosuppressive medications should have a gynecologic examination, including a breast examination and a pap smear, every 6 months or at a minimum yearly. Women with a history of genital condylomata (or papilloma virus) are particularly at risk. Very careful consideration should be given to the gynecologic history, with particular attention to abnormal pap smears or a history of condylomata prior to starting such therapy.

Will Termination of Pregnancy Affect My Disease? Pregnant MS patients should not terminate their pregnancies solely because of their MS. There is some risk of exacerbation following termination of pregnancy at any time during gestation.

Will MS Affect My Delivery? Labor management should be routine. Analgesia with parenteral narcotics should be used as needed. There is no evidence that MS patients would benefit from shortening the second stage of labor. Maternal exhaustion may necessitate the use of instruments to assist vaginal delivery in some cases. One needs to consider the need for steroid coverage during labor and delivery in patients who have taken more than 10–20 mg of prednisone for more than 2 weeks in the preceding year. A number of regimens have been used when there is concern for possible adrenal insufficiency. A simple and commonly recommended course is 100 mg of hydrocortisone intramuscularly upon admission to the labor room, followed by 100 mg of hydrocortisone intramuscularly every 8 hours for 24 hours or until complications are not anticipated.

What Anesthetics are Safe During Labor or Cesarean Section? Cesarean section should be used only for the usual obstetric indications. There are fewer options for anesthesia for labor analgesia or cesarean section for MS patients than the general population.[44] Epidural anesthesia during labor is becoming increasing popular, although there are few reports of epidural regional anesthesia in MS patients.[45] Precluding incidental lumbar puncture, epidural anesthesia is thought to be safer than spinal anesthesia. Spinal anesthesia has traditionally been avoided in MS patients because of the high incidence of relapse in the postpartum period, although it is not known to change the frequency or severity of postpartum exacerbation. The relative safety of spinal or epidural anesthesia compared with general anesthesia is unknown.

Can I Breastfeed with MS? Multiple sclerosis doesn't affect a woman's ability to breastfeed. While many women believe that breastfeeding can prevent postpartum exacerbations,[46] this belief is not supported by data. Nelson et al.[47] reported that breastfeeding was not associated with any change in the likelihood, timing, or severity of postpartum exacerbations. We routinely encourage breastfeeding by women with MS who wish to do so. To avoid exhaustion, however, a schedule to accommodate a full night of sleep can be achieved by augmenting nursing with formula or with pumped, refrigerated breast milk fed to the infant by a helper.

Which Drugs are Safe During Pregnancy or During Breastfeeding? Teratogenic potential of many drugs in humans is uncertain or is only presumed based on case reports or animal studies. In general, treatment regimens should be reviewed and drugs eliminated when possible prior to conception.[48–54]

Prednisone and ACTH are both commonly used to treat MS exacerbations. Both drugs should be avoided if possible. The risk of teratogenicity or virilization of female fetuses is highest in the first trimester, while the risk of fetal adrenal suppression is greatest with high doses of corticosteroids late in gestation. Limited data show no teratogenic effects of ACTH. ACTH should be avoided in the first trimester when its use may stimulate androgen production by maternal adrenal glands and result in virilization of female fetuses. Studies in rodents showed prednisone to be associated with an increased rate of spontaneous abortions, placental insufficiency, and cleft palate. These effects, however, have not been confirmed in humans. Antenatal steroids, commonly betamethasone, are used to enhance fetal lung maturity when preterm delivery is threatened and postnatal studies on the infants have shown no adverse effects. Studies in women with various autoimmune diseases, particularly SLE and in renal transplant patients, have failed to demonstrate any adverse effects of prednisone, other than neonatal adrenal suppression. If steroids are considered absolutely necessary for treating MS during pregnancy, we would recommend using as low a dose of prednisone as possible to stabilize symptoms. We commonly use 30 mg qAM for 7 days for this purpose.

Less information is available for immunosuppressive or cytotoxic drugs. Azathioprine and cyclophosphamide are classified as Category D risks, meaning that there is evidence of fetal risk but that use in some circumstances may be acceptable despite this. Cyclophosphamide is associated with amenorrhea and azoospermia, and there is probably some risk of permanent sterility. Use of these drugs during pregnancy has usually been associated with a good outcome, but fetal malformations have been reported. For example, a number of pregnancies have been reported in women with SLE or following renal transplants who took azathioprine, often in association with prednisone. In the largest study, 4 of 44 liveborn infants had major congenital anomalies, 23% of the infants were born prematurely and 24% had low birth weights when born at term.[54] Amniocentesis and fetal ultrasound may play a role in assessing fetal development when pregnancy occurs in women treated with these drugs.

The use of diazepam, phenytoin and carbamazepine should be avoided, if possible, particularly in the first trimester. All three drugs have been implicated in fetal malformations in some pregnancies.

A few studies have been done documenting the presence of prednisone in breast milk after small doses (5–10 mg).[49] No studies are available on significantly higher doses that may be used in MS relapses. Infants that have been followed after chronic exposure in mothers taking low doses of steroids have shown no adverse effects but little data is available. Renal transplant patients taking azathioprine, known to be excreted in breast milk as 6-mercaptopurine, have breastfed with no apparent adverse outcomes. We advise against breastfeeding when immunosuppressive drugs are used, because of concerns over neonatal bone marrow suppression and other adverse effects of corticosteroids. Similarly, the use of diazepam by nursing mothers should be avoided, due to the possible side effects of infant lethargy, hypoventilation, and weight loss. If the use of diazepam is necessary, we recommend against breastfeeding.

<u>Should My MS Treatments Be Altered?</u> There is no reason to change routine management for MS. For example, physical therapy programs for improving balance, strength, endurance, or for decreasing spasticity should be continued.

References

1. Poser CM, Paty DW, Scheinberg L, et al: New diagnostic criteria for multiple sclerosis. *Ann Neurol* 13:227–231, 1983.
2. Chiappa KH: Pattern-shift visual, brainstem auditory and short-latency somatosensory evoked potentials in multiple sclerosis. *Ann NY Acad Sci* 436:315–326, 1984.
3. Johnson KP, Nelson BJ: Multiple sclerosis: diagnostic usefulness of cerebrospinal fluid. *Ann Neurol* 2:425–431, 1977.
4. Tourtellotte WW, Potvin AR, Fleming JO, et al: Multiple sclerosis: measurement and validation of central nervous system IgG synthesis rate. *Neurology* 30:240–244, 1980.
5. Rudick RA, French CA, Breton D, et al: Relative diagnostic value of cerebrospinal fluid kappa chains in MS. *Neurology* 39:964–968, 1989.
6. Kurtzke JF: MS from an epidemiological view-point. In *MS: A Critical Perspectus*. Edited by EJ Field. Lancaster, PA. MTP Press, 1977.
7. Rudick RA, Schiffer RB, Herndon RM: Drug treatment of multiple sclerosis. *Semin Neurol* 7:150–159, 1987.
8. Tillman A: The effect of pregnancy on multiple sclerosis and its management. *Res Publ Ass Res Nerv Ment Dis* 28:548–582, 1950.
9. Shapira K, Poskanzer DC, Newell DJ, et al: Marriage, pregnancy and multiple sclerosis. *Brain* 89:419–428, 1966.
10. Poser S, Poser W: Multiple sclerosis and gestation. *Neurology* 33:1422–1427, 1983.
11. Sweeney WJ: Pregnancy and multiple sclerosis. *Am J Obstet Gynecol* 66:124–130, 1955.
12. Sadovnick AD, Baird PA: Reproductive counselling for multiple sclerosis patients. *Am J Med Genetics* 20:349–354, 1985.
13. Leibowitz U, Antonovsky A, Kats R, et al: Does pregnancy increase the risk of multiple sclerosis? *J Neurol Neurosurg Psych* 30:354–357, 1967.
14. Thompson DS, Nelson LM, Burns A, et al: The effects of pregnancy in multiple sclerosis: a retrospective study. *Neurology* 36:1097–1099, 1986.
15. Miller JHD, Allison RS, Cheeseman EA, et al: Pregnancy as a factor influencing relapse in disseminated sclerosis. *Brain* 82:417–426, 1959.
16. Ghezzi A, Caputo D: Pregnancy: a factor influencing the course of multiple sclerosis? *Eur Neurol* 20:517–519, 1981.
17. Korn-Lubetzki I, Kahana E, Cooper G, et al: Activity of multiple sclerosis during pregnancy and puerperium. *Ann Neurol* 16:229–231, 1984.
18. Birk K, Ford C, Smeltzer S, et al: The clinical course of multiple sclerosis during pregnancy and the puerperium. *Arch Neurol* 47:738–742, 1990.
19. Birk K, Rudick R: Pregnancy and multiple sclerosis. *Arch Neurol* 43:719–726, 1986.
20. Hauser, SL, Dawson DM, Lehrich JR, et al: Intensive immunosuppression in progressive multiple sclerosis. A randomized, three-arm study of high-dose intravenous cyclophosphamide, plasma exchange, and ACTH. *N Engl J Med* 308:173–180, 1983.

21. Cook SD, Troiano R, Zito G, et al: Effect of total lymphoid irradiation in chronic progressive multiple sclerosis. *Lancet* i:1405–1409, 1986.
22. Panitch HS, Hirsch RL, Schindler J, et al: Treatment of multiple sclerosis with gamma interferon: exacerbations associated with activation of the immune system. *Neurology* 37:1097–1102, 1987.
23. Gall S: Maternal adjustments in the immune system in normal pregnancy. *Clin Obstet Gynecol* 26(3):521–536, 1983.
24. Weinberg E: Pregnancy-associated depression of cell-mediated immunity. *Rev Infect Dis* 6(6):814–831, 1984.
25. Rocklin RE, Kitzmiller JL, Kaye MD: Immunobiology of the maternal-fetal relationship. *Ann Rev Med* 30:375–404, 1979.
26. Adelsberg BR: Immunology of pregnancy. *Mt. Sinai J Med* 52:5–10, 1985.
27. Wegmann T, Gill T: *Immunology of Reproduction*. New York, NY. Oxford University Press. 1983, pp. 365–380.
28. Stahn R, Fabricius HA, Hartleitner W: Suppression of human T-cell colony formation during pregnancy. *Nature* 276:831–832, 1978.
29. Maroulis GB, Buckley RH, Younger JB: Serum immunoglobulin levels during normal pregnancy. *Am J Obstet Gynecol* 109:971–976, 1971.
30. Hogarth PJ: *Immunological Aspects of Mammalian Reproduction*. Glasgow, Blackie. 1982, pp. 83–449.
31. Evron S, Brenner T, Abramsky O: Suppressive effect of pregnancy on the development of experimental allergic encephalomyelitis in rabbits. *Am J Reprod Immunol* 5:109–113, 1984.
32. Abramsky O, Lubetzki-Korn I, Evron S, et al: Suppressive effect of pregnancy on MS and EAE. *Prog Clin Biol Res* 146:399–406, 1984.
33. Abramsky O, Brenner T, Mizrachi R, et al: Alpha-fetoprotein suppresses experimental allergic encephalomyelitis. *J Neuroimmunol* 2:1–7, 1982.
34. Arnason BG, Richman DP: Effect of oral contraceptives on experimental demyelinating disease. *Arch Neurol* 21:103–108, 1969.
35. Greig ME, Gibbons AJ, Elliott GA: A comparison of the effects of melengestrol acetate and hydrocortisone acetate on experimental allergic encephalomyelitis in rats. *J Pharm Exp Ther* 173(1):85–93, 1970.
36. Kurtzke JF: Rating neurologic impairment in multiple sclerosis: an expanded disability status scale (EDSS). *Neurology* 33:1444–1452, 1983.
37. Bornstein, MB, Miller A, Slagle S, et al: A pilot trial of COP 1 in exacerbating-remitting multiple sclerosis. *N Engl J Med* 317:408–414, 1987.
38. Weinshenker BG, Bass B, Rice GPA, et al: The natural history of multiple sclerosis: a geographically based study. 1. Clinical course and disability. *Brain* 112:133–146, 1989.
39. Sadovnick AD: Empiric recurrence risks for use in the genetic counselling of multiple sclerosis patients. *Am J Med Genet* 17:713–714, 1984.
40. Sadovnick AD, Baird PA, Ward RH: Multiple sclerosis: updated risks for relatives. *Am J Med Genet* 29(3):533–541, 1988.
41. Birk KA, Rudick RA: Caring for the obstetric patient with multiple sclerosis. *Contemp Obstet Gynecol* 1989.
42. Sillman F, Stanek A, Sedlis A, et al: The relationship between human papillomavirus and lower genital intraepithelial neoplasia in immunosuppressed women. *Am J Obstet Gynecol* 150:300–308, 1984.

43. Schneider V, Kay S, Lee HM: Immunosuppression as a high-risk factor in the development of condyloma acuminatum and squamous neoplasia of the cervix. *Acta Cytologica* 27(3):220–224, 1983.
44. Bamford C, Sibley W, Laguna J: Anesthesia in multiple sclerosis. *Can J Neurol Sci* 5(1):41–44, 1978.
45. Warren TM, Datta S, Ostheimer GW: Lumbar epidural anesthesia in a patient with multiple sclerosis. *Anesth Analg* 61(12):1022–1023, 1982.
46. Smeltzer S. Personal communication.
47. Nelson LM, Franklin GM, Jones, MC, et al: Risk of multiple sclerosis exacerbation during pregnancy and breast-feeding. *JAMA* 259:3441–3443, 1988.
48. Stern L: *Drug Use In Pregnancy.* ADIS Health Sci Press (Aust), 1984.
49. Briggs GG, Bodendorger TW, et al: *Drugs in Pregnancy and Lactation.* Baltimore, MD. Williams and Wilkins. 1983.
50. Lawrence RA. *Breast Feeding—A Guide for the Medical Profession.* Second Edition. St. Louis, MO. CV Mosby Co., 1985.
51. IARC Working Group: Antineoplastic and immunosuppressive agents: azathioprine. *IARC Monographs: Evaluation of Carcinogenic Risk* 26:47–78, 1981.
52. Symington GR, Mackay IR, Lambert RP: Cancer and teratogenesis: infrequent occurrence after medical use of immunosuppressive drugs. *Aust NZ J Med* 7:368–372, 1977.
53. Sieber SM, Adamson H: Toxicity of antineoplastic agents in man: chromosomal aberrations, antifertility effects, congenital malformations, and carcinogenic potential. *Adv Ca Res* 22:57–155, 1975.
54. Penn I, Makowski EL, Harris P: Parenthood following renal transplantation. *Kidney Int* 18:221–233, 1980.

8

Movement Disorders in Pregnancy

Christopher F. O'Brien, M.D.
Roger Kurlan, M.D.

Introduction

The relationship between movement disorders and pregnancy has three levels of importance. Most fundamental is the impact of a particular disorder on the health of the mother and child. This encompasses both the influence of the pregnancy on the movement disorder and the effect of the disorder and its treatment on the pregnancy. Secondly, the onset of a movement disorder during pregnancy poses special issues regarding differential diagnosis, evaluation, and treatment. Finally, insight into pathogenetic mechanisms for movement disorders may be gained in the setting of the complex physiological changes of pregnancy. Progestational and estrogenic hormones have documented influence on central neuronal systems, including effects on membrane activity[1] and dopamine receptor function.[2,3] Amphetamine or apomorphine-induced stereotyped behavior in rats, which reflects central dopamine activity, is significantly reduced following oophorectomy. Postoophorectomy treatment with estradiol valerate or progesterone will eliminate this reduction. These observations suggest that these hormonal compounds directly increase dopamine receptor sensitivity.[2,3] Increased receptor numbers

From Goldstein PJ, Stern BJ, (eds): *Neurological Disorders of Pregnancy. Second Revised Edition.* Mount Kisco NY, Futura Publishing Co., Inc., © 1992.
Supported by a Veola S. Kerr Fellowship of the Parkinson's Disease Foundation, New York.

have also been demonstrated after estrogen treatment in rat striatum.[4] We will attempt to address each of the three aforementioned areas in relationship to specific movement disorders occurring during pregnancy.

Chorea

Chorea, from the Latin word *chorus* (to dance), consists of brief, arrhythmic, involuntary dance-like movements. This hyperkinetic activity may affect small muscles around the face and mouth, the extremities, or trunk. When interwoven with normal actions chorea may take on a semipurposeful character.

Historically, the term "chorea gravidarum" has been used for chorea with onset during pregnancy and with an association with rheumatic fever. We now know, however, that chorea in the setting of pregnancy can have multiple etiologies with differing treatments and prognoses. Table I lists the general approach to differential diagnosis.

Chorea and Infection

The most common form of infectious chorea is Sydenham's, a manifestation of rheumatic fever. The involuntary movements appear

---

Table I.
Approach to Differential Diagnosis of Chorea in Pregnancy

1. Prior episodes of chorea (with or without pregnancy)?
2. Family history of chorea?
3. Prior rheumatic fever?
4. Drug or toxin exposure?
5. Associated neurological signs?
6. Presence of systemic disease?
7. Classify:
   Infectious
   Genetic
   Immune mediated
   Cerebrovascular
   Toxic/metabolic
   Other

weeks to months after group A streptococcal infection of the pharynx. It does not occur after streptococcal infection of the skin. An elevated antistreptolysin O titer (ASO) remains the best diagnostic test, although it is not specific because individual titers may be increased in populations with a high prevalence of streptococcal infection. Furthermore, the ASO titer declines if the interval between infection and rheumatic fever is greater than 2 months. Anti-DNAse-B titers may remain elevated up to 1 year after pharyngitis. Throat cultures are not adequate to document rheumatic chorea because normal individuals may harbor the organism and true cases of Sydenham's chorea may have cleared the antecedent infection.

An alteration in sensorium may be observed in patients with Sydenham's chorea. Lethargy, confusion, or coma may coincide with the movement disorder and resolve with the disappearance of the movements. No specific abnormalities are generally found with neuroimaging or following lumbar puncture. Electroencephalography (EEG) may show generalized slowing but no focal changes or epileptic discharges.

Immune-mediated mechanisms appear to underlie the development of chorea in the setting of rheumatic fever. Antibodies to neuronal cytoplasm antigens in the caudate and subthalamic nuclei have been demonstrated in patients with rheumatic fever. These antibodies cross react with group A streptococcal membranes.[5] Several lines of evidence suggest that susceptibility to rheumatic fever and chorea after streptococcal infection is due to HLA-linked antigen expression.[6] This would place specific individuals at risk for chorea in the setting of rheumatic fever though it remains unknown why pregnancy is associated with the later emergence of this immune-mediated syndrome as chorea gravidarum. Symptom precipitation may occur in susceptible women with the influence of estrogen and progestational hormones.

Wilson and Preece[7] undertook the earliest comprehensive review of chorea gravidarum in 1932, and concluded that "chorea occurring during pregnancy is identically the same disease as Sydenham's chorea in adolescence, modified slightly, in certain respects, by its association with pregnancy". This view is still held today. While the incidence at that time was close to 1:3,500 pregnancies, the decline in rheumatic fever cases correlates strongly with a dramatic decrease in chorea gravidarum over the past 50 years. While the true incidence is difficult to ascertain, an estimate of 1:139,000 was reported in 1968.[8]

Prompt treatment of streptococcal pharyngitis with penicillin has markedly reduced the incidence of rheumatic fever and its sequelae of carditis, valvular heart disease, arthritis, and Sydenham's chorea.

Wilson and Preece reported 253 choreic pregnancies in 99 patients without evidence of acute streptococcal infection. A history of rheumatic fever with chorea was present in over one third of the women and over one half reported prior episodes of chorea. Of those patients that came to autopsy, carditis was found in 87%. Recent reports of multiple choreic pregnancies demonstrate underlying susceptibility without evidence of recurrent streptococcal infection.[9,10]

Haloperidol (0.5–15 mg/day),[11] tetrabenazine,[12] and sodium valproate[13] have been used effectively as antichoreic agents. The neuroleptic drug haloperidol, which blocks dopamine receptors, is generally free of embryotoxicity if its use is restricted to the second and third trimesters. Fetal limb deformity has been reported with the use of haloperidol during the limb genesis period of the first trimester,[14,15] although sufficient evidence to prove cause and effect is lacking. Tetrabenazine, a drug that depletes presynaptic stores of dopamine and has receptor dopamine blocking effects, has been used to suppress chorea during pregnancy[12] although it remains an investigational drug in the United States. While sodium valproate has been beneficial in decreasing Sydenham's chorea,[13] this medication is not used during pregnancy due to its potential embryotoxicity.[16] Unless active streptococcal infection is present, penicillin therapy is not required.

Other forms of infectious chorea are much less common. Herpes simplex encephalitis may lead to choreiform activity although seizures are more likely to accompany the illness. Table II lists other reported infectious choreas mediated by bacterial toxins, cytotoxic antibodies, immune complexes or direct cerebral invasion by the pathogen that could occur during pregnancy.[17]

Chorea and Immune Disease

The immune system is implicated in the production of chorea associated with systemic lupus erythematosus (SLE) and antiphospholipid (lupus anticoagulant) syndromes.[18-26] Neuropathological studies of cases with chorea associated with SLE have failed to consistently identify structural lesions in the basal ganglia.[27] The likely mechanism of chorea is an immune-related process, probably me-

Table II.
Infectious Choreas

Post-streptococcal (Sydenham's)
Viral encephalitis:
    Influenza
    Mumps
    Measles
    Varicella
    Human immunodeficiency virus (HIV)
    Epstein-Barr (mononucleosis)
    Cytomegalovirus
Subacute bacterial endocarditis
Neurosyphilis

diated by a variety of antistriatal antibodies that my be present, including antiphospholipid[24,26,28] and several antineuronal types.[28,29]

Antiphospholipid (including anticardiolipin and lupus anticoagulant) can be associated with SLE and related diseases, though they seem capable of producing chorea in patients without any other identifiable disease process. Systemic immune dysfunction (e.g., renal impairment, skin rash) does not appear to correlate well with the presence or severity of neurological symptoms. No specific marker of disease activity (e.g., sedimentation rate, ANA titer, or complement level) is a reliable measure of central nervous system (CNS) involvement. Patients with antiphospholipid antibodies are predisposed to cerebral infarction, a process that may contribute to the development of choreas as well.[23]

Chorea and Metabolic Disease

Disruptions of metabolic homeostasis are capable of producing chorea during pregnancy, including hypoglycemia,[30] hyperglycemia,[31] hyponatremia,[32] hypernatremia,[33] hypocalcemia,[34] hyperthyroidism,[35] hypoparathyroidism,[36] and rarely, thiamine and nicotinic acid deficiencies.[17] Hypocalcemia, hyperglycemia and thiamine deficiency are particularly associated with pregnancy. Resolution of chorea generally follows correction of the underlying disorder, although in some instances associated complications (e.g., cerebral infarction with nonketotic hyperglycemia[37] or central pontine myelinolysis with rapidly corrected hyponatremia[38]) may lead to more long-lasting symptoms.

Chorea and Cerebrovascular Disease

Chorea, and the related phenomenon of ballism (high-amplitude chorea involving more proximal limb musculature), is occasionally associated with cerebrovascular disease.[39] As the risk of cerebral infarction increases during pregnancy, the clinician may need to investigate the heart, the clotting system, or the cerebral circulation for patients presenting with chorea. In general, large vessel occlusions rarely produce chorea; small vessel involvement with infarction of the posterior thalamus, basal ganglia, or the subthalamic nuclei is more likely in this setting. Clues that chorea is due to cerebral infarction include abrupt onset, presence of other deficits or signs on examination, a unilateral (i.e., hemichorea) pattern, and associated headache. Appropriate investigations and treatment approaches have been outlined in Chapter 4. Special consideration should be given to cerebrovascular complications of autoimmune disease as treatment of the underlying illness may reduce fetal and maternal mortality.[12]

Drug- and Toxin-Induced Chorea

A wide array of medications may produce chorea (Table III).[17] Most common are neuroleptics, anticonvulsants, antiparkinsonian agents, and hormonal preparations. Discontinuation of the offending drug usually results in improvement or resolution of the movement disorder. Drug-induced chorea, such as occurs with oral contraceptives,[40] is likely related to alterations in dopamine receptor sensitivity or number. Tardive dyskinesia, the development of involuntary movements (typically chorea) during long-term treatment with neuroleptic drugs is likely due to dopamine receptor up-regulation that occurs in response to chronic drug-induced receptor blockade. Involuntary movements may also appear immediately following discontinuation or dosage reduction of such drugs (withdrawal emergent syndrome).[41] The newborn is not free of such risk either. Infants have

Table III.
Drug-Induced Chorea

Neuroleptics	Lithium
Levodopa	Methadone
Bromocriptine	Metoclopramide
Pergolide	Methylphenidate
Amphetamines	Phenytoin
Theophylline	Carbamazepine
Caffeine	Anticholinergics
Oral contraceptives	Antihistamines
Tricyclic antidepressants	Cocaine

had transient involuntary movements following birth to mothers treated with neuroleptics.[42] In addition to antipsychotics, other drugs that block dopamine receptors, such as metoclopramide (Reglan® [A.H. Robbins, Richmond, VA, USA]) or prochlorperazine (Compazine® [Smith, Kline & French, Philadelphia, PA, USA]) may lead to tardive dyskinesia and other movement disorders. Tardive dyskinesia is best treated by withdrawing the offending agent if possible.

Drugs such as cocaine and its increasingly common potent derivative "crack", amphetamines, alcohol, and methadone can produce chorea.[17] Moreover, cocaine, amphetamines, and alcohol may also lead to cerebral infarction or hemorrhage as other potential etiologies for chorea.

Genetic Choreas

Heredofamilial choreas may emerge during the gravid state. Huntington's disease is an autosomal dominant disorder with an age at onset that typically corresponds to the reproductive years. Characteristic features include psychiatric dysfunction (depression, personality change), dementia, and chorea. Diagnosis is based on identifying a family history for the disorder. The identification of a genetic marker closely linked to the gene for Huntington's chorea on chromosome 4 has led to the availability of accurate and reliable genetic testing for the illness. With up to about 95% certainty, one can determine whether or not a fetus, or an adult contemplating pregnancy,[43] carries the disease gene. A sufficient number of relatives must be available to allow accurate genetic characterization. The psychosocial issues related to such genetic testing are complex and referral to experienced centers is recommended.

Neuroacanthocytosis is a hereditary syndrome characterized by involuntary movements (chorea and tics), peripheral neuropathy, and circulating acanthocytes.[44]. Muscle atrophy, parkinsonism, pes cavus, and seizures may also occur. Autosomal recessive inheritance is most common although sporadic and autosomal dominant patterns have been described.[45] Treatment of the involuntary movements associated with neuroacanthocytosis has been strikingly unsatisfying to this point so that the use of potentially toxic antichoreic drugs does not seem warranted during pregnancy.

Tics and Tourette's Syndrome

Tourette's syndrome is defined as the presence of multiple motor tics and one or more vocal tics for at least 1 year.[46] Motor tics are brief involuntary movements, such as eyeblinking or head jerks, and vocal (or phonic) tics are involuntary sounds, such as throat clearing or grunting. Tics occur from a background normal activity and are often voluntarily suppressible for brief periods. Current evidence suggests that tics are related to dopamine receptor supersensitivity as evidenced by the tic suppressing effects of dopamine antagonists (e.g., haloperidol) and tic worsening effect of dopaminergic agents (e.g., amphetamines). It is now recognized that almost all cases of Tourette's syndrome occur on a hereditary basis with an autosomal dominant pattern of transmission. Behavioral abnormalities, including obsessive compulsive symptoms and attentional difficulties, are frequently associated with tics.

Tourette's syndrome has an onset before age 21 years and is generally a chronic, lifelong condition. Very little information is available in the literature regarding pregnancy in Tourette's syndrome despite the overlapping ages of peak incidence. It has been our experience that tic disorders are frequently unrecognized. Waxing and waning of the severity of tics is the rule in Tourette's syndrome and worsening during pregnancy has been observed, though not predictably. The influence of estrogens on dopamine receptor sensitivity may underlie the effects of pregnancy on this disorder. Premenstrual intensification of Tourette's syndrome has been reported with beneficial response following conjugated estrogens as adjunct treatment.[47] The mainstay of therapy for disabling tics is the dopamine receptor blocking drug haloperidol. Use of this agent should be restricted to the second and third trimesters due to potential embryotoxicity as discussed above. Newer therapies such as pimozide and clonidine have not been evaluated in pregnancy.

Tremor

Tremor is a rhythmic, involuntary oscillation of part of the body. In the setting of pregnancy, four varieties of action tremor are likely to be encountered. Action tremor occurs during intended voluntary activities of the hands and differs from tremor at rest that is characteristic of Parkinson's disease (see below).

Accentuated physiological tremor is common and may arise in nearly anyone given the appropriate stress. Anxiety, fatigue, exercise, and caffeine are common factors that may exacerbate normal physiological tremor. The frequency is 10–12 Hz and the amplitude is usually small. The tremor will improve following correction of contributing factors.

Drug-induced tremor may occur with medications used during pregnancy, labor and delivery. Any sympathomimetic (e.g., epinephrine, aminophylline) or oxytocin may cause tremor. β_2-Adrenergic stimulants used to decrease uterine contractions, such as the tocolytic terbutaline, may also produce tremor. Occasionally, general anesthetics have produced rhythmic myoclonus that may resemble tremor.

Essential tremor is most often familial and has a similar appearance to physiological or drug-induced tremor. Onset is usually during adolescence or early adulthood and amplitude increases with age. The movement most often involves the distal limbs during voluntary activity. The head, face, tongue and vocal cords (essential voice tremor) may also be affected. Any condition that can accentuate physiological tremor will do the same for essential tremor. Patients often note that ingestion of 1–2 ounces of alcohol markedly suppresses the tremor, although this therapy is not recommended during pregnancy. While tremor itself has little impact on pregnancy, the condition may worsen during the gravid state. Therapy is usually not indicated unless the severity of tremor is disabling. The mainstays of medical treatment are drugs that block β-adrenergic receptors (e.g., propranolol, 60–180 mg/day) and primidone (25–250 mg q hs). Both medications have potential adverse effects on the fetus. Propranolol crosses the placenta and has caused bradycardia and hypotension in neonates.[48] Primidone's major metabolite phenobarbital has been associated with various types of birth defects when used during pregnancy (see Chapter 2). It should also be kept in mind that primidone, like phenobarbital, may decrease the effectiveness of oral contraceptives.[49]

Multiple sclerosis (MS) occurs with greatest incidence during the reproductive years. Multiple sclerosis lesions in the subcortical, brainstem, and cerebellar white matter sometime lead to a coarse intention (rubral, cerebellar outflow) tremor. Medical therapy of this type of tremor is disappointing and includes drugs not acceptable in pregnancy (e.g., isoniazid). Stereotactic lesions placed in the ventral lateral thalamus and the nucleus ventralis intermedius[50] have been beneficial in selected nonpregnant patients. The natural history of MS is quite variable, and since pregnancy and especially the postpartum period are associated with symptom fluctuations, it is difficult to predict the clinical course of tremor during this time period.

Parkinson's Disease

Although idiopathic Parkinson's disease has a mean age at onset of about 60 years, it is not uncommon to see patients present with the illness in their thirties or forties. The parkinsonian syndrome (bradykinesia, rigidity, tremor, imbalance) that occurs in association with a variety of other neurological conditions includes a broader range of ages and encompasses atypical parkinsonian variants (e.g., multisystem atrophy, striatonigral denegeration, olivopontocerebellar atrophy), drug-induced parkinsonism, postinfectious parkinsonism, post-traumatic parkinsonism, Hallervorden-Spatz disease, and other rare forms.[51]

Parkinson's disease and pregnancy do not commonly coexist, although recent estimates predict that 400 women under the age of 50 will be diagnosed with Parkinson's disease annually in the United

States.[52] Within this subgroup will be women who are pregnant or contemplating pregnancy. Golbe.[52] reported on 24 pregnancies among 18 women with Parkinson's disease. Mean age at conception was 34.7 years. There were 3 spontaneous abortions, 4 elective abortions, and 17 term pregnancies. Ten of the 17 completed pregnancies were associated with permanent worsening of Parkinson's disease symptoms but overall disability was not changed. Each of 4 women taking amantadine reported some form of complication (miscarriage, first trimester vaginal bleeding, hydatiform mole, pre-eclampsia). Although this is a small, selected series and a specific cause and effect for this medication cannot be accurately assessed, the findings do suggest that amantadine should be avoided during pregnancy. Levodopa use during pregnancy does not appear to cause problems although the total number of such treated pregnant women is small. Both decreased and increased levodopa effect has been reported during pregnancy, including worsened Parkinson's disease symptoms and heightened drug-induced involuntary movements.[52–54]

Experience with bromocriptine therapy for pregnant Parkinson's disease patients is very limited. The drug has been used during pregnancy in doses lower than that used to treat Parkinson's disease to prevent enlargement of pituitary microadenomas and hyperprolactinemia. Several hundred pregnant women have been followed on bromocriptine without reported fetal abnormalities.[55] While the impact of associated decreased amniotic fluid prolactin is unknown, no adverse effect on postnatal development has been found. Newer antiparkinsonian medications such as selegiline (deprenyl) or pergolide have not been studied with respect to pregnancy.

Postencephalitic parkinsonism, related to the epidemic of encephalitis lethargica in 1916–1926, is of historical interest. Roques[56] reported on the relationship between pregnancy and epidemic encephalitis in 1928 and his report included 200 pregnant women. Sixteen of 20 women who suffered acute encephalitis during pregnancy went on to develop parkinsonism, an increased rate compared to nonpregnant women. Exacerbation of existing parkinsonism was also common during pregnancy, especially in the first or second trimester. There were no specific complications for infants born to parkinsonian mothers. Infants born to mothers with acute encephalitis had increased mortality and epidemic encephalitis neonatorum was noted as a distinct clinical entity, with documentation of transplacental passage of the virus.

Dystonia

Dystonia refers to sustained, involuntary twisting movements. The disorder may be localized to specific body regions, such as writer's cramp, blepharospasm, or torticollis, or it may be generalized. During pregnancy, problems that may arise include acute reversible dystonia, genetic counseling for familial dystonias, and treatment issues in pregnant women with chronic dystonia.

The acute dystonias are most often drug-induced and the agents are almost invariably dopamine receptor antagonists. Many of the agents capable of producing chorea (Table II) may also produce dystonia. The pathophysiology is not well understood, although acute presynaptic dopamine receptor blockade with resultant increased postsynaptic dopamine activity has been implicated. Acute dystonic reactions can be quite terrifying for patients, but fortunately respond quickly to treatment with antihistamines (diphenhydramine; [Benadryl®; Parke Davis, Morris Plains, NJ, USA]] 25–75 mg IV/IM) or anticholinergics (benzotropine; [Cogentin®; Merck Sharp & Donne, West Point, PA, USA] 2 mg IV/IM). Acute dystonia may also occur as part of one of the paroxysmal dystonia syndromes, including kinesiogenic (movement-induced) and nonkinesiogenic types.[57,58] These disorders may be hereditary. The kinesiogenic form generally responds well to anticonvulsant drugs, although treatment should probably be delayed until after completion of the pregnancy given the potential embryotoxicity of these agents.

Most cases of childhood-onset dystonia are inherited, including dominant, recessive and sex-linked forms.[59] Considerable controversy exists regarding classification, etiology, and treatment of hereditary dystonias. The gene for autosomal dominant hereditary dystonia has been localized to chromosome 9[60] and genetic testing may become available for this disorder. No literature is available discussing pregnancy in women with familial dystonia. Perinatal injury (e.g., anoxia) may also result in dystonia that may be first encountered during adolescence or early adulthood. The mechanism for this phenomenon is unclear.

Focal dystonias (e.g., torticollis) are usually without an obvious etiology. No specific relationship to pregnancy has been reported. Women with dystonia who are planning pregnancy should be cautioned as to the relative risks of two of the most common classes of therapeutic agents: anticholinergics and benzodiazepines. Anticholinergics appear free of embryotoxicity although side effects (e.g., heat intolerance, dry mouth) may be exacerbated during pregnancy. Benzodiazepines were initially thought to increase the risk of cleft palate,[61] but subsequent controlled large scale trials have failed to document an increase in fetal abnormalities.[62] Benzodiazepine use during the third trimester can produce neonatal depression and the "floppy infant syndrome". Local intramuscular injections of botulinum toxin may become the therapy of choice for focal dystonias such as torticollis[63] and blepharospasm[64] though little information is available on this treatment approach in pregnant women. However, the rare complication of generalized weakness and the occasional appearance of botulinum toxin antibodies are reasons to avoid exposure to the toxin during pregnancy.

Wilson's Disease

Hepatolenticular degeneration (Wilson disease) is a rare disorder of copper metabolism characterized by progressive cirrhosis of the liver, neurological impairment, and Kayser-Fleischer rings in the cornea. DNA markers indicate that the genetic mutation is localized to chromosome 13.[65] Ceruloplasmin, a circulating polypeptide involved in several aspects of copper transport and metabolism, is usually low or nearly undetectable in patients with Wilson's disease. Fifty to 70% of patients initially present with neurological problems, nearly 20% to 30% with hepatic dysfunction, and the remainder with rheumatologic, ophthalmologic, hematopoietic and other problems.[66] While Kinnier-Wilson described the classic "wing beating" tremor in 1912, dysarthria and loss of coordination are the most common initial neurological manifestations. Parkinsonism, dystonia, and cognitive dysfunction occur not uncommonly. To counter the excessive accumulation of copper in brain, therapy is directed at decreasing dietary copper and increasing copper excretion. Care must be exercised as aggressive decoppering with chelating agents can be associated with worsening neurological symptoms and other organ system damage.

The use of D-penicillamine, the most commonly used chelating agent, has dramatically altered the prognosis for this disorder. Pregnancy in untreated patients had been uncommon due to dysmenorrhea with infertility and increased spontaneous abortions. However, since D-penicillamine therapy was introduced for the treatment of Wilson's disease in 1956, several reports have described successful pregnancies for patients with the illness.[67,68] Scheinberg and Sternleib[67] reviewed 29 pregnancies in 18 women with Wilson's disease who received penicillamine before or during pregnancy and found 29 normal infants resulted. Their review was prompted by a case report of a connective tissue abnormality (cutis laxa, hyperextensible skin without joint involvement) in one infant born to a mother with cystinuria who was receiving 2 g of penicillamine daily. Since that time, over 100 normal pregnancies have been reported in patients receiving the drug for Wilson's disease and other conditions.[68] However, there is emerging evidence that maternal exposure to penicillamine may indeed be embryotoxic, as cutis laxa was reported in five human births and mircrognathia with ear defects in 3 births. The observed connective tissue problem suggests that penicillamine may interfere with collagen cross linking.[69] Strikingly, cutis laxa appears to depend on continued exposure, as the abnormalities in infants tend to resolve over several weeks of life. The micrognathia and ear defects may reflect interference with normal neural crest migration in early embryogenesis. Although no specific dose relationship is appreciable, it seems prudent to use the lowest possible dose of penicillamine during pregnancy. Patients should be counseled as to the potential risks to both fetus and the mother regarding any change in therapy. Discontinuation of therapy may result in permanent neurological dysfunction, hepatitis, and rarely, death.

A newer decoppering agent, trientine (triethylene tetramine dihydrochloride; formerly Cuprid®, now Syprine® [Merck Sharp & Dohme, West Point, PA, USA]) may prove superior to penicillamine for patients with Wilson's disease. Eleven pregnancies were reported in seven Wilson's disease patients treated with trientine.[70] Eight of the nine children were normal at birth (including normal cord ceruloplasmin). One spontaneous abortion was associated with a retained IUD, one therapeutic abortion was performed, and one 31-week delivery of a female infant with isochrome X occurred. Wilson's disease symptoms were not unfavorably affected by pregnancy and no consistent effects on serum copper or ceruloplasmin were found. Trientine doses of 1–2 g/day were used. Adjunctive therapies, such as zinc supplementation, help decrease copper absorption but have not been studied in pregnant women.

Myoclonus

Myoclonic movements are rapid lightning-like involuntary jerks that are usually asynchronous and asymmetric. Amplitude may vary and movements are often stimulus (e.g., touch, sound) or action sensitive. The condition has been linked to disordered central serotonin neurotransmission. Myoclonus may be physiological (e.g., nocturnal myoclonus), inherited (e.g., hereditary essential myoclonus) and often accompanies epileptic disorders. This involuntary movement is most commonly seen in the setting of metabolic derangements, such as hypoxia and uremia, associated with encephalopathy. In the setting of pregnancy, gestational diabetes may produce hyperglycemic myoclonus. Structural brain or spinal cord lesions may also lead to myoclonus. The wide range of etiologies for myoclonus have been reviewed by Fahn et al.[71]

Treatment for myoclonus is directed at the underlying condition whenever possible. The movements can be suppressed by clonazepam and valproate, although both medications have potential embryotoxicity. Treatment with 5-hydroxytryptophan and carbidopa has been of benefit for patients with postanoxic and other forms of myoclonus but this remains an investigational form of therapy and use in pregnancy has not been evaluated.

Restless Legs Syndrome and Akathisia

Restless legs syndrome (RLS) is characterized by dysesthesias and restlessness of the lower limbs that occurs during relaxed states and when attempting to sleep.[72] Partial relief is found in moving the legs or walking. There is an increased incidence of associated involuntary periodic movements of sleep which are stereotyped, repetitive movements of the legs that occur in the sleeping state.[73] Electromyographically, the periodic movements resemble the Babinski and triple flexion response with dorsiflexion of the ankle, great toe and occasionally flexion at the hip and knee. While sometimes described as nocturnal myoclonus, more detailed studies suggest that periodic movements differ from true myoclonus. Restless legs syndrome appears commonly during pregnancy. Patients often describe "pins and needles", cramping or coldness. Onset is typically during the second or third trimester and symptoms disappear after delivery. A history of RLS or periodic movements within the family or with previous pregnancies may help clarify the diagnosis. Restless legs syndrome is transmitted as an autosomal dominant gene in some families.[74]

The pathophysiology of RLS and periodic movements of sleep is unknown, although disturbances of central dopamine and opioid systems have been suggested.[75] While many different medical problems have been associated with RLS—including peripheral neuropathy, lumbar stenosis, anemia and uremia—subcortical, basal ganglia, and spinal cord origins seem most likely.

Treatment of RLS during pregnancy varies depending on symptom severity. Conservative measures such as leg stretching exercises, muscle massage, and walking are most suitable for mild cases. Restless legs syndrome and periodic movements that interfere with sleep may prompt medical intervention. Carbidopa/levodopa 25/100 or 25/250 mg at bedtime has been very effective[72,75] and appears to be safe during pregnancy. Codeine (30–120 mg at bedtime) may be used safely in the third trimester with good results. Propoxyphene (Darvon®, 65–130 mg [Eli Lilly and Company, Indianapolis, IN, USA]) has also been used successfully but much less is known about its safety in pregnancy. Correction of underlying folate deficiency, hypocalcemia or iron deficiency anemia if present may provide additional benefit.

Akathisia represents an uncomfortable sensation of extreme restlessness, often accompanied by difficulty in sitting still. Akathisia is a common side effect of neuroleptic drugs and can occur during treatment with other medications including estrogens.[76] No clear descriptions of akathisia specifically associated with pregnancy (in the absence of neuroleptics) have come to our attention.

Neuroleptic Malignant Syndrome

Neuroleptic malignant syndrome (NMS) is a potentially fatal idiosyncratic reaction to neuroleptic (dopamine receptor blocking) drugs. It is characterized by hyperthermia, muscular rigidity, tremor, and altered consciousness. Evidence of disordered autonomic function is common. The syndrome can occur at any time during the course of neuroleptic therapy but typically appears following initiation of treatment or increasing drug dosage. Symptoms intensify rapidly over a few days and may last up to 1 month. Central dopamine receptor blockade at several sites (hypothalamus, striatum, spinal cord) has been implicated in the pathogenesis of the disorder. Prompt discontinuation of neuroleptic therapy, immediate institution of measures to control body temperature, and treatment with dopaminergic agents (bromocriptine or levodopa) and the skeletal muscle relaxant dantroline constitute appropriate treatment. Possible NMS has been reported in the postpartum state for one patient treated with droperidol during cesarean section.[77] In addition to antipsychotics, drugs used for nausea (e.g., prochlorperazine [Compazine®; Smith Kline & French, Philadelphia, PA, USA], metaclopramide [Reglan®; Smith Kline & French, Philadelphia, PA, USA], hiccoughs (e.g., chlorpromazine [Thorazine®; Smith Kline & French, Philadelphia, PA, USA] or agitation (e.g., haloperidol [Haldol®; McNeil Pharmaceuticals, Spring House, PA, USA] may precipitate NMS.

References

1. Datta S: Sex hormone effects on excitable membranes. In *Neurological Disorders of Pregnancy*. Edited by P Goldstein. Mt. Kisco, NY. Futura Publishing Company, Inc., 1986, pp. 265–277.
2. Nausieda P, Koller W, Weiner W: Modification of post-synaptic dopaminergic sensitivity by female sex hormones. *Life Sci* 25:521–526, 1979.
3. Hruska R, Silbergeld R: Estrogen treatment enhances dopamine receptor sensitivity in the rat striatum. *Eur J Pharmacol* 61:397–400, 1980.
4. Cogen PH, Simmerman EA: Ovarian steroid hormones and cerebral function. *Adv Neurol* 26:123–133, 1979.
5. Husby G, Van De Rijn U, Zabriskie JB, et al: Antibodies reacting with cytoplasm of subthalamic and caudate nuclei neurons in chorea and acute rheumatic fever. *J Exp Med* 144:1094–1110, 1976.
6. Ayoub EM, Barrett DJ, Maclaren NK, et al: Association of class II human histocompatibility leukocyte antigens with rheumatic fever. *J Clin Invest* 77:2019–2026, 1986.
7. Wilson P, Preece A: Chorea gravidarium. *Arch Intern Med* 49:671–697, 1932.
8. Zegart KN, Schwarz RH: Chorea gravidarium. *Obstet Gynecol* 32:24–27, 1968.
9. Ghanem Q: Recurrent chorea gravidarum in four pregnancies. *Can J Neurol Sci* 12:136–138, 1985.
10. Jonas S, Spagnvolo M, Kloth H: Chorea gravidarium and streptococcal infection. *Obstet Gynecol* 39:77–79, 1972.

11. Donaldson J: Control of chorea gravidarium with haloperidol. *Obstet Gynecol* 59:381–382, 1982.
12. Lubbe WF, Walker EB: Chorea gravidarum associated with circulating lupus anticoagulant: successful outcome of pregnancy with prednisone and aspirin therapy. Case report. *Br J Obstet Gynaecol* 90:487–490, 1983.
13. Dhanaraj M, Radharrishran AR, Srinivas K, et al: Sodium valproate in Syndenham's chorea. *Neurology* 35:114–115, 1985.
14. Hanson J: Haloperidol and limb deformity (letter). *JAMA* 231:26, 1975.
15. Kopelman A, McCullar F, Heggeness L: Limb malformations following maternal use of haloperidol. *JAMA* 231:62–64, 1975.
16. Gram L, Drachman Bentsen K: Valproate: an updated review. *Acta Neurol Scan* 72:129–139, 1985.
17. Shoulson I: On Chorea. *Clin Neuropharmacol* 9:585–599, 1986.
18. Thomas D, Byrne PD, Travers RL: Systemic lupus erythematosus presenting as post-partum chorea. *Aust NZ J Med* 9:568–570, 1979.
19. Ginnetti RA, Bredfeldt RC, Pegg EW: Chorea gravidarum. A case report including magnetic resonance imaging results. *J Fam Pract* 29:87–89, 1989.
20. Bruyn GW, Padberg G: Chorea and systemic lupus erythematosus. A critical review. *Eur Neurol* 23:278–290, 1984.
21. Wolf RE, McBeath JG: Chorea gravidarum in systemic lupus erythematosus. *J Rheumatol* 12:992–993, 1985.
22. Hayslett J, Reece E: Systemic lupus erythmatosus in pregnancy. *Clin Perinatol* 12:539–550, 1985.
23. Levine S, Welch K: The spectrum of neurologic disease associated with antiphospholipid antibodies: lupus anticoagulants and anticardiolipin antibodies. *Arch Neurol* 44:876–883, 1987.
24. Asherson R, Hughes G: Antiphospholipid antibodies and chorea. *J Rheumatol* 15:377–379, 1988.
25. Agrawal B, Foa R: Collagen vascular disease appearing as chorea gravidarum. *Arch Neurol* 39:192–193, 1982.
26. Asherson R, Derksen R, Harris E: Chorea in systemic lupus erythematosus and "lupus-like disease": association with antiphospholipid antibodies. *Semin Arthritis Rheum* 16:253–259, 1987.
27. Ichikawa K, Kim R, Givelber H: Chorea gravidarum: report of a fetal case with neuropathological observations. *Arch Neurol* 37:429–432, 1980.
28. Asherson RA, Hughes GR, Gledhill R: Absence of antibodies to cardiolipin in patients with Huntington's chorea, Sydenham's chorea and acute rheumatic fever. *J Neurol Neurosurg Psychiatry* 51:1458, 1988.
29. Bonfa E, Golombek S, Kaufman L: Association between lupus psychosis and antiribosomal P protein antibodies. *N Engl J Med* 317:265–271, 1987.
30. Newman RP, Kinkel WR: Paroxysmal choreoathetosis due to hypoglycemia. *Arch Neurol* 41:341–342, 1984.
31. Tortoritis M, Cornish D, Thompson F: Nonketotic hypergylcemia. *Arch Intern Med* 142:1405, 1982.
32. Tang WY, Gill DS, Chuan PS: Chorea, a manifestation of hyponatremia? *Singapore Med J* 22:92–93, 1981.
33. Sparacioo RR, Anziska B, Schutta HS: Hypernatremia and chorea. *Neurology* 26:46–50, 1976.

34. Howde PD, Bone I, Losowsky MS: Hypocalcaemic chorea secondary to malabsorption. *Postgrad Med J* 55:561–563, 1979.
35. Fidler SM, O'Rourke RA, Buehsbaum HM: Choreoathetosis as a manifestation of thyrotoxicosis. *Neurology* 21:55–57, 1971.
36. Salti I, Paris A, Tannir N, et al: Rapid correction by I-alpha-hydroxycholecalceferal of hemichorea in surgical hypoparathyroidism. *J Neurol Neurosurg Psychiatry* 40:692–694, 1977.
37. Gaffney J, Kurlan R, Goldblatt D, et al: Hemichorea and hyperglycemia. *Ann Neurol* 24:180, 1988.
38. Kurlan R, Shoulson I: Dystonia and akinetic-rigid features in central pontine myelinolysis. *Ann Neurol* 26:141, 1989.
39. Hoogstraten MC, Lakke JP, Zwarts MJ: Bilateral ballism: a rare syndrome. Review of the literature and presentation of a case. *J Neurol* 233:25–29, 1986.
40. Bedard P, Langelier P, Villeneuve A: Oestrogens and extrapyramidal system. *Lancet* 1:1367–1368, 1977.
41. Gardos G, Cole JO, Tarsy D: Withdrawal syndromes associated with antipsychotic drugs. *Am J Psychiatry* 135:1321–1324, 1978.
42. Sexson WR, Barak Y: Withdrawal emergent syndrome in an infant associated with maternal haloperidol therapy. *J Perinatol* 9:170–172, 1989.
43. Hayden MR, Hewitt J, Kastelein JJ, et al: First-trimester prenatal diagnosis for Huntington's disease with DNA probes. *Lancet* 1:1284–1285, 1987.
44. Weiner W, Lang AE: Other choreas and miscellaneous dyskinesias. In *Movement Disorders: A Comprehensive Survey*. Edited by W Weiner, AE Lang. Mt. Kisco, NY, Futura Publishing Company, Inc. 1989, pp. 569.
45. Vance JM, Pericak-Vance MA, Bowman MH, et al: Chorea-acanthocytosis. A report of three new families and implications for genetic counseling. *Am J Med Genetics* 28:403–410, 1987.
46. Kurlan R: Tourette's syndrome: current concepts. *Neurology* 39:1625–1630, 1989.
47. Sandyk R, Banford CR: Estrogen as adjuvant treatment of Tourette syndrome. *Pediatr Neurol* 3:122, 1987.
48. Niebyl J: *Drug Use in Pregnancy*. Philadelphia, PA. Lea and Febiger, 1988, pp. 58–59.
49. Mattson RH, Cramer JA, Darney PD, et al: Use of oral contraceptives by women with epilepsy. *JAMA* 256:238–240, 1986.
50. Narabayashi H: Stereotaxic Vim thalamotomy for treatment of tremor. *Eur Neurol* 29:29–32, 1989.
51. Jankovic J: Parkinsonian disorders. In *Current Neurology*. Edited by S Appel. New York, NY. John Wiley and Sons, 1984, pp. 1–49.
52. Golbe LI: Parkinson's disease and pregnancy. *Neurology* 37:1245–1249, 1987.
53. Cook DG, Klawans HL: Levodopa during pregnancy. *Clin Neuropharmacol* 8:93–95, 1985.
54. Allain H, Bentue-Ferrer D, Milon D, et al: Pregnancy and parkinsonism. A case report without problem. *Clin Neuropharmacol* 12:217–219, 1989.
55. Weil C: The safety of bromocriptine in long-term use: a review of the literature. *Curr Med Res Opin* 10:25–51, 1986.

56. Rogues F: Pregnancy and epidemic encephalitis. *Proc Royal Soc Med* 17:1053–1063, 1928.
57. Lance JW: Familial paroxysmal dystonic choreoathetosis and its differentiation from related syndromes. *Ann Neurol* 2:285–293, 1977.
58. Weiner W, Lang AE: Other choreas of miscellaneous dyskinesias. In *Movement Disorders: A Comprehensive Survey*. Edited by W Weiner, AE Lang. Mt. Kisco, NY, Futura Publishing Company, Inc., 1989, pp. 581.
59. Fahn S: Concept and classification of dystonia. *Adv Neurol* 50:1–8, 1988.
60. Ozelius L, Kramer PL, Moskowitz CB, et al: Human gene for torsion dystonia located on chromosome 9 q^{32}-q^{34}. *Neuron* 2:1427–1434, 1989.
61. Rosenberg L: Lack of relation of oral clefts to diazepam use in pregnancy. *N Engl J Med* 311:919, 1984.
62. Safra M, Oakley G: Association between cleft lip with or without cleft palate and prenatal exposure to diazepam. *Lancet* 26:478, 1975.
63. Jankovic J, Schwartz K: Botulinum toxin for cervical dystonia. *Neurology* 40:277–280, 1990.
64. Scott AB: Botulinum toxin for blepharospasm. In *Current Therapy in Ophthalmic Surg*. Edited by GL Spaeth, LJ Katz, KW Parker. B.C. Decker, Inc., 1989, pp. 322–324.
65. Frydman M, Bonne-Tamin B, Farrer LA, et al: Assignment of the gene for Wilson's disease to chromosome 13: linkage to the esterase-D locus. *Proc Natl Acad Sci* 82:1819–1821, 1985.
66. Starosta-Rubinstein S, Young A, Kluin K, et al: Clinical assessment of 31 patients with Wilson's disease: correlations with structural changes on magnetic resonance imaging. *Arch Neurol* 44:365–368, 1987.
67. Scheinberg IH, Sternlieb I: Pregnancy in penicillamine-treated patients with Wilson's disease. *N Engl J Med* 293:1300–1302, 1975.
68. Biller J, Swiontoniowski M, Brazis PW: Successful pregnancy in Wilson's disease: a case report and review of the literature. *Eur Neurol* 24:306–309, 1985.
69. Rosa FW: Teratogen update: penicillamine. *Teratology* 33:127–131, 1986.
70. Walshe JM: The management of pregnancy in Wilson's disease treated with trientine. *Q J Med* 58:81–87, 1986.
71. Fahn S, Marsden CD, VanWoert MH: Definition and classification of myoclonus. In *Advances in Neurology, Myoclonus*. Edited by S Fahn, CD Marsden, W VanWoert. New York, NY. Raven Press, 1986, pp. 1–5.
72. Lugaresi E, Cirignatta F, Coccagna G, et al: Nocturnal myoclonus and restless legs syndrome. In *Advances in Neurology, Myoclonus*. Edited by S Fahn, CD Marsden, W VanWoert. New York, NY. Raven Press, 1986, pp. 295–307.
73. Montplaisir J, Godbout R: Restless leg syndrome and periodic movements during sleep. In *Principals and Practice of Sleep Medicine*. Edited by MH Kryger, T Roth, WC Dement. Philadelphia, PA. WB Saunders Company, 1989, pp. 402–409.
74. Boghen D, Beyronnard JM: Myoclonus in familial restless leg syndrome. *Arch Neurol* 33:368–370, 1976.

75. Walters AS, Hening W: Clinical presentation and neuropharmacology of restless legs syndrome. *Clin Neuropharmacol* 10:225–237, 1987.
76. Krishnan KR, France RD, Ellinwood EA: Tricyclic-induced akathisia in patients taking conjugated estrogens. *Am J Psychiatry* 141:696–697, 1984.
77. Weinger MB, Swerdlow NR, Millar WL: Acute postoperative delirium and extrapyramidal signs in a previously healthy parturient. *Anesth Analg* 67:291–295, 1988.

9

Spinal Cord Injured Women: Sexuality, Fertility and Pregnancy

Gary M. Yarkony, M.D.

Spinal Cord Injury

Introduction

Trauma to the spinal cord resulting in paralysis occurs most frequently in younger males. The ratio of injury of males to females is generally considered to be 4:1. Approximately 10,000 spinal cord injuries occur in the United States each year. Males are considered more susceptible to these injuries due to their higher exposure to motor vehicles, fire arms, sporting activities, and propensity for taking risks.[1]

Data collected from the Model Spinal Cord Injury Systems[1] on 9,647 individuals, 18% of whom are female, reveal some important data. The mean age of injury was 29.7 years (median 25, mode 19) with the 16 to 30 age group more likely to suffer a spinal cord injury than all other age groups combined. Seventy-four percent of injuries occur in whites, notably less than their 83% representation in the population. In females, the leading cause of injury is motor vehicle accidents (60.1%), followed by falls (17.3%), acts of violence (12.8%), and sporting injuries (7.1%). The proportion of falls increases with

From Goldstein PJ, Stern BJ, (eds): *Neurological Disorders of Pregnancy. Second Revised Edition.* Mount Kisco NY, Futura Publishing Co., Inc., © 1992.

advancing age. Males are twice as likely to be injured in sporting accidents than females. Most injuries occur in July and the other summer months with Saturday and Sunday the common days of injury. It is estimated that there are 200,000 individuals in the United States surviving with a spinal cord injury.

Due to the complex nature of these injuries, Model Systems of Care has been developed to care for spinal cord injuries. They provide a coordinated system from point of injury to lifelong follow-up. This process is necessary as sufficient expertise among staff members and provision of specialized services can only be developed in a regional center. The team includes a physician, nurse therapist, physical therapist, occupational therapist, psychologist, social worker, vocational rehabilitation counselor, speech pathologist, chaplain, recreation therapist, care sponsor (insurer, case manager), and the patient and family.[2]

Types of Injuries

Spinal cord injuries[3] are injuries that occur to the nervous system within the spinal canal from the foramen magnum to the conus medullaris, including the nerves of the cauda equina. Quadriplegia refers to damage within the cervical canal resulting in varying degrees of functional impairment to the arms, trunk, legs, and bowel and bladder. Paraplegia refers to damage to the thoracic, lumbar, or sacral segments including the conus medullaris and cauda equina. Both of these definitions exclude injuries outside the canal, such as injuries to the lumbar or brachial plexus.

The standards of the American Spinal Injury Association[3] are generally used to define the level and extent of injury. Motor level is defined by the last normal level with antigravity motor strength assuming normal function above that level. The key motor levels are listed in Table I. Sensory level is determined by pinprick examination. The dermatome chart of Figure 1 pictures the dermatomes with a black dot indicating the key area to test for each dermatome. Examples of important sensory areas are the xyphoid for T-6 and T-10 at the umbilicus.

Lesions may be defined as complete or incomplete. After the last normal level is determined, the zone of partial preservation is considered three segments below that level. If any sensory or motor func-

Table 1.
Muscles for Motor Level Classification

C1-3	Sensory level
C-4	Diaphragm
C-5	Elbow flexors
C-6	Wrist extensors
C-7	Elbow extensors
C-8	Finger flexors
T-1	Intrinsic muscles of the hand
T2-L1	Use sensory level/Beevor's Sign
L-2	Hip flexors
L-3	Knee extensors
L-4	Ankle dorsiflexors
L-5	Long to extensors
S-1	Ankle plantar flexors
S2-S5	Sensory level

From American Spinal Injury Association Standards for Neurological Classification, 1989.

tion exists below the zone of partial preservation the injury is considered incomplete. The wide variations of incomplete lesions include sacral sparring with preservation of rectal sensation, trace movements of a distal muscle, or significant strength that allows the individual to walk. The Frankel classification is frequently used to define the extent of injury. A Frankel grade A is a complete lesion, grade B a sensory incomplete lesion, and grade C has nonuseful motor function. A Frankel classification of D indicates the presence of an incomplete lesion with useful motor function and grade E indicates complete recovery although brisk reflexes may still be present.

Damage limited to certain areas of the spinal cord may result in commonly recognized syndromes. The central cord syndrome results from damage to the central part of the cervical cord with arm paralysis greater than leg paralysis. These individuals may walk, but have partial or complete paralysis of the arms. In the Brown-Séquard syndrome, a hemisection of the spinal cord presents with paralysis on one side with contralateral loss of pain sensation. The anterior cord syndrome spares posterior column function. Incomplete syndromes not following any pattern are called mixed syndromes.

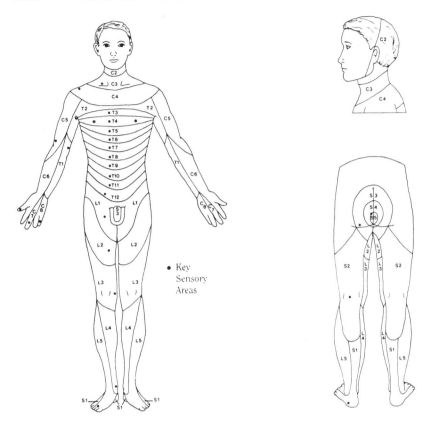

Figure 1: Dermatome Chart. Key Sensory Areas Indicated by Black Dot (Reprinted with permission from the American Spinal Injury Association).

Functional Outcomes After Spinal Cord Injury

Pregnancy may further interfere with an individual's ability to perform daily activities. Therefore, it is important for the obstetrician to be aware of the functional abilities at the various levels of quadriplegia and paraplegia. Motor function is the primary determinant of functional abilities, although other factors such as age, physique, and motivation will impact. The descriptions of the common levels below are guidelines of what can be expected of common complete motor levels of functioning.

The C-5 quadriplegic[4] has good strength in the deltoid and bicep muscles. This individual eats and drinks food provided and cut up with the assistance of static hand splints and utensil cuffs. A manual wheelchair with projections on the rims may be used for short distances, but electric wheelchairs are generally required for long distances. Upper extremity dressing may be completed as well as oral facial hygiene. Transfer assistance is required.

The C-6 level adds radial wrist extensors and improved proximal strength.[5] The presence of wrist extensors allows for grasp using tenodesis, the relative shortening of the finger flexors with wrist extension that results in the thumb and index finger coming together. This allows for greater independence in feeding, and increased likelihood of performing upper and lower body dressing. Individuals at this level may transfer from the wheelchair to the bed and some may perform intermittent catheterization. Manual wheelchairs may be propelled in the community.

The C-7 level adds on triceps and the ability to transfer to more complex surfaces such as the toilet or tub bench. At this level total independence becomes more likely with less need for attendant care. The presence of long finger flexors at C-8 and intrinsics at T-1 further enhances independence, particularly in relation to bowel and bladder management.

At the thoracic levels, total independence is possible.[6] The majority of thoracic paraplegics use wheelchairs for mobility. This is due to the excessive energy requirements to use long leg braces and crutches that can range from 6 to 12 times as much energy per unit distance as is normally required. As motor function improves in the lumbar segments ambulation is more likely, particularly in those individuals with improved hip control and knee extension.

Common Medical Problems After Spinal Cord Injury

Neurogenic Bowel and Bladder

The neurogenic bladder presents a difficult challenge to the physician caring for spinal cord injured individuals. The goal of maintaining normal renal function while preventing complications such as renal and bladder stones, infection, and hydronephrosis must be balanced against the individual's desire for a practical system that will not interfere with community reintegration. Because the pregnant woman is at increased risk for asymptomatic bacteriuria, and because pregnancy-related urologic anatomical changes occur, attention to the urological management in spinal cord injured patients must be enhanced. Many options exist for bladder management. Many cervical and thoracic injuries will have reflex bladder functioning and void with sufficiently small residual urine volumes to be catheter free. Men in this situation will wear an external (condom-type) catheter as they are generally not able to detect when they will void or lack the ability to transfer and undress quickly enough. As there is no suitable external catheter for women, they generally opt for an indwelling catheter. A suprapubic catheter may be preferred as it is easier to change and a larger bore catheter may be used.

Intermittent catheterization is an option at all levels of injury. Lack of a foreign body in the bladder decreases the risk of infection and stones. In general, spinal cord injured individuals are started on this technique as soon after injury as possible. Those most likely to continue on this technique have good hand function and sufficient motivation to perform the procedure every 4 to 6 hours or adequate attendant care. Measures to keep the individual dry between catheterizations include the use of medications such as probanthine and oxybutynin (Ditropan®; Marion Merrell Dow, Inc., Kansas City, MO, USA).

The neurogenic bowel is generally easier to manage. Regulation in upper motor neuron lesions is generally obtained with suppositories or digital stimulation daily or every other day. Stool softeners or fiber preparations are used frequently. The individual is encouraged to maintain a high-fiber diet with adequate fluid intake. Distal lower motor neuron lesions may require manual removal.

Pressure Ulcers

Skin breakdown due to pressure and shear is a common complication of spinal cord injury.[7] Incontinence, poor nutrition, and cigarette smoking may exacerbate the risk of pressure ulcers. "Bed sores" and "decubitus ulcers" are terms often used to describe these lesions.

During the initial phase after injury, pressure ulcers most commonly occur on the sacrum or the heels. As the individuals become more active the skin over the ischial tuberosities and greater trochanters is at greater risk. Pregnancy may further decrease mobility, and increase the risk of skin breakdown. Pressure relief techniques such as push-ups, leaning from side to side in the wheelchair, and turns in bed may diminish with pregnancy.

The first step in the management of these lesions is to remove pressure. This is often resisted by the patient as it limits mobility. Debridement can generally be accomplished surgically or with wet to dry dressings. Once the wound is clean and the pressure removed, the moist wound environment allows healing and decreased frequency of dressing changes.[8] Chronic ulcerations with exposure of bone will generally require a musculocutaneous flap performed by an experienced plastic surgeon.

Pulmonary Dysfunction

The loss of the chest wall musculature and immobilization result in decreased vital capacity, inability to cough, and a greater risk of atelectasis and pneumonia. Initial management includes frequent position changes, postural drainage, and respiratory therapy. Tracheostomy may be required.

In quadriplegics, gravity will have an adverse affect in the sitting position. The flaccid abdominal muscles allow the abdominal contents to protrude and the diaphragm to lower, resulting in a shorter descent of the diaphragm during inspiration. During expiration the diaphragm does not have the assistance of abdominal rebound to return it to a better resting position. Therefore, the supine position improves ventilation as the diaphragm is pushed by the cephalad movement of abdominal contents during expiration, decreasing end-expiratory volume. Spasticity of the abdominal wall enhances expiration. With time, pulmonary function improves. Spasticity of the abdominal and intercostal muscles decreases end-expiratory volume and improves diaphragmatic function.[9]

To enhance pulmonary function, exercises are performed to strengthen inspiratory musculature through use of incentive spirometry or inspiration against graded resistance. Assistive cough helps to clear secretions. At higher levels of injury, home and portable suctioning equipment may be needed.

Spasticity

Spasticity may be both beneficial and problematic to the spinal cord injured patient. Beneficial effects include maintenance of muscle bulk, decreased lower extremity edema, and enhanced pulmonary functioning. Spasticity may interfere with functional skills, result in falls during ambulation or transfers, and be uncomfortable.

The foundation of management of spasticity is sound basic medical care.[10] As spasticity may be exacerbated by urinary tract infections, bladder stones, ingrown toenails, bowel impactions, or pressure ulcers, proper prevention and care of these conditions is essential. An adequate range of motion program is an essential ingredient in the treatment of spasticity.

Four medications are generally used either alone or in combination for treatment of spasticity.[11,12] Baclofen (Lioresal®; Geigy Pharmaceuticals, Summit, NJ, USA), a γ-aminobuteric acid derivative acting directly on the spinal cord, is generally the first line drug. There are no studies of its usage in pregnant women and the manufacturer advises that its usage in pregnancy should be considered only if the benefit clearly justifies the potential risk to the fetus. Adverse effects have been seen in animal studies.[13] A single case report demonstrates that baclofen is excreted in breast milk at one thousandth of the ingested dose and should not reach toxic levels in the newborn.[14] Baclofen should be tapered when discontinuing its use to avoid hallucinations, anxiety, and tachycardia that may occur with sudden cessation.

Diazepam (Valium®; Roche Products, Inc., Manati, Puerto Rico) is another centrally acting drug indicated for spasticity. Diazepam and its metabolies cross the placenta and accumulate in the fetal circulation.[15] Although the association between diazepam and oral clefts has been questioned,[16] other malformations demonstrated include inguinal hernia, cardiac defects, pyloric stenosis, and hemangiomas.[15] The floppy infant syndrome occurs as well.[17] Diazepam is excreted in breast milk and may reach high levels in breast-fed infants.

Clonidine, a centrally acting α-adrenergic agonist used to treat hypertension has been shown to be beneficial in the treatment of spasticity.[11] Clonidine crosses the placenta extensively and is generally considered free of teratogenic risk. It is not known to be deleterious for fetal growth, mortality, and morbidity. There may be a long-term behavioral teratogenicity manifesting as hyperactivity and sleep disturbances. No data exist on fetal hemodynamics.[18] Clonidine is excreted in breast milk. In a small series there were no adverse effects on newborns.[19]

Dantrolene (Dantrium®; Norwich Eaton Pharmaceuticals, Inc., Norwich, NY, USA) acts directly on muscle to decrease release of calcium from the sarcoplasmic reticulum. A major drawback of its usage is hepatoxicity. Its safety in pregnancy has not been established and it should not be used by nursing mothers.[13] Dantrolene has been studied in pregnant women as a prophylactic agent to prevent malignant hyperthermia. When given 5 days before and 3 days after delivery it was not felt to be deleterious to the fetus and newborn. There was no long-term follow-up on the newborn.[20]

Surgical intervention may be necessary if conservative measures fail. Tendon lengthening procedures may be necessary or local nerve blocks such as obturator neurectomy can allow for perineal care. Rhizotomy has been performed frequently. The baclofen pump is now being tested.[21] This pump delivers baclofen to the spinal fluid in microgram dosages and has been shown to greatly diminish spasticity.

Autonomic Dysreflexia

Autonomic dysreflexia is a syndrome characterized by exaggerated autonomic responses to stimuli that are innocuous in normal individuals.[22,23] The group at risk for this syndrome is generally considered to be spinal cord injured individuals with lesions at or above T-6. However, there are reports of this syndrome occurring in a male of T-8 and a T-10 paraplegic during the postpartum period, indicating that caution should be used in ascribing its signs and symptoms to other causes based on level of injury alone.[24,25] It is often referred to as autonomic hyperreflexia, and by those suffering from it as "going hyper".

The first description of this syndrome is attributed to Bowlby in 1890. It was further clarified by Head and Riddoch in 1917[26] and Guttmann and Whitteridge in 1947.[27] Its incidence has been reported to range from 48% to 85% of those susceptible.[28,29] The syndrome occurs because the hypothalamic control of the sympathetic spinal reflexes is lost as the splanchnic outflow is isolated in lesions at T-6 and above. The primary differential diagnosis is with pheochromocytoma[30] or other catecholamine secreting tumors[31] and toxemia of pregnancy. The hypertension of toxemia is not transient and episodic like that of autonomic dysreflexia. Autonomic dysreflexia does not respond to magnesium sulfate.

Onset generally occurs after the first 2 months postinjury and 92% of those who develop the syndrome do so within the first year. However, there are reports indicating that it may occur for the first time as late as 15 years postinjury. It can occur in complete and incomplete lesions.

The syndrome generally results from distension of a pelvic viscus such as the bladder,[32] colon, or rectum or from uterine contractions during labor.[33] When associated with uterine contractions, hypertension begins within a few seconds of the onset of a contraction and may diminish or dissipate completely between contractions.[34] Numerous stimuli that produce the syndrome include bladder catheterization, urinary tract infection, hemorrhagic cystitis, testicular torsion, sexual intercourse, intra-abdominal catastrophies, surgical manipulation of the pelvis or abdomen, pressure ulcers and tight clothing, shoes, or leg bag strapping. Bladder distension is the most common stimulus followed by rectal distention (fecal impaction). Unusual causes reported in females include ovarian cysts[35] and breast feeding.[36]

Symptoms include headache, hyperhydrosis, cutaneous vasodilation, nasal obstruction, piloerection (gooseflesh), paresthesias, and splotches on the face and neck. Anxiety and the desire to void may be experienced.

Examination reveals hypertension, hyperhydrosis and, in general, bladder distension, fecal impaction, or uterine contractions. Bradycardia may be found, particularly if the patient is evaluated early in the course of the episode. Tachycardia or a normal pulse rate is more common. Other findings include a prominent Horner's syndrome. ECG changes may be found and have been reported during labor.

The hypertension associated with the syndrome is the primary cause of the morbidity and mortality associated with autonomic dysreflexia. It may result in loss of consciousness, seizures, intracranial bleeding, and death.[37] Patients may present with seizures and be treated for a primary seizure disorder with the autonomic dysreflexia being unrecognized.[38]

Prevention is the primary goal of management of autonomic dysreflexia. Optimal general medical management and annual genitourinary evaluations are essential. When an episode does occur, the patient should have the head of the bed elevated or be raised to a sitting position, tight clothing removed, and a cause sought. Generally, a distended bladder is found and relieved by performing a straight catheterization, unkinking a catheter, emptying a leg bag, or changing a clogged indwelling catheter. Episodes due to rectal distension may resolve, but if rectal examination is required an anesthetic ointment should be used.

Pharmacological intervention during the acute episode is directed toward decreasing blood pressure.[39] Agents that have generally been successful include nifedipine, diazoxide, nitroprusside, hydralazine, chlorpramazine, and amyl nitrate. Recurrent episodes not responsive to successful bladder or bowel management are generally treated with α blockers such as phenoxybenzamine, mecamylamine, and guanethidine. Specific reports during labor will be discussed.

Autonomic dysreflexia is a well recognized complication of urologic and other surgeries in spinal cord injured individuals. Numerous anesthetic approaches have been attempted. These techniques either attempt to prevent the syndrome from occurring, which is preferred, or treat the resultant hypertension.

Ganglionic blocking agents such as hexamethonium or tetraethylammonium chloride were reported to be effective.[40] More recently trimethaphan (Arfonad®; Roche Laboratories, Nutley, NJ, USA) has been shown to be useful in several case reports.[41] This approach allows the dysreflexia to develop as opposed to preventing its onset. Bilateral paravertebral sympathetic blocks are insufficient to prevent dysreflexia. Spinal anesthesia has been shown to prevent the reflex and eliminate the associated hypertension and headache.[42] Bradycardia is unpredictable and may occur suddenly with spinal anesthesia. Technical difficulties with spinal anesthesia occur primarily with lumbar injuries. Epidural anesthesia may also be effective.[32] With epidural anesthesia there is also the danger of inadvertent subarachnoid injection and acute apneic episodes may occur.[42] The height of the block with these techniques may be difficult to determine and hypotension may occur.[41]

General anesthesia may pose a problem due to decreased vital capacity, bronchial secretions, and diminished cough. Nitrous oxide plus narcotics are less effective than halothane or enflurane anesthesia with assisted ventilation. Arrythmias have been reported in patients receiving general anesthesia without assisted ventilation. Hypotension is also a risk, but may be diminished with preoperative hydration. Nondepolarizing muscle relaxants should be used as succinyl chloline has been shown to induce hyperkalemia and subsequent cardiac arrest.[43]

Sexuality, Adjustment, and Menstruation

Sexual adjustment after a spinal cord injury is an important part of the person's psychological and social rehabilitation.[44,45] Women have been reported to have less impairment in sex role function and identification after disability than men.[46] This adjustment may take several years postinjury. Disability may lead to postinjury divorce, further complicating adjustment.[47]

The woman's self concept and degree of perceived independence postinjury may impact on a woman's participation as a sexual partner.[48] Counseling[49–52] may play an important part in the adaptation process. A woman must acknowledge that sexuality is an integral part of her being and be encouraged to experiment with her sexual expression. Counseling may be needed on a short- or long-term basis. Issues in counseling may be related to problems such as positioning, contractures, management of menstrual periods, or dealing with bladder and bowel incontinence. Other areas that may require long-term counseling include presentation and perception of self and social skills, communication and cueing during sexual activity, and the impact of the injury on the marriage and family.[51] Counseling may be helpful prior to conception to help the spinal cord injured woman prepare for the difficulties she may encounter in caring for a child.

In spite of the absence of genital sensation, other erogenous areas such as the breasts, shoulders, neck, or mouth may enhance the sexual experience.[52] Women report orgasm in spite of reports that it is not possible with complete lesions of the spinothalamic tracts.[53] Phantom orgasms have been reported in the dreams of paraplegics.[54] Orgasm[55] may be described as similar to that of able-bodied women or as a wide variety of psychological experiences such as pleasant, relaxful, and glowing feelings.[45] Vaginal lubrication may occur reflexly with lesions with T-9, not at all with lesions between T-10 and T-12, and psychogenic lubrication may occur in lesions below T-12.[44]

Amenorrhea may occur following a spinal cord injury although its occurrence is not uniform and menstruation generally returns in 1 year.[49] Reports of secondary amenorrhea after a spinal cord injury range from 50% to 60%.[56,57] Axel[56] reported a mean return of menses in 5 months. Axel's report contradicted Comarr's[57] report that dysmenorrhea will cease. Comarr reported that the majority will have return of menses within 6 months although one woman's delay was 30 months. Women at or near the climacteric may become menopausal.

Birth control is a complex issue after spinal cord injury.[49] Intrauterine device usage is limited by the lack of pain sensation. The use of a diaphragm is limited by dexterity. Oral contraceptive use may further increase the risk of deep venous thrombosis.

Pregnancy, Labor, and Delivery

There are numerous reports of pregnancy occurring in spinal cord injured women. These reports date back to 1906 and note painless labor and caesarean section without anesthesia.[58] Unfortunately, these generally are in the form of case studies[24,59–78] and reviews,[44,53,79,80] as opposed to controlled studies resulting in guidelines for optimum management.

It is not unusual for women to sustain a spinal cord injury during their pregnancy. Unfortunately they may not be aware that they are pregnant or be unable to inform the staff of this due to associated brain injury. Pregnancy during the acute phase may limit radiological evaluation and surgical treatment of the injured spine necessitating conservative spine management.

Goller and Paeslack[81] have reported two cases in which the unborn child may have sustained cranial injuries at the time of the accident in which the mother was rendered paraplegic. This may have been due to direct trauma, anoxia, or hypoxemia. In a second series[64] based on a questionnaire of 45 pregnancies at the time of injury there were 31 healthy babies. There were 5 children were born with malformations or disability; 5 spontaneous abortions; 2 induced abortions; 1 death due to lung immaturity, and 1 stillbirth due to placenta previa. Insufficient data exist to analyze the abnormalities in these births that are likely to be multifactorial. They also reported a series of 130 spinal cord injured women with 147 normal children whose pregnancies began after injury, and which included 13 abortions (10 spontaneous) and 5 stillbirths. They noted an increase in premature and small for date children in this group, but no problems with malformations.

Robertson and Guttmann[82,83] have reported their experience of 25 spinal cord injured women giving birth to 33 children. Several of their observations are generally well accepted. It is well known that the uterus can contract with the nerve supply severed. As labor will be painless with lesions above T-10, examination may be necessary to determine the onset of labor. Premature labor is more common and premature delivery may occur in unfavorable surroundings without competent medical care. They recommended examination beginning at the 28th week with admission if the cervix is effaced and routine admission by the 35th week. Home tokadynamometry and patient instruction in uterine palpation may be helpful as well.[84]

Spinal cord injury is not by itself an indication for cesarean section.[72] Indications for surgery are the same as in nonspinal cord injured women. Breast feeding was successful as well, although there is a case report of it stimulating autonomic dysreflexia.[36]

Greenspoon and Paul[84] recommend a team approach in dealing with these pregnancies. A team including the primary care physician, neurologist, rehabilitation personnel, obstetrician, anesthesiologist, and urologist is recommended. The delivery facility should be able to perform invasive hemodynamic monitoring and the neonatal unit should be able to care for a premature infant. The management of the patient includes: (1) recognition and treatment of autonomic dysreflexia; (2) the ability to support respiration in cervical lesions; (3) prevention of unsupervised delivery; (4) surveillance for urinary tract infections· (5) treatment of anemia; (6) skin care to prevent pressure ulcers; (7) maintenance of normal bowel function; (8) counseling, and (9) contraception and sterilization.

Autonomic dysreflexia during labor has generated numerous reports and much controversy. Obviously the first step is awareness of this condition by the labor and delivery team. There are recent reports of intraventricular hemorrhage with resultant neurological deficits[69,76] and death[59,76] indicating that unrecognized autonomic dysreflexia still results in morbidity and mortality.

Although autonomic dysreflexia generally occurs in lesions at T-6 and above, one case in labor is reported at T-10.[24] Monitoring the situation may require an intra-arterial catheter, cardiac monitoring, the ability to administer antihypertensive medication, fetal monitoring as maternal hypotension may cause fetal hypoperfusion, and appropriate anesthesia. Cardiac arrythmias may occur in the mother due to the dysreflexia, although they are considered a general manifestation of the dysreflexia and not solely due to the pregnancy.[65]

Reserpine 2 weeks prior to the expected date of delivery has been suggested as a means to prevent the occurrence of autonomic dysreflexia.[73] Based on a cystometrogram in the same patient Saunders et al.[73] suggested that cystometrograms can predict dysreflexia during delivery but guidelines were lacking. Nitroglycerine has been given intravenously during cesarean section in hypertensive women, but it has not been studied in spinal cord injury. Nitroprusside has been used, but an epidural was required and concerns exist about the metabolic effects of cyanide that has been detected in fetal blood after maternal exposure to nitroprusside.[15,85] Young[86] reported the use of diazepam, diphenhydramine, and promethazine, none of which are commonly used to treat dysreflexia. This report resulted in numerous letters suggesting that continuous epidural anesthesia or spinal anesthesia would have been more appropriate.[68,74] This suggestion was based on reports by Stirt,[75] Ciliberti,[40] and Abouleish[59] of success with epidural anesthesia. Many believe epidural anesthesia to be the method of choice as it blocks the reflex arc. It is easy to perform and control and beneficial in that it prevents the syndrome. Epidural anesthesia has been reported to improve patient comfort[78] and to be preferable to spinal anesthesia because of difficulties in controlling the level of block and the increased risk of hypotension.[75] There are reports of epidural anesthesia failing with spinal anesthesia succeeding, probably due to epidural catheter placement difficulties. Nath[71] suggested that if autonomic dysreflexia cannot be controlled, prompt delivery by cesarean section may be the most expedient method of management.

Other suggestions to prevent autonomic dysreflexia include avoidance of external restraints, an indwelling catheter to prevent bladder distenion particularly during the later stages of pregnancy, and use of anesthetic ointments during examinations and catheter manipulation.

Early mobilization after delivery is encouraged to prevent deep venous thrombosis. Physical therapy to assist lower extremity function should be available.

Urologic complications have been noted as a result of pregnancy. Although ileal conduits are not used frequently, obstruction may occur.[61] Urinary infection may lead to pyelonephritis or septicemia.[60] It should not be assumed that normal patterns of voiding will resume after delivery. Increased residual urine volumes have resulted and the loss of reflex bladder function has occurred with the need for indwelling catheters.[58] An indwelling catheter may facilitate bladder management as pregnancy progresses.

Management of anemia with oral iron may exacerbate constipation and require modification of the bowel program.[34] Folate deficiencies may be present in women being treated for seizure disorders with phenytoin.

The rehabilitation team may be helpful to the obstetrician. Consultation may be obtained in regard to positioning for comfort and treatment of pressure ulcers. The rehabilitation facility may be an appropriate site to manage the patient during pregnancy.[67] After delivery, our center has admitted the mother and child to the same room. This facilitates bonding and allows the mother to learn to care for the infant as part of her rehabilitation.

Summary

Pregnancy associated with spinal cord injury represents a challenge to the obstetrician. A team approach in caring for these women may result in optimum outcomes. Further study is needed in this area to determine optimal management during pregnancy and delivery.

References

1. Stover SL, Fine PR, (eds): *Spinal Cord Injury: The Facts and Figures.* Birmingham, AL. The University of Albama at Birmingham, 1986.
2. Yarkony GM, Roth EJ, Heinemann AW, et al: Benefits of rehabilitation for traumatic spinal cord injury: multivariate analysis in 711 patients. *Arch Neurol* 44:93–96, 1987.
3. American Spinal Injury Association: *Standards for Neurological Classification of Spinal Injury Patients.* Chicago, IL. American Spinal Injury Association, 1989.

4. Yarkony GM, Roth E, Lovell L, et al: Rehabilitation outcomes in complete C₅ quadriplegia. *Am J Phys Med Rehabil* 67:73–76, 1988.
5. Yarkony GM, Roth EJ, Heinemann AW, et al: Rehabilitation outcomes in C₆ tetraplegia. *Paraplegia* 26:177–185, 1988.
6. Yarkony GM, Roth EJ, Meyer PR Jr, et al: Rehabilitation outcomes in patients with complete thoracic spinal cord injury. *Am J Phys Med Rehabil* 69:23–27, 1990.
7. Yarkony GM, Kramer E, King R, et al: Pressure sore management: efficacy of a moisture reactive occlusive dressing. *Arch Phys Med Rehabil* 65:597–600, 1984.
8. Gorse GJ, Messner RL: Improved pressure sore healing with hydrocolloid dressings. *Arch Dermatol* 123:766–771, 1987.
9. McMichan JC, Michel L, Westbrook PR: Pulmonary dysfunction following traumatic quadriplegia. *JAMA* 243:528–531, 1980.
10. Merritt JL: Management of spasticity in spinal cord injury. *Mayo Clin Proc* 56:614–622, 1981.
11. Donovan WH, Carter RE, Rossi D, et al: Clonidine effect on spasticity: a clinical trial. *Arch Phys Med Rehabil* 69:193–194, 1988.
12. Young RR, Delwaide PJ: Drug therapy: spasticity. *N Engl J Med* 304:28–33, 96–99, 1981.
13. Huff BB, (ed): *Physicians Desk Reference*. 43 ed. Oradel, NJ, Medical Economics Company, 1989.
14. Erikkson G, Swahn CG: Concentrations of baclofen in serum and breast milk from a lactating woman. *Scand J Clin Lab Invest* 91:185–187, 1981.
15. Petrie RH, (ed): *Perinatal Pharmacology*. Oradell, NJ, Medical Economics Company, Inc. 1989.
16. Rosenberg L, Mitchell AA, Parsells JL, et al: Lack of relation of oral clefts to diazepam use during pregnancy. *N Engl J Med* 309:1282–1285, 1983.
17. Schlumpf M, Ramseier H, Abriel H, et al: Diazepam effects on the fetus. *Neurotoxicology* 10:501–516, 1989.
18. Boutroy MJ: Fetal effects of maternally administered clonidine and angiotensin-converting enzyme inhibitors. *Dev Pharmacol Ther* 13:199–204, 1989.
19. Hartikainen-Sorri AL, Heikkinen JE, Koivisto M: Pharmokinetics of clonidine during pregnancy and nursing. *Obstet Gynecol* 69:598–600, 1987.
20. Shime J, Gare D, Andrews T, et al: Dantrolene in pregnancy: lack of adverse effects on the fetus and newborn infant. *Am J Obstet Gynecol* 159:831–834, 1988.
21. Penn RD, Savoy SM, Corcos D, et al: Intrathecal baclofen for severe spinal spasticity. *N Engl J Med* 320:1517–1521, 1989.
22. Erickson RP: Autonomic hyperreflexia: pathophysiology and medical management. *Arch Phys Med Rehabil* 61:431–440, 1980.
23. Kewalramani LS: Autonomic dysreflexia in traumatic myelopathy. *Am J Phys Med* 59:1–21, 1980.
24. Gimovsky ML, Ojeda A, Ozaki R, et al: Management of autonomic hyperreflexia associated with a low thoracic spinal cord lesion. *Obstet Gynecol* 153:223–224, 1985.

25. Moeller BA, Scheinberg D: Autonomic dysreflexia in injuries below the sixth thoracic segment. *JAMA* 224:1295, 1973.
26. Head H, Riddoch G: The automatic bladder, excessive sweating and some other reflex conditions in gross injuries of the spinal cord. *Brain* 46:188–263, 1917.
27. Guttmann L, Whitteridge D: Effects of bladder distension on autonomic mechanisms after spinal cord injuries. *Brain* 70:362–404, 1947.
28. Kurnick NB: Autonomic hyperreflexia and its control in patients with spinal cord lesions. *Ann Intern Med* 44:678–686, 1956.
29. Lindan R, Joiner E, Freehafer AA, et al: Incidence and clinical features of autonomic dysreflexia in patients with spinal cord injury. *Paraplegia* 18:285–292, 1980.
30. Manger WM, Davis SW, Chu D: Autonomic hyperreflexia and its differentiation from pheochromocytoma. *Arch Phys Med Rehabil* 60:159–161, 1979.
31. Wright KC, Agre JC, Wilson BC, et al: Autonomic dysreflexia in a paraplegic man with catecholamine-secreting neuroblastoma. *Arch Phys Med Rehabil* 67:566–567, 1986.
32. Neider RM, O'Higgins JW, Aldrete JA: Autonomic hyperreflexia in urologic surgery. *JAMA* 213:867–869, 1970.
33. Tabsh K, Brinkman CR, Reff RA: Autonomic dysreflexia in pregnancy. *Obstet Gynecol* 60:119–121, 1982.
34. Rossier AB, Ruffieux M, Ziegler WH: Pregnancy and labour in high traumatic spinal cord lesion. *Paraplegia* 7:210–216, 1971.
35. Kumar VN, Mullican CN: Ovarian cyst and autonomic dysreflexia. *Arch Phys Med Rehabil* 70:547–548, 1989.
36. Devenport JK, Swenson JR: An unusual cause of autonomic dysreflexia (abstract). *Arch Phys Med Rehabil* 64:485, 1983.
37. Guttmann L: *Spinal Cord Injuries Comprehensive Management and Research.* 2nd ed. Boston, MA. Blackwell Scientific Publications Inc., 1976.
38. Yarkony GM, Katz RT, Wu Y: Seizures secondary to autonomic dysreflexia. *Arch Phys Med Rehabil* 67:834–835, 1986.
39. McGuire EJ, Rossie AB: Treatment of acute autonomic dysreflexia. *J Urol* 129:1185–1186, 1983.
40. Ciliberti BJ, Goldfein J, Rovenstein EA: Hypertension during anesthesia in patients with spinal cord injuries. *Anesthesiology* 15:273–279, 1954.
41. Thorn-Alquist A: Prevention of hypertensive crises in patients with high spinal lesions during cystoscopy and lithotripsy. *Acta Anaesth Scand* 57(Suppl):79–82, 1975.
42. Schonwald G, Fish KJ, Perkash I: Cardiovascular complications during anesthesia in chronic spinal cord injured patients. *Anesthesiology* 55:550–558, 1981.
43. Brooke MM, Donovon WH, Stolov WC: Paraplegia: succinycholine induced hyperkalemia and cardiac arrest. *Arch Phys Med Rehabil* 59:306–308, 1978.
44. Berard EJT: The sexuality of spinal cord injured women: physiology and pathophysiology, a review. *Paraplegia* 22:99–112, 1989.
45. Bregman S, Hadley RG: Sexual adjustment and feminine attractiveness

among spinal cord injured women. *Arch Phys Med Rehabil* 57:448–450, 1976.

46. Weiss AJ, Diamond MD: Sexual adjustment, identification and attitudes of patients with myelopathy. *Arch Phys Med Rehabil* 47:245–250, 1966.
47. DeVivo MJ, Fine PR: Spinal cord injury: its short-term impact on marital status. *Arch Phys Med Rehabil* 66:501–504, 1985.
48. Fitting MD, Salisbury S, Davies NH, et al: Self-concept and sexuality of spinal cord injured women. *Arch Sex Behav* 7:143–156, 1978.
49. Cole TM: Sexuality and physical disabilities. *Arch Sex Behav* 4:389–403, 1975.
50. Griffith ER, Trieschmann RB: Sexual functioning in women with spinal cord injury. *Arch Phys Med Rehabil* 56:18–21, 1975.
51. Romano MD: Counseling the spinal cord injured female. In Sha'ked A (ed) *Human Sexuality and Rehabilitation*. Edited by A. Sha'ked. Baltimore, MD. Williams & Wilkins, 1981, pp. 157–166.
52. Thorton CE: Sexual counseling of women with spinal cord injuries. *Sex Disability* 2:267–277, 1979.
53. Ohry A, Deleg D, Goldman J, et al: Sexual function, pregnancy and delivery in spinal cord injured women. *Gynecol Obstet Invest* 9:281–291, 1978.
54. Money J: Phantom orgasm in the dreams of paraplegic men and women. *Arch Gen Psych* 3:373–382, 1960.
55. Geiger RL: Neurophysiology of sexual response in spinal cord injury. *Sex Disability* 2:257–266, 1979.
56. Axel SJ: Spinal cord injured women's concerns: menstruation and pregnancy. *Rehab Nurs* 7:10–15, 1982.
57. Comarr AE: Observations on menstruation and pregnancy among female spinal cord injury patients. *Paraplegia* 3:263–272, 1966.
58. Wanner MB, Rageth CJ, Zach GA: Pregnancy and autonomic hyperreflexia in patients with spinal cord lesions. *Paraplegia* 25:482–490, 1987.
59. Abouleish E: Hypertension in a paraplegic parturient. *Anesthesiology* 53:348–49, 1980.
60. Bradley WS, Walker WW, Searight MW: Pregnancy in paraplegia: a case report with urologic complication. *Obstet Gynecol* 10:573–575, 1957.
61. Daw E: Pregnancy problems in a paraplegic patient with an ileal conduit bladder. *Practitioner* 211:781–784, 1973.
62. Dickinson FT: Paraplegia in pregnancy and labor: report of case and review of literature. *J Am Obstet Assoc* 76:537–539, 1977.
63. Ferguson JE, Catanzorite VA: Clinical management of spinal cord injury. *Obstet Gynecol* 64:588–589, 1984.
64. Goller H, Paeslack V: Our experiences about pregnancy and delivery of the paraplegic women. *Paraplegia* 8:161–166, 1970.
65. Guttmann L, Frankel HL, Paeslack V: Cardiac irregularities during labour in paraplegic women. *Paraplegia* 3:144–151, 1965.
66. Hardy AG, Worrell DW: Pregnancy and labour in complete tetraplegia. *Paraplegia* 3:182–186, 1965.
67. Letcher JC, Goldfine LJ: Management of a pregnant paraplegic patient in a rehabilitation center. *Arch Phys Med Rehabil* 67:477–488, 1986.

68. McCunniff DE, Dewon D: Pregnancy after spinal cord Injury. *Obstet Gynecol* 63:757, 1984.
69. McGregor JA, Meeuwsen J: Autonomic hyperreflexia: a mortal danger for spinal cord-damaged women in labor. *Am J Obstet Gynecol* 151:330–333, 1985.
70. Mulla N: Vaginal delivery in a paraplegic patient. *Am J Obstet Gynecol* 73:1346–1348, 1957.
71. Nath M, Vivian JM, Cherny WB: Autonomic hyperreflexia in pregnancy and labor: a case report. *Am J Obstet Gynecol* 134:390–391, 1979.
72. Oppenhimer WM: Pregnancy in paraplegic patients: two case reports. *Am J Obstet Gynecol* 110:784–786, 1971.
73. Saunders D, Yeo J: Pregnancy and quadriplegia—the problem of autonomic dysreflexia. *Aust NZ J Obstet Gynaecol* 8:152–154, 1968.
74. Spielman FJ: Parturient with spinal cord transection: complications of autonomic hyperreflexia. *Obstet Gynecol* 64:147, 1984.
75. Stirt JA, Marco A, Conklin KA: Obstetric anesthesia for a quadriplegic patient with autonomic hyperreflexia. *Anesthesiology* 51:560–562, 1979.
76. Verduyn WH: A deadly combination: induction of labor with oxytocin/pitocin in spinal cord injured women, T_6 and above. Proceedings American Spinal Injury Association, Fifteenth Annual Meeting, pp 37, 1989.
77. Ware HH: Pregnancy after paralysis—report of three cases. *JAMA* 102:1833–1834, 1934.
78. Watson DW, Downey GO: Epidural anesthesia for labor and delivery of twins of a paraplegic mother. *Anesthesiology* 52:259–261, 1980.
79. Turk R, Turk M, Assejeu V: The female paraplegic and mother-child relations. *Paraplegia* 21:186–191, 1983.
80. Verduyn WH: Spinal cord injured women, pregnancy and delivery. *Paraplegia* 24:231–240, 1986.
81. Goller H, Paeslack V: Pregnancy, damage and birth-complications in the children of paraplegic women. *Paraplegia* 10:213–217, 1972.
82. Robertson DNS: Pregnancy and labour in the paraplegic. *Paraplegia* 10:209–212, 1972.
83. Robertson DNS, Guttmann L: The paraplegic patient in pregnancy and labour. *Proc Royal Soc Med* 56:381–387, 1963.
84. Greenspoon JS, Paul RH: Paraplegia and quadriplegia: special considerations during pregnancy and labor and delivery. *Am J Obstet Gynecol* 155:738–741, 1986.
85. Ravindran RS, Cummins DF, Smith IE: Experience with the use of nitroprusside and subsequent epidural analgesia in a pregnant quadriplegia patient. *Anesth Analg* 60:61–63, 1981.
86. Young BK, Katz M, Klein SA: Pregnancy after spinal cord injury: altered maternal and fetal response to labor. *Obstet Gynecol* 62:59–63, 1983.

10

Peripheral Nervous System Disorders and Pregnancy

Gerald Felsenthal, M.D.

Introduction

The peripheral nervous system or lower motor neuron unit begins with the anterior horn cell and extends through nerve root, plexus, peripheral nerve, and across the myoneural junction to terminate at the muscle. Any lesions of the peripheral nervous system that may affect a nongravid female patient may affect a pregnant patient of the same age. Although at one time a specific peripheral nerve abnormality of pregnancy was proposed,[1] careful review of the literature has not documented the existence of such an entity.[2] Pregnancy may, however, exacerbate pre-existing diseases of the peripheral nervous system. Additionally, some conditions of the peripheral nervous system may be precipitated during pregnancy, parturition, or the puerperium, apparently due to altered nutritional and/or changes in hormonal, fluid, and electrolyte levels.[3] Emphasis will be placed on those disorders reported as being exacerbated or precipitated by pregnancy. A differential diagnosis of non-neurological conditions in the evaluation of peripheral nervous system disorders will be included in the discussions.

From Goldstein PJ, Stern BJ, (eds): *Neurological Disorders of Pregnancy. Second Revised Edition.* Mount Kisco NY, Futura Publishing Co., Inc., © 1992.

Table I.
Level of Lesion: Differential Diagnosis

	Central Nervous System	Peripheral Nervous System
Sensation	Decreased throughout involved extremity	Decreased in dermatomal or peripheral nerve distribution
Strength	Decreased in hemiplegic, para-, or quadriplegic distribution	Decreased in portion of extremity according to innervation involved, i.e., root, peripheral nerve, etc.
Reflexes	Increased	Decreased
Tone	Increased	Decreased

General Considerations

A careful history and physical examination are essential to confirm the presence of a peripheral nervous system disorder; to localize the level of the lesion; to identify the etiology; and to guide specific and supportive treatment. The usual presenting complaints suggesting a lesion of the peripheral nervous system are pain, paresthesia, or weakness. Pain may be intense or burning. Paresthesias are described as tingling, numbness, or a "peculiar feeling" rather than anesthesia. Weakness may present as fatigability.

In general, sensory and motor abnormality follow the distribution of the affected part of the peripheral nervous system rather than involving an entire extremity. Reflexes and tone both tend to be decreased in peripheral nervous system disorders in the distribution of the involved portion of the system. Table I indicates those physical findings that, when combined with history, enable the clinician to distinguish a lesion of the peripheral nervous system from that of the central nervous system.

Myopathy Versus Neuropathy

In general, weakness located in the proximal portion of the extremity is suggestive of a myopathy. Distal weakness usually indicates a neuropathy. Some exceptions are myotonic dystrophy and Landry-Guillain-Barré-Strohl neuropathic syndrome. The former involves the distal portions of the extremities and the latter often involves the proximal portions of the extremities prior to the distal. Symptoms suggesting sensory neuropathy include paresthesias, dysesthesias, and hyper-, or hypoalgesia. Sensory loss in the presence of peripheral neuropathy is usually noted distally in a stocking-glove distribution. When dealing with a root lesion or a compression or entrapment lesion of a peripheral nerve, a sensory loss is noted in the particular dermatomal or peripheral distribution of the involved nerve. In myopathy, there is no associated sensory loss or sensory symptoms except for complaints of pain in involved muscles. Reflexes are decreased in neuropathy, affecting first the distal reflexes such as the ankle jerk. In myopathy, reflexes are usually uninvolved until late in the clinical course. Physical examination findings that differentiate between neuropathy and myopathy are indicated in Table II.

Electromyography and nerve conduction studies are the prime electrodiagnostic methods utilized to confirm the presence of abnormalities of the peripheral nervous system and to localize the level or extent of involvement. These diagnostic methods are extensions of the history and physical examination. Blood or urine tests as well as radiological procedures or muscle or nerve biopsy may be indicated and will be discussed as appropriate under specific disorders in this review. Electromyography and nerve conduction studies have a general diagnostic application and are not contraindicated during pregnancy. There is no significant predictable morbidity to these procedures, and the only concern during pregnancy is to accommodate the patient in positioning.

Electromyography is the study of the pattern of electrical activity of the muscles. A coaxial or monopolar needle electrode is inserted into a suspected involved muscle, and the response of the muscle to

Table II.
Level of Lesion: Differential Diagnosis

	Neuropathy	Myopathy
Sensation	Decreased	Unaffected
Strength	Decreased in distal muscles	Decreased in proximal muscles
Reflexes	Decreased	Usually uninvolved until late in course

the insertion while at rest and the electrical activity with minimal and maximal activity is noted. In normal muscles, there is minimum insertional activity and silence is noted at rest. Voluntary units are bi- and triphasic, and the summation pattern is usually complete. Disorder of the peripheral nervous system may be reflected by abnormal insertional activity and lack of silence of the muscles at rest. Voluntary units may be either larger or smaller than normal, and summation patterns may reveal an abnormality characteristic of myopathy or neuropathy.

Nerve conduction studies, which can investigate either sensory or motor components of nerves, involve the supramaximal electrical stimulation of a nerve at a given site and recording of the configuration of the evoked response and of the time from the electrical stimulation until the nerve or muscle response is noted on the monitor. These techniques allow diagnosis of peripheral neuropathy affecting multiple nerves as opposed to entrapment or compression syndromes that may affect just a portion of a nerve. Modifications of these techniques are used to evaluate the neuromuscular junction. In order to accurately localize the level of a peripheral nervous system disorder, both electromyography and nerve conduction studies are usually needed.[4] Table III summarizes the electrodiagnostic findings in peripheral nervous system disorders.

When considering treatment of the peripheral nervous system disorders associated with pregnancy, one should keep in mind the general statement made by Graham that disorders precipitated by pregnancy mostly remit naturally in the puerperium.[5] Disorders antedating pregnancy may worsen during the pregnancy and then remit after parturition. Some progressive disorders, such as amyotrophic lateral sclerosis, may continue to progress during pregnancy the same as they would in a nonpregnant patient. If the specific etiology of the disorder can be determined, then appropriate treatment can be given, (i.e., thiamine for nutritional polyneuritis). However, surgical intervention, such as for carpal tunnel syndrome or lumbosacral root lesions, should be delayed in the absence of a clear-cut indication for intervention until it can be determined that the symptoms will not resolve in the puerperium. Fetal morbidity due to a peripheral nervous system disorder is rare in pregnancy unless respiratory compromise or aspiration pneumonia develop. The physiology and the clinical management of respiratory disorders known to occur in pregnancy have been reviewed by Leontic.[6] A rehabilitation program,

Table III.
Electrodiagnosis of Lower Motor Neuron Disorders

	NCV	EMG	Comments
Anterior Horn Cell	− [1]	+	EMG positive in at least three extremities and cranial nerve innervated muscles
Nerve Root	− [2]	+	EMG positive in extremity muscles innervated by root and paraspinal muscles
Plexus	+ [3]	+	EMG and NCV localize abnormality to plexus and indicate normal paraspinal muscles
Polyneuropathy	+	±	NCV indicates multiple nerve involvement
Mononeuropathy	+	±	Single nerve involved
Mononeuropathy Multiplex	+	±	Few nerves involved with others normal
Entrapment/Compression Syndrome peripheral nerve	+	±	Segment of nerve involved
Myopathy	− [1]	+	Usually proximal muscles involved
Neuromuscular Junction	±	±	Repetitive testing (incremental or decremental responses)

Code: − = Normal.
  + = Abnormal.
  ± = May be normal or abnormal.

[1] Unless atrophy advanced which may be associated with slight slowing of motor conduction.
[2] Except for H reflex positive in S1 lesions.
[3] Helpful if able to stimulate nerve proximal to lesions, or if nerve accessible to techniques testing proximal portion of nerve.

based on the individual evaluation of each patient, should be offered to the pregnant patient. This program, within the limitations of the disease process and without overtaxing the patient's residual neuromuscular function, should emphasize functional ability, compensate for disability, and prevent complications, such as pressure ulcers, contractures, and deconditioning. Specific treatment recommendations will be discussed as pertinent to each disorder.

Back Pain

Mechanical Back Pain

Fast and associates[7] report that more than half (56%) of pregnant women interviewed 24–36 hours postpartum had experienced back pain during pregnancy beginning most frequently between the fifth and seventh month. Nearly half of the affected patients had pain radiating down one or both legs. One third of the patients noted that the pain increased during the course of the day (conversely, one third reported worsening at night). The most common explanation of this back pain is the musculoskeletal theory and relates to the enlarging uterus shifting the body's center of gravity anteriorly. Lumbar lordosis increases and concomitantly, the paraspinal muscles are placed in a shortened position while the abdominal muscles are in a lengthened position. Thus, both sets of muscles are not at their optimal functional position. Excessive stress is placed on the facet joints and posterior ligaments of the lumbar spine. Involvement of these posterior segments of the spinal unit produces pain with frequent radiation into the buttocks and the posterior thighs.[8] Physical findings include tenderness in the low back area and spasm of the paraspinal muscles as well as the increase in lumbar lordosis. Neurological examination of the lower extremities under these circumstances is within normal limits.

Fast et al.[9] subsequently reported a 67% incidence of night backache in a survey of 100 pregnant women. They "hypothesize that (in the recumbent position) hypervolemia combined with obstruction of the inferior vena cava, caused by the enlarging uterus, is the underlying pathomechanism". This leads "to engorgement and increased back pressure in the veins (venous channels and vertebral bodies) distal to the obstructed area". Consequently, "edema and stasis may develop in the nerve roots and vasa nervorum, leading to stagnant hypoxemia and metabolic disturbances of the neural elements" thus explaining the night backache.

Pelvic Relaxation Syndromes

Peculiar to pregnancy and ascribed to hormonal changes are pelvic girdle relaxation syndromes (pubic symphysis separation, sacroiliac relaxation, and osteitis condensans ilii). Widening of the symphysis pubis to a distance of more than 5 mm and, to a lesser degree, of the sacroiliac joints, occurs early in the pregnancy and disappears within 3 months after delivery. There is increased rotary motion at the sacroiliac joints and consequent mechanical instability. The sacrum is displaced anterior to its iliac articulations. This movement is facilitated by the greater anterior width of the sacrum and by the increasing anterior weight of the enlarging uterus. The anterior pelvic tilt and increasing lumbar lordosis exaggerate the forces on the posterior segment and facet joints.[10] Again, with increased facet stress, pain is not limited to the area of compression but radiates to the buttocks and often to the posterior thighs. Pain usually does not extend distally below the knees and neurological deficit is absent. The pain may be severe enough that the patient cannot walk or stand. The pain is relieved frequently by lying in bed with the hips abducted. During pregnancy, pelvic relaxation syndromes may be suggested by the patient's symptoms and clinical examination.[11] Stress maneuvers affecting the sacroiliac joint and/or symphysis pubis are helpful when they reproduce the pain, e.g., sacroiliac joint fixation test, Patrick's test (FABERE), and compression or distraction of the joints. Confirmation of these syndromes as etiology of the patient's complaints and differentiation of the types of syndrome are dependent upon x-ray studies. The potential risks for these studies should be weighed against the diagnostic benefits. Examination, in the case of pubic symphysis separation, may show a diastasis of the pubic rami of greater than 10 mm[12] and a vertical mobility of greater than 2 mm on films taken while standing alternately on each leg.[13] Sacroiliac relaxation may be associated with x-ray findings of sclerosis and widening of the sacroiliac joints. Barsony and Polgar[14] found para-articular sclerosis of the sacroiliac joint in the medial and distal part of the ilium and termed this condition osteitis condensans ilii.

The back pain associated with mechanical instability can often be relieved during pregnancy by restricting activity, localized heat, a trochanteric belt, or a gestational corset. Local injection with lidocaine alone or with a long-acting steroid, may produce temporary or somewhat longer lasting relief. A firm mattress or bedboard may be helpful in decreasing symptoms while at rest. Mobilization of the sacroiliac joint has been reported useful.[11] In the presence of a pelvic girdle relaxation syndrome, the lax pelvic joints cannot be protected by voluntary muscle control if the patient is being delivered under anesthesia. Thus, modification of the delivery position may be indicated, specifically using the Sims rather than the lithotomy position.[15] Following delivery, even though there may be resolution of lower back symptoms, attention should be paid to the muscular status of the abdominal, pelvic, and gluteal muscles in order to restore strength and prevent recurrence of the symptoms at a later time. In most cases, the symptoms of pelvic girdle relaxation syndrome disappear spontaneously or with appropriate conservative measures within a year of delivery (mean four months, range 0.5–12 months).[11] Favorable prognostic factors include first occurrence of relaxation, early treatment, and a younger age group.

Transient Osteoporosis of the Hip

A rare but potentially dangerous disorder of pregnancy is transient osteoporosis of the hip. The symptoms are vague and may involve pelvic, hip, thigh, or groin pain. Symptoms usually develop in the last trimester of pregnancy and may be misinterpreted as being due to pelvic girdle relaxation syndrome. If undetected and untreated, fracture of the femoral neck may occur. This condition, which may be a variant of reflex sympathetic dystrophy, has a gradual onset with pain slowly increasing in intensity and eventually interfering with weight-bearing on the affected limb. An x-ray film is necessary to confirm the diagnosis of transient osteoporosis.[8] The syndrome is usually self-limited with full recovery in 3 months to 1 year. Treatment is symptomatic with bed rest, protected weight-bearing, and analgesics as necessary.[16]

Other Causes of Back Pain

Postpartum back or sciatic pain may be the result of abscess formation, either retropsoas or subgluteal. This may result from paracervical and/or pudendal anesthesia.[17] In the reported cases, the only common symptom was pain. It tended to localize in the hip, buttock, back, leg, perineum, or abdomen. Radiographic studies have shown dispersal or infiltration of anesthetic agents via the paracervical and pudendal route dorsally along the roots of the pudendal nerve to involve the retropsoas space and the lower lumbosacral plexus. Further spread may continue caudally to involve the sciatic nerve. Immediate and direct therapy is necessary when the diagnosis of abscess is established, with complete drainage, cultures, and appropriate antibiotic treatment.

Lumbosacral Root Lesions

When back pain occurs during pregnancy and is accompanied by radicular complaints, etiologies other than musculoskeletal or mechanical back pain must be considered. There are reports of intervertebral disc protrusion occurring for the first time during pregnancy, or, having pre-existed, becoming symptomatic again during pregnancy.[18] Symptoms and signs of herniated intervertebral discs do not differ in pregnancy patients from those that occur in nonpregnant patients. These include back pain with radiation into one or both extremities, often exacerbated by coughing, sneezing, or straining. Paresthesias may be present in the feet. Muscular weakness may occur and there may be loss of sensation within the root distribution. The most common root levels involved in lumbosacral intervertebral disc disease are the fourth and fifth lumbar and the first sacral roots. The physical findings for each of these root levels are summarized in Table IV. Thus, a decreased knee jerk and decreased sensation along the medial aspect of the leg combined with weakness in muscles of L-4 root origin such as the quadriceps and hip adductors are suggestive of an L-4 lesion. An L-5 lesion is suggested by dimin-

Table IV.
Radicular Lesions: Lumbo Sacral Intervertebral Disc Syndromes

Root	Refex	Sensation	Muscles Involved
L4	Knee jerk	Decreased Medial leg	Adductors (except adductor magnus) (L2, 3, 4) Quadriceps (L2, 3, 4)
L5	Medial Hamstring	Decreased Lateral leg and dorsal foot	Extensor hallucis longus (L5–S1) Posterior Tibialis (L5–S1)
S1	Ankle jerk	Decreased Lateral foot	Soleus (S1–2), gluteus maximus (L5–S1–2)

ished medial hamstring reflexes and the presence of symmetric normal knee and ankle jerks,[19] as well as by decreased sensation along the lateral aspect of the leg extending onto the dorsum of the foot. Muscles of L-5 root origin such as the extensor hallucis longus and tibialis posterior may be weak. First sacral root involvement is indicated by a diminished ankle jerk and diminished sensation along the lateral aspect of the foot and the plantar surface of the foot. Muscles innervated from the first sacral root are the soleus and gluteus maximus. Other root level lesions are less common. Magnetic resonance imaging may be useful in the pregnant patient.[20] Radiological evaluation is usually deferred until after delivery.

Electrodiagnostic studies are physiological diagnostic procedures used to evaluate the patient with possible disc disease. Electromyography of the extremity muscles and the paravertebral muscles in the lumbosacral region is of value in detecting abnormalities and assisting in their localization. Nerve conduction studies are usually normal. A special technique of value in studying S-1 root lesions is the H-reflex, which is the electrophysiological equivalent of the ankle jerk. The H-reflex is usually abnormal in the presence of an S-1 root lesion. Other etiologies of lower back pain discussed in this section would not be associated with electromyographic or nerve conduction abnormalities.[4]

For most cases of lumbar disc disease with radiculopathy, conservative therapy is the treatment of choice. Exceptions would be indicated by bowel and bladder abnormalities suggesting cauda equina lesions and rapidly progressing neurological deficits, which do not improve, despite bed rest. Most authorities now agree that for most cases, a period of bed rest for up to 6 weeks is indicated. For this reason, with the few exceptions noted, there is no great urgency to proceed with invasive diagnostic procedures or surgical intervention. If, with complete bed rest, 80% to 85% relief is achieved, the patient can be carefully mobilized and fitted with a corset, and other methods of pain management can be used such as heat and, sometimes, transcutaneous electrical nerve stimulation. For those patients in whom symptoms persist or recur following ambulation but who do not present with urgent findings indicating a potential need for immediate surgery, further bed rest is suggested, with investigation and treatment after delivery. Several excellent algorithms have been developed for treatment of low back pain, with and without sciatica.[21,22] Surgery for patients, incapacitated with pain, is usually reserved until after the first trimester.

Cervical Root Lesions

Cervical radiculopathy may occur during pregnancy. In most instances, this is secondary to degenerative disc disease that may become symptomatic during the childbearing years. Acute cervical disc herniation is an uncommon finding except in cases of severe injury. Most neck complaints following automobile accidents are musculoligamentous in nature. In a number of instances, neck pain may be postural. As with low back pain, patients with cervical pain should be carefully examined in order to determine whether the problem is postural/mechanical, whether it represents soft tissue injury, or whether radiculopathy with neurological deficit is present. Table V indicates the patterns of abnormality that are found at the various root levels. Electrodiagnostic studies may confirm the presence of a nerve root lesion.[4] Radiographic studies of the cervical spine are not contraindicated in pregnancy provided that shielding of the abdomen and lumbosacral area is done. Except where urgently indicated, however, these studies are best deferred until the postpartum period.

Table V.
Radicular Lesions: Cervical Intervertebral Disc Syndromes

Reflex	Sensation	Additional Muscles Involved—See Reflex
C5 Biceps (C5–6)	Decreased lateral arm	Deltoid (C5–6)
C6 Brachioradialis	Decreased lateral forearm-thumb	Extensor carpi Radialis (C6–7)
C7 Triceps (C7–8)	Decreased middle finger	Long finger flexors (C7–8)
C8	Decreased medial forearm-little finger	Thenar, hypothenar, and hand intrinsics (C8–T1)
T1	Decreased medial arm	Thenar, hypothenar, and hand intrinsics (C8–T1)

Plexus Disorders

Acute brachial plexus neuritis (also called Parsonage-Turner Syndrome or neuralgic amyotrophy) has been reported both as sporadic and familial variants. Both types can occur in females of childbearing age and have been reported during pregnancy. The familial variant is rare, with only about 10 families reported and only 20 cases involving female patients.[23-26] In those families in which females were in the childbearing years, 13 experienced attacks during pregnancy, or, more commonly, immediately postpartum. The condition, when recurrent, has a good prognosis for the individual attack. The sporadic variant is even rarer in pregnancy with only two cases reported—one in the third trimester[27] and the other immediately postpartum.[28] Both patients had bilateral involvement and recovery was variable. The neuritis is usually in the brachial plexus but may involve cranial nerves as well. The plexus involvement causes sensory loss, pain, and paresthesias and weakness and atrophy. Recovery takes place over many months. Prognosis depends on the extent of axonal damage as evidenced by membrane instability on electromyography. Nerve conduction studies, except for an abnormality in the specific nerve involved such as the axillary or radial nerve, are within normal limits. Because reinnervation occurs at a rate of about 1 mm per day, proximal improvement will occur first. If the electromyographic evaluation is within normal limits, a more rapid recovery may be noted. There is no specific treatment and no reports of adverse effects on the pregnancy. Physical and occupational therapy is indicated to strengthen the involved muscles, prevent contractures, insure use of the uninvolved muscles in the weakened extremity, and teach compensation techniques for performance of activities of daily living.

King[29] describes brachial plexus lesions secondary to malpositioning of the arm during delivery. Depending upon positioning or compression, any portion or all of the plexus may be involved. Prognosis depends upon the degree of axonal damage.

Dysesthesias in Pregnancy

During pregnancy, many patients present with complaints of dysesthesias involving the fingers. These complaints tend not to follow a dermatomal or peripheral nerve distribution. Five percent or more of all pregnant women have been reported to be affected.[30] This syndrome has been called brachialgia statica dysesthetica, acrodysesthesia, acroparesthesia, or the droopy shoulder syndrome.

Patients may develop complaints at any stage during pregnancy or postpartum. Benson and Inman[30] describe the symptoms as occurring in the first trimester, while Soferman et al.[31] describe the onset as occurring in the fifth to ninth months of gestation, with an average of 7.2 months. Nocturnal or early morning numbness, tingling, and stiffness of all the fingers of one or both hands are noted. There may be temporary anesthesia and a slight decrease in proprioceptive acuity. In general, however, there are no objective neurological or vascular findings and electrodiagnostic studies are normal. Low set, droopy shoulders and a long swan neck may be noted in some patients. Other patients are thickset with heavy breasts. Symptoms may be provoked by downward traction on the arm with concomitant forced flexion of the head to the opposite side. A Tinel's sign may be found over the brachial plexus. X-rays in certain "long-necked" individuals reveal a visible second thoracic vertebra above the shoulders on lateral cervical spine films. Normally, only six and one-half to seven cervical vertebrae are seen on this view.[32]

There has been speculation as to the etiology of this syndrome. Faulty posture and other factors that place a downward pull on the cervical roots and brachial plexus have been implicated. Enlargement of the breasts and abdomen, edema, and carrying of heavy objects may play a role. Some of the cases reported as having dysesthesias of pregnancy undoubtedly include patients with carpal tunnel syndrome or ulnar nerve compression. Thoracic outlet compression involving muscular or bony structures may produce similar symptoms. In these cases, the presence of a cervical rib may be detected on radiographs, and scalenus muscle and costoclavicular compressions may be suggested by the various thoracic outlet maneuvers for vascular compression[33] or electrodiagnostic evaluation.

Therapy is based on defining the etiologic factors. Postural correction is helpful in many cases. An exercise program is designed to strengthen the shoulder girdle muscles and correct the forward-thrust head and the "droopy" shoulders. Support to heavy breasts by means of strapless, supported brassieres may be helpful. About half of the patients benefit by these measures. In others, the symptoms improve following delivery. Where symptoms persist in the postpartum period, relief of breast engorgement[34] and attention to postural and mechanical factors as well as additional diagnostic studies may be necessary.

Maternal Obstetric Palsies

Lumbosacral plexus lesions are usually secondary to trauma caused by the direct compression of the plexus in the pelvis either by the fetal head or by obstetrical forceps. At greatest risk is the primipara with a large baby or an abnormal pelvis leading to cephalopelvic disproportion and a difficult, often instrumental, delivery.[5] The incidence of maternal obstetric paralysis has been calculated as 1:2,600 to 1:6,400.[35,36] Radiographically, the pelvis may show a straight sacrum, flat and wide posterior pelvis, prominent sacroiliac joint, posterior displacement of the transverse diameter of the inlet, prominent ischial spines, or wide sacroiliac notches.[37]

Anatomically, the most susceptible portion of the lumbosacral plexus is the posterior portion composed of the fourth and fifth lumbar roots. Next at risk are the higher sacral roots. These roots supply the sciatic nerve (peroneal more than tibial division) and the superior gluteal nerve. The upper lumbar plexus and its femoral nerve are protected by the psoas muscle and are distant from the true pelvis. The femoral nerve, however, may be involved by other obstetrical complications. The obturator nerve may be compressed intrapelvically in its course along the lateral pelvic wall to the obturator canal.

The clinical picture reflects the specific portion of the plexus that is compressed. There may be pain or sensory loss in the appropriate dermatomal distributions. There may be foot drop if muscles of the anterior compartment of the leg are weakened, or weakness of the calf muscles if roots responsible for their innervation are compressed. There is weakness of the hip musculature if the gluteal, femoral, or obturator nerve is affected.

Pain during delivery is the dominant complaint and increases with uterine contraction. Specific complaints of either weakness or hypoesthesia may be delayed until after delivery. Management should be individualized and may include cesarean section, epidural anesthesia, or shortening of the second stage of labor by forceps or vacuum extraction. If the pathological mechanism is conduction block (neuropraxia), recovery can be anticipated within weeks to a few months. With more significant compression, axonal degeneration may occur and recovery is delayed while reinnervation proceeds. Sensory symptoms may persist, and some patients may be left with significant disability.[31] King is more pessimistic, saying that "we have never seen complete recovery . . . when outspoken physical signs were discovered on examination. . . ."[29]

The most common residual deficit noted is weakness of ankle dorsiflexion. Postpartum foot drop is most commonly secondary to compression of the lumbosacral trunk (L4-5) in the true pelvis. It occurs in a small woman who is carrying a large fetus, has prolonged labor, and midforceps rotation after a transverse arrest. Foot drop is unilateral and on the same side as the infant's brow during descent through the pelvis.[38] Almost identical symptoms can be produced by compression of the peroneal nerve as it crosses the fibular head. This can be caused by poorly positioned leg holders.[39] Bilateral foot drop has been reported secondary to prolonged squatting in natural childbirth with positional compression or stretch of the peroneal nerve.[40] An L-5 root level lesion or sciatic nerve lesion can also present as foot drop.

Electrodiagnostic evaluation differentiates among the possible causes of foot drop by indicating a root, plexus, or sciatic nerve abnormality, or localized compression of the peroneal nerve. Also, electrodiagnostic evaluation aids prognosis by showing the extent of axonal damage. In addition, prognosis would be influenced by the level of the lesion as determined on the electrodiagnostic study, with the more proximal lesion having the worse prognosis.[4]

Treatment includes the use of an orthosis in order to control foot drop. Physical therapy is prescribed to strengthen paretic muscles as they recover, and to prevent contracture and disuse atrophy of the other muscles in the involved extremity.

The femoral nerve, which is derived from the second, third, and fourth lumbar roots through the lumbar plexus, may be injured in the lithotomy position. Strong flexion of the thighs on the abdomen with abduction and outward rotation produces pressure on the nerve by Poupart's ligament or the iliopsoas muscle.[29] Use of self-retaining retractors in gynecologic surgery has also been associated with injury to the femoral nerve. The causative factor has been described as pressure on the nerve and thus on the vaso nervorum, or on the external iliac artery, either directly or through the psoas muscles. The nerve is most susceptible to this type of injury as it passes over the pelvic brim or under Poupart's ligament.[41] Bilateral postpartum femoral neuropathy has also been associated with hypotension and ischemia of the femoral nerve during prolonged labor.[42] Clinically, patients exhibit weakness of knee extension and loss of the knee jerk. Sensory loss will be over the anterior thigh and medial leg. Hip flexion will be weakened but present. Prognosis for complete functional recovery is good, although it may take several months. Electrodiagnostic testing can confirm that the lesion is limited to the distribution of the femoral nerve.

Obturator nerve compression may occur intrapelvically as mentioned previously. This nerve may also be compressed in the obturator canal.[5,43] Tight application of foot straps can result in damage to the small cutaneous branches of the foot.[38,39]

Sixth cranial (abducens) nerve palsy following a subarachnoid block for obstetrical anesthesia has been reported. This is thought to be the consequence of a dural leak and low cerebrospinal fluid pressure. The nerve is vulnerable to pressure when it courses over the petrous portion of the temporal bone. Complaints include blurring of vision as well as diplopia. Headaches frequently precede the palsy. Prognosis is excellent for a complete return of normal vision.[44] An associated fourth cranial (trochlear) nerve palsy has been reported.[45]

Anterior Horn Cell Disorders

Amyotrophic Lateral Sclerosis

Amyotrophic lateral sclerosis (ALS) is a disease of unknown etiology. It affects the anterior horn of the spinal cord, the cranial nerve nuclei of the pons and medulla, and the cortical upper motor neurons. Because the condition is rare (prevalence 4 per 100,000) and occurs more frequently in males and the older population, case reports in pregnancy in the United States are rare. However, in Guam and the Mariana Islands, the prevalence is 100 times greater. Although there are a number of different clinical presentations,[46] the classic presentation is weakness, atrophy, and fasciculations affecting the distal musculature of the extremities. Bulbar signs and symptoms may be present. Electromyography typically reveals involvement of at least three extremities as well as muscles innervated by cranial nerves.

Motor nerve conductions might be slowed somewhat, but sensory nerve conductions are normal.[4]

Levine and Michels[47] report a woman who developed clinically typical ALS in the sixth month of her second pregnancy. She had a progressive course, and when seen in her third pregnancy was wheelchair-bound with atrophy and weakness of all extremities and severe bulbar palsy. This pregnancy proceeded uneventfully, and a normal infant was delivered vaginally under local pudendal anesthesia. Her postpartum course was uneventful. They make the point that uterine musculature is never involved, and the weakness of the perineal floor actually reduces resistance to parturition. Delivery is usually normal, spontaneous, and associated with an uneventful postpartum course.

Huston et al.[48] studied the effect of ALS on pregnancy and delivery in 17 patients on the island of Guam. They noted there was no specific effect of pregnancy on the course of the disease and that pregnancy did not seem to be altered in any specific way by the disease. Patients who became pregnant late in the course of the disease died prior to delivery. Patients who had advanced disease and survived to term found that motor function, already severely impaired by the illness, frequently became inadequate and that they became bedridden. Enlargement of the uterus impaired respiration and swallowing problems impaired nutrition. Seventeen patients carried to term and delivery was usually spontaneous and uneventful. Infants in all but two instances were normal and showed normal development.

There is no specific medical treatment for ALS. An effective rehabilitation program should be initiated with a goal of maintaining performance at a submaximal level of the patient's endurance to save energy and avoid fatigue, to teach the patient energy conservation, and to assist the patient and family in the selection and utilization of assistive devices. The patient should be kept as active as possible throughout the course of the disease.[49] Long-term management of respiratory failure is discussed by Sivak et al.[50]

Poliomyelitis

Acute poliomyelitis during pregnancy has nearly been eliminated in the Western world by immunization. Dawn and Chandler[51] have reviewed 49 pregnancies in 37 patients who had suffered from childhood poliomyelitis. They found that the obstetric complications were proportional to the clinical disabilities of the patient. Pelvic asymmetry was the main complicating factor and was noted in association with lumbosacral scoliosis, unilateral weight-bearing especially as influenced by the use of external appliances, and reconstructive procedures. Other factors noted include leg muscle imbalance, particularly paralysis of the pelvifemoral and pelvispinal muscles, and paralysis of muscles below the hip. In cases of significant pelvic asymmetry, delivery was by cesarean section. Respiratory difficulties appear to be due to uterine enlargement, which takes up abdominal space so that diaphragmatic excursion is restricted. Respiratory management initially consists of intensive physical therapy and occasionally of positive pressure assistance. When this is no longer adequate, intubation or tracheostomy with intermittent positive pressure ventilation may be necessary. Noninvasive respiratory assistance with the old tank ventilator remains an alternative.[52] Local anesthesia or pudendal block is recommended at delivery rather than other anesthesia in view of the compromised respiration due to the respiratory changes of pregnancy and poliomyelitis.

If an unimmunized pregnant woman is identified, it is recommended that she be immunized. "There is no increase in abortion rate in women vaccinated during the first trimester, and no teratogenic effects attributable to the administration of the vaccine have been encountered."[53] In patients with acute poliomyelitis, the rate of abortion is increased, especially in the first trimester. Krieger[54] states that the determination of the best mode and time for delivery of the patient with acute poliomyelitis is guided by the state of the patient's respirations. "In nonrespirator cases, spontaneous labor and vaginal delivery can be awaited even if all four extremities are involved. In patients with acute, severe, progressive bulbar and spinal poliomyelitis who are 4 to 6 weeks before term, cesarean section is probably indicated to relieve stress on the mother and to ensure a live infant. . . . The danger of respiratory embarrassment makes the anesthesia of choice for vaginal delivery pudendal block, and for cesarean section, local infiltration."[54] In modern obstetrics, regional anesthesia is probably the method of choice.

Peripheral Neuropathies

Any peripheral neuropathy that may present in a nonpregnant patient may present in a pregnant patient. Many peripheral neuropathies are described, but this discussion will be limited to those reported to occur in pregnant patients or those that may occur in association with medical conditions commonly found in women in the childbearing years. Presenting complaints suggestive of neuropathy usually include distal paresthesias or dysesthesias more commonly starting in the lower rather than in the upper extremities. Weakness may be a presenting feature. Physical examination reveals altered distal sensation, loss of reflexes, usually initially at the ankle, and weakness and atrophy of distal muscles. Electrodiagnostic evaluation demonstrates abnormalities of motor or sensory conduction, particularly in conditions that cause demyelination. In diseases affecting the axons, the amplitude of the evoked nerve conduction response is diminished, and electromyography reveals evidence of membrane instability or abnormal motor units and summation patterns. Specific laboratory abnormalities depend on the etiology of the peripheral neuropathy.

Hereditary Neuropathy

Charcot-Marie-Tooth Disease

Charcot-Marie-Tooth disease (hereditary motor and sensory neuropathy type 1) is an autosomal dominant hypertrophic neuropathy with slowly progressive, symmetric, muscular atrophy first involving the feet and legs (stork-leg appearance) and then hands and forearms. Peripheral sensory loss also occurs. Electrodiagnostic studies reveal remarkably slow nerve conduction velocities. Bellina and Deming[55] reported on a patient who completed six pregnancies without obstetric complications but who had an exacerbation of the neuropathy with each pregnancy and no progression between pregnancies. They mention that a sibling also had experienced an exacerbation during pregnancy. Pollock et al.[56] reported on a previously asymptomatic patient who had subclinical Charcot-Marie-Tooth disease exacerbated in the third trimester. Following cesarean section, there was immediate improvement. Biopsy revealed neural edema. They conclude that "affected women can be reassured that recovery will follow pregnancy".[11] There is a risk of earlier onset and more severe exacerbations in subsequent pregnancies. Each attack increases the likelihood of permanent neurological disability.

Familial Dysautonomia

Familial dysautonomia or Riley-Day syndrome[57] is an autosomal recessive genetic disorder. The autonomic nervous system and certain portions of the sensory nervous system are affected. Clinical presentation includes lack of overflow tears, short stature, postural hypotension, absent deep tendon reflexes, and impaired sensation of pain, temperature, and taste. Other features include vomiting attacks, pneumonia, spinal curvature, abnormal histamine tests, lack of fungiform papillae on the tongue, and pupillary supersensitivity to methacholine chloride.

Prognostically, 50% of patients die by age 4, but a number also reach adulthood. Puberty is delayed, with 50% of women having menarche after 16 years of age. The two patients in the report by Porges et al.[57] are the first known to have conceived. They carried the pregnancies to near term and had phenotypically normal heterozygous infants. Uterine contractions and labor were initiated normally, and vaginal delivery occurred. Cardiovascular, gastrointestinal, and renal dysfunction related to the primary disease presented complicated but not insurmountable clinical problems.

Metabolic Neuropathy

Porphyria

The acute porphyrias include acute intermittent porphyria, porphyria variegata, and hereditary coproporphyria. They are the result of an inborn error of heme biosynthesis. The usual clinical presentation of acute intermittent porphyria is acute abdominal pain, often with vomiting and constipation. Neuropathy, when it occurs following the abdominal symptoms[34] may be motor, sensory, and autonomic and may even progress to quadriplegia with bulbar and respiratory paralysis. The central manifestations include mental disturbance, convulsions, hypothalamic dysfunction, and extrapyramidal signs. All of the clinical manifestations of the acute attack have been explained as being caused by neurogenic dysfunction within the central and peripheral nervous systems.[58] Two unusual clinical features suggestive of porphyric neuropathy are the preservation of the ankle jerk with loss of tendon reflexes elsewhere, and a trunk or bathing suit distribution of superficial sensory loss. Laboratory findings include increased urinary excretion of δ-aminolevulinic acid and porphobilinogen in acute intermittent porphyria. Burgundy-colored urine is described, and the Watson-Schwartz test will show the characteristic color change.

There have been several reviews of the effect of the acute porphyrias on pregnancy. Brodie et al.[59] reviewed the obstetric histories of 50 woman with acute porphyria of whom 39 had acute intermittent porphyria, 3 had variegate porphyria, and 8 had hereditary coproporphyria. Fifty-four percent of the women with acute intermittent porphyria had an attack during pregnancy or in the puerperium. One maternal death was recorded. One patient with variegate porphyria and two with hereditary coproporphyria had attacks related to the pregnancy. There was 13% fetal loss and the infants born to mothers who sustained attacks of acute intermittent porphyria were smaller than those who remained healthy.[59] Donaldson, in his review of reported cases of exacerbation of acute intermittent porphyria during pregnancy, noted that 60% of exacerbations occurred in early pregnancy and that the majority of these episodes did not affect a successful pregnancy outcome. Fifteen percent of exacerbations occurred later in pregnancy and were associated with prematurity and high maternal and fetal mortality rates. Postpartum cases accounted for 25%, and it was thought that intrapartum administration of barbiturates precipitated the attacks. Respiratory paralysis was a serious complication.[60]

In general, pregnancy seems to precipitate attacks, possibly due to hormonal changes. A number of drugs have been implicated, notably barbiturates, sulfonamides, phenytoin, estrogens and progesterone, as well as fasting, febrile illness, and surgical procedures.

The best treatment is prevention and thus avoidance of precipitating factors. Symptomatic treatment is important in the management of abdominal symptoms and chlorpromazine or other phenothiazines may be used for this purpose. Propranolol can be used to treat sinus tachycardia and hypertension.[39] Treatment with hematin has been effective in approximately 50% of cases.[58]

Toxic Neuropathy

Peripheral neuropathies may occur as toxic reactions to certain medications such as phenytoin, sulfanomides, or nitrofurantoin. Lane and Routledge[61] have extensively reviewed drug-induced neurological disorders including those causing peripheral neuropathy, myasthenia gravis and myasthenic syndromes, and myopathies. King[29] reviewed the use of some historical abortifacients that may cause peripheral neuropathies and present either as polyneuropathy or mononeuropathy superimposed on an underlying subclinical peripheral neuropathy. Electrodiagnostic studies have also revealed evidence of peripheral neuropathy in drug abusers using heroin or LSD.[62] Neuropathies due to heavy metal exposure or exposure to organic compounds have been reported in cases of personal abuse and also related to employment. Review of the recent medical literature has not revealed any specific reports of pregnancy associated with any of these causes of peripheral neuropathy.

A case of ingestion of a food toxin (ciguatoxin) from eating reef fish by a pregnant patient near term has been published.[63] Symptoms developed in 4 hours and included nausea, weakness, and paresthesias and hyperesthesias of the fingers, lips, scalp, and tongue. Bizarre fetal movements were noted. Cesarean section delivered a male infant with a left-sided facial palsy and possible myotonia of small hand muscles. Meconium was present in the fluid and the baby required intensive care for respiratory distress syndrome. At 6 weeks, the infant had not smiled, but was otherwise normal. The mother had residual hyperesthesia, including that of the nipple during attempted breast feeding. Ciguatea fish poisoning is not uncommon, with 129 cases occurring in the Miami area in 1980.[64]

Diabetic Neuropathy

Although pregnancy is diabetogenic, diabetic neuropathy is not usually a condition that begins or is exacerbated in pregnancy.[65,66] Neuropathic abnormalities from various etiologies tend to be additive and neuropathies from other causes may, of course, appear in the pregnant diabetic as in other pregnant patients. White[66] found that most of the neuropathies in her pregnant diabetics were sensory and, if dysesthetic, responded to analgesics. Neuropathy in diabetics tends to affect sensory before motor nerves, and legs before arms.

Diabetic amyotrophy is clinically defined by the sudden onset of pain over the anterior thigh with resolution of the pain as weakness develops. Either one or both legs may be involved at different times. Lumbar root, lumbar plexus, or femoral nerve variants of this syndrome, with different distributions of weakness, have been described.[67] Diabetic polyradiculoneuritis (of which diabetic amyotrophy is one variant) may also produce thoracic[68] or abdominal[69] pain that must be considered in the differential diagnosis of acute abdominal complaints. Treatment of these diabetic neurological syndromes includes good diabetic management and symptomatic support.[70] During pregnancy, improvement of the postural hypotension associated with diabetic autonomic neuropathy has been reported. This was ascribed to the increase in blood volume that begins in the first trimester.

Nutritional Neuropathy

Gestational or nutritional neuropathy associated with pregnancy is now rare in the Western world, since emphasis on proper nutrition, including vitamin supplements, has been instituted in the care of the pregnant patient. Etiologic factors include alcoholism, hyperemesis gravidarum, and fad diets.[71]

Mild neuropathy with encephalopathy and severe neuropathy without encephalopathy have been described.[60] Transient subjective sensory complaints are most common, although severe paralysis with pronounced cognitive disturbances may develop. Polyneuritis symptoms may include painful burning with hyperesthesias and hypersensitive skin.[5] Numbness and tingling begin in the extremities and extend to the trunk or face. Muscular weakness with loss of tendon reflexes occurs. Less characteristic features are optic neuritis, central deafness, choreiform movements of the head, and involuntary urination.

Mortality rates vary from 18% to 68% in different series.[72] When recovery from paralysis occurs, it is usually reasonably complete but slow. Death is usually due to intercurrent disease or respiratory paralysis. The fetal death rate is high. Treatment should include prophylactic use of thiamine or vitamin B complex. After the onset of symptoms, vitamin treatment is less effective, especially in cases with advanced disease. Breast feeding should be avoided in all but the mildest forms. There are different opinions with regard to terminating the pregnancy, with suggested indications for abortion including vagus or phrenic nerve involvement, ascending paralysis, severe hyperemesis, psychosis, and lack of response to conservative therapy.

Wernicke's encephalopathy with ataxia and gaze palsies can occur. Korsakoff's psychosis can develop with confusion and severe memory deficits with confabulation. Severe or late manifestations of thiamine deficiency (wet form of beriberi) include anorexia, serous effusion, edema, and cardiac insufficiency with tachycardia or dyspnea.[29]

Infectious Neuropathy

Leprosy

The most common cause of neuropathy worldwide is leprosy. Neuritis in pregnancy and the puerperium caused by leprosy has been reported by Duncan and Pearson.[73] Causation is ascribed to the ability of the organsim to enter nerves and multiply within Schwann cells. In their series, the authors describe the condition as occurring in patients with active leprosy and in those who had discontinued treatment because of assumed cure. Overt neuritis, with pain and nerve tenderness was encountered. Silent neuritis, with progressive loss of sensory and motor function, occurs more frequently than overt neuritis. Patients should be examined for motor and sensory loss clinically and by means of nerve conduction studies and treated with appropriate medications for the disease.

HIV-Associated Neuropathies

A discussion of HIV-associated neuropathies is found in Chapter 6.

Idiopathic Neuropathies

Landry-Guillain-Barré-Strohl Syndrome

Landry-Guillain-Barré-Strohl syndrome, or acute inflammatory polyradiculoneuritis, is an immunologically mediated demyelinative neuropathy.[74] The reported incidence in the female population is 0.4 per 100,000.[75] Sixty-seven percent of patients have been reported as having had an antecedent illness within 8 weeks prior to onset of symptoms. The peak period of onset of Guillain-Barré syndrome is in the second week after the onset of the prior illness. Five percent of patients report having undergone surgery prior to onset, and 4.5% report having received vaccinations.

Clinical criteria required for diagnosis[74] include the following: rapid progression of the symptoms and signs of motor weakness, reaching a maximum by 4 weeks into the illness; relative symmetry of weakness; mild sensory symptoms or signs; involvement of cranial nerves including the facial, which occurs in approximately 50% of cases, and less often cranial nerves innervating the tongue, and muscles of deglutition. Autonomic dysfunction can occur including arrhythmias and extremes of blood pressure. Recovery usually begins within 2 to 4 weeks after maximum weakness has been reached.

The incidence of the syndrome during pregnancy is low, with approximately 30 cases reported in the obstetric literature over the past 70 years.[76,77] Furthermore, there is no evidence that the incidence is dissimilar in pregnant and nonpregnant women.[78] There is no evidence that pregnancy affects the severity of the syndrome, and the pregnancy appears to be unaffected.[5] Early spontaneous abortion has been reported once in the literature. There is too little information to suggest an increase in the frequency of abortion.[77] In patients with the onset of symptoms during the first or second trimester, pregnancy proceeded without complications in most cases, and parturition was normal.[77] As with other neurological diseases, uterine contractility is not impaired but with paresis of abdominal muscles, second stage assistance may be necessary. In the third trimester, there is a risk of premature labor, and Bravo et al.[76] have warned that "the pregnant woman . . . may not be able to perceive or report the presence or absence of uterine contractions and fetal movements. Weekly pelvic examinations and nonstress testing should be routinely performed."

The three cases of maternal mortality reported in the literature occurred with onset of symptoms in the third trimester and were associated with respiratory difficulties and aspiration pneumonia.[79–81]

Fetal prognosis is generally favorable. Most infants born to mothers with Guillain-Barré syndrome are normal, and no associated fetal anomaly has been reported in the literature.[81] Of the 30 pregnancies reported between Ahlberg and Ahlmark's study[77] and the subsequent case reported by Bravo et al.,[76] the infant survival rate exceeded 88%. Three babies died shortly after parturition from complications that were not related to the syndrome.[77]

When the diagnosis is made, the patient should be hospitalized and monitored. At present, there are no preventive or curative treatments available for the patient. Plasmapheresis decreases the duration of respirator dependence and hastens functional recovery.[82] However, plasmapheresis is associated with hypovolemia and vasovagal reactions may occur.[83] The goal is to provide supportive treatment, prevent musculoskeletal contractures and peripheral nerve compressions, protect the skin, and prevent venous thrombosis.[84]

Pulmonary function and blood gases should be closely monitored and, with a decline in respiratory function, the patient should be placed in an intensive care unit. Early intubation is indicated if there is difficulty in maintaining an adequate airway and if there are problems with secretions. If respiratory paralysis occurs, and the patient is near term, cesarean section is probably the treatment of choice. Otherwise, delivery may be vaginal. Analgesia that can interfere with respiratory function should be minimized; thus, prepared childbirth techniques and local anesthetics are preferred. Delivery, because of inadequate propulsive forces and a prolonged second stage, may require vacuum or forceps extraction.[76]

Chronic Relapsing Polyneuritis

A chronic relapsing polyneuritis associated with pregnancy has been described,[85] with a sensorimotor polyneuropathy of slow onset, reaching a maximum disability after 6 to 12 months. The course is usually steadily progressive, and/or relapsing-remitting, thus distinguishing it from the Guillain-Barré syndrome. A significant increase in the number of relapses during pregnancy may occur, and there is a tendency for the symptoms to worsen in the third trimester or immediately postpartum.[86] There is marked slowing of nerve conduction velocities. Cerebrospinal fluid protein is elevated. Other than an association with HIV infection, there is no evidence of other etiologic causes of this neuropathy, and serum immunoglobulin electrophoresis is normal.[87] Sural nerve biopsy reveals segmental demyelination. Pregnancies in patients with this condition were carried to term, and deliveries were normal, either vaginal or cesarean. In one case, a third episode of recurrent polyneuropathy occurred while taking oral contraceptives.[88] One patient responded to corticosteroid management.[89]

Entrapment/Compression Syndromes

Carpal Tunnel Syndrome

Carpal tunnel syndrome is the most common compression syndrome. Patients usually complain of burning dysesthesias or numbness affecting the fingers. Symptoms are frequently bilateral. There are frequently sensations of swelling. Symptoms may arouse the patient from sleep and may be relieved by shaking the hands. The symptoms typically involve the thumb and adjacent two and one-half fingers, or may be described as involving the whole hand. Not uncommonly, there are complaints of aching pain in the forearm, which may extend to the shoulder. Repetitive activities that place the wrist in extension or flexion, such as driving or holding a book, may elicit symptoms.

Physical findings include diminished sensation over the thumb and adjacent two and one-half fingers. Thenar eminence sensation is usually normal. Weakness of the median nerve innervated abductor pollicis brevis and opponens pollis may be noted, but atrophy of these muscles is rarely found in carpal tunnel syndrome associated with pregnancy. Tinel's sign can be positive over the median nerve at the wrist. There may be symptoms when the wrist is placed in either hyperextension or hyperflexion (Phalen's manuever).

Association of DeQuervain's tenosynovitis, carpal tunnel syndrome, and pregnancy has been reported. Additional physical findings include those associated with thumb and ulnar deviation of the wrist (Finkelstein's sign).[90] Conservative treatment includes splinting of the thumb and wrist in slight extension leaving the interphalangeal joint free, nonsteroidal anti-inflammatory drugs, or local steroid injection.[91]

Many systemic illnesses are associated with carpal tunnel syndrome,[92] including diabetes mellitus, other endocrine disorders, and infections. Frequently, median nerve irritation is associated with jobs that require repetitive activity. In many cases, no etiologic factor is found.

The carpal tunnel anatomically has a floor made up of the carpal bones and the roof is formed by the transverse carpal ligament. Contents, in addition to median nerve, are the tendons of the long finger flexors. Computed tomography has shown that in patients with carpal tunnel syndrome, the cross-sectional area is reduced as compared to normal controls.[93] Diagnosis is usually suspected clinically, and then confirmed by nerve conduction studies. Melvin et al.[94] were able to diagnose' the presence of carpal tunnel syndrome in 15 of 36 pregnant women complaining of symptoms. Recently reported modifications of nerve conduction techniques are more sensitive and allow electrodiagnostic confirmation in a higher percentage of clinically suspected cases of carpal tunnel syndrome.[95,96]

Voitk et al.[97] interviewed 1,000 consecutive postpartum patients by questionnaire. Twenty-five percent had symptoms of carpal tunnel syndrome. Onset most often is between the fourth and ninth month of gestation. Symptoms may be unilateral or bilateral but most frequently appear first in the dominant hand.[42] Edema has been one postulated etiology, and it has been shown that the rate of ring removal because of swelling in pregnancy was twice as great for women with symptoms of carpal tunnel syndrome as for asymptomatic women.[97] Possibly, the height of the carpal tunnel is reduced in pregnancy because of relaxation of the transverse carpal ligament. This ligament is stretched, allowing the arch of the carpal bones to flatten. The decreased height leads to increased compression of the median nerve in the carpal tunnel.[94,98]

Massey,[92] in his review on carpal tunnel syndrome in pregnancy, stated that symptoms may persist for as long as 12 weeks postparum, with gradual disappearance. Occasionally, symptoms may disappear as rapidly as in the first 48 hours after parturition.[99] Sometimes symptoms do not disappear and may even recur with succeeding pregnancies. Tobin[100] found that 85% of cases of carpal tunnel syndrome associated with pregnancy cleared spontaneously. Fifteen percent of his series required surgical decompression, and all of these patients obtained complete relief. Five of his patients had recurrence of the syndrome with subsequent pregnancies.[100] Because such a high proportion of cases of carpal tunnel syndrome resolves spontaneously after delivery, initial symptomatic treatment appears to be indicated. Patients with mild symptoms and minor electrodiagnostic abnormalities appear to respond well to conservative management.[101] Analgesics and diuretics have also been used for treatment.[102] Patients who do not benefit from conservative treatment should be considered for surgical decompression of the carpal tunnel. It should be pointed out that there can be morbidity associated with this surgical procedure. Partial to complete division of the median nerve may occur, repeat surgery may be necessary because the distal border of the transverse carpal ligament or flexor retinaculum has not been devided, and misdiagnosis can occur with symptoms not relieved by decompression of the median nerve.[103,104] Between 5% and 30% of patients complain of postoperative complications.[103]

There has been one case report of reflex sympathetic dystrophy associated with carpal tunnel syndrome and pregnancy. Hand symptoms and signs included severe burning and aching pain, itching and redness, edema, and hyperhidrosis. Management required a series of stellate ganglion blocks in order to alleviate signs and symptoms; postpartum findings resolved.[105]

Ulnar Nerve Compression

In a study of 1,216 consecutive postpartum patients, McLennon et al.[106] found that 2% complained of symptoms of ulnar nerve compression. The most common site of compression of the ulnar nerve is at the elbow over the ulnar sulcus (olecranon groove) and, more rarely, at the wrist in Guyon's tunnel. External compression of the nerve is the usual etiology in this age group. Symptoms include paresthesias in the little and ulnar half of the ring fingers if the lesion is at the level of the wrist. If the lesion is more proximal, the hypothenar eminence and dorsum of the ulnar aspect of the hand may be involved. Weakness, depending on the level of the lesion, involves the ulnar innervated forearm muscles, particularly the flexor digitorum profundus to the ring and little fingers, as well as the ulnar innervated muscles of the hand. Tinel's sign can be positive either across the elbow or at the wrist. Atrophy may be seen. Nerve conduction studies confirm the presence of a lesion, either at the elbow or at the wrist. Treatment is usually symptomatic particularly involving protection of the nerve so that further compression does not occur. It is rarely necessary to transpose the ulnar nerve.[92]

Compression or entrapment syndromes have been reported for most of the other nerves of the upper extremity, but not in association with pregnancy and will not be discussed further in this review. Thoracic outlet syndromes may also present with ulnar nerve symptoms (see section on *Dysesthesias in Pregnancy* in this chapter).

Tarsal Tunnel Syndrome

The equivalent of the carpal tunnel syndrome in the lower extremities is the tarsal tunnel syndrome. Symptoms inlcude tingling, numbness, burning, and pain in the foot, particularly on the sole of the foot and dorsal and volar aspects of the toes. Complaints may extend up the leg. Symptoms are aggravated by prolonged standing or walking and frequently occur at night. The underlying cause of this problem is compression of the posterior tibial nerve beneath the flexor retinaculum at the ankle. Helm et al.[107] examined 164 pregnant women. Abnormalities of nerve conduction of the tibial nerve were found in 92 patients (56.1%). Of these 92 subjects, 57.6% had symptoms of leg cramps or burning feet. An additional 11.9% had other leg complaints. Thirteen subjects who had abnormal conduction studies of tibial nerves were examined 6 weeks postpartum, with 12 showing reversion to normal values. The authors concluded that "there appears to be a correlation between tibial nerve dysfunction during pregnancy and the many symptoms pregnant women have related to their legs and feet." Thus, tibial nerve dysfunction, including tarsal tunnel syndrome, should be considered in the differential diagnosis of leg complaints, including leg cramps.

Meralgia Paresthetica

Meralgia paresthetica is a syndrome caused by compression of the lateral femoral cutaneous nerve of the thigh, either under the inguinal ligament, medial to the anterior superior iliac spine,[108,109] or retroperitoneally where the proximal components of the nerve angulate over the sacroiliac joint.[21] Symptoms may be severe pain, numbness, tingling, or hyperesthesia in the anterolateral aspect of the thigh. There are no motor findings because this is a pure sensory nerve. Symptoms are exaggerated in the standing position by extending the hip and are relieved by sitting or lying down.

In pregnant women, symptoms occur beginning about the 30th week of pregnancy[110] and may be bilateral. There can be a recurrence with subsequent pregnancies.[111] The underlying cause is the increasing girth of the abdomen and the exaggerated lumbar lordosis of pregnancy, both of which tend to stretch the nerve and make it more vulnerable to compression. After delivery, improvement in symptoms can be expected.[112] A diagnostic test and symptomatic treatment is the injection of a local anesthetic near the anterior superior iliac spine where the nerve may be compressed under the inguinal ligament, or infiltration about the sacroiliac joint.[21] Surgery is seldom advised.

Intercostal Neuralgia

Intercostal neuralgia of pregnancy has been described.[113] Painful dysesthesias were noted in the right hypochondrium. In one case study, these occurred in each of two pregnancies. The occurrence was in the sixth to eighth months of gestation. There was abatement of symptoms in the immediate postpartum period, leaving a small hypoesthetic zone just to the right of the xyphoid process. The area of involvement encompassed the anterior divisions of the eighth through the eleventh intercostal nerves. Full term infants were delivered without incident. Intercostal neuralgia may be misdiagnosed as pain due to intra-abdominal disease. It should be recognized as a benign entity, so that unnecessary measures are not used in treatment. Other neurological conditions that can mimic intra-abdominal disease include acute porphyria and diabetic polyradiculoneuritis.

Facial or Bell's Palsy

The frequency of a peripheral facial palsy in pregnant women is 45.1 per 100,000 births. For nonpregnant women of the same age group, the frequency is 17.4 per 100,000 per year. Per year of exposure, the risk to pregnant women is 3.3 times the risk to nonpregnant women of the same age group. The greatest incidence is in the third trimester and early puerperium where Hilsinger[3] calculated a frequency of 118.2 per 100,000 per year of exposure. Recurrence in subsequent pregnancies has been reported, as has bilateral involvement.[114]

The onset of Bell's palsy is usually sudden. The patient awakens in the morning and finds that one half of the face is paralyzed. She may be concerned that she has had a stroke, but facial weakness secondary to an upper motor neuron lesion usually affects principally the lower portion of the face, sparing the forehead. The patient with Bell's palsy cannot raise her eyebrow, completely close her eye, or purse her lips to kiss, whistle, or smile. Food accumulates between teeth and cheek. Sensation of the face is unimpaired. If the lesion is proximal to the branching of the chorda tympani from the facial nerve, taste sensation over the anterior two thirds of the tongue on the same side is lost. Hyperacusis and increased tearing can be noted. Bilateral facial palsy is rare; in such cases it should be remembered that Guillain-Barré syndrome may present as facial palsy.[115] Pain can occur with some aching posterior to the ear.

Electrodiagnostic study allows localization of the lesion to the facial nerve. In addition, if the patient is seen within days of onset, progression or lack of progression of the lesion can be determined. If the lesion is severe, treatment with corticosteroids may be indicated. Hilsinger et al.[3] used methylprednisolone treatment during pregnancy and each of their patients delivered a normal infant. One worthwhile caveat is "that steroids should not be given to pregnant women with Bell's palsy unless concurrent viral infection has been excluded."[116]

If the paralysis remains incomplete, and there is no evidence of denervation on electromyography, recovery can be expected in 3 to 6 weeks. If partial denervation has occurred, partial function might return in 3 weeks but it is likely to take up to 12 weeks for maximum recovery.[117] In the presence of a complete lesion, our experience is that recovery will be partial and that patients may develop synkinesis of facial movements and tearing with eating. Adour[115] has stated that, in his patients, facial nerve decompression has not been performed since 1970.

While waiting for recovery from facial nerve palsy, symptomatic treatment should be initiated. In particular, if eye closure is not complete, the conjunctiva should be examined. Conjunctival irritation can be prevented by patching of the eye and using artificial tears. Ophthalmologic referral is indicated if irritation is present. Use of facial muscle massage and exercises in a home program may help prevent contractures while waiting for reinnervation of the muscles. Electrical stimulation has been shown to delay atrophy in muscles following nerve injury and may have some value. Its use requires frequent application, several times daily, and is best done as a home program with a portable stimulator until there is either electrodiagnostic or clinical evidence of partial recovery.

The etiology of Bell's palsy remains unclear. Some studies have shown an associated increased incidence with pre-eclampsia/toxemia. There is speculation about a relationship to edema or hormonal changes in pregnancy.[117] A viral etiology has been postulated.[3,116,117] Other causes of facial paresis may need to be excluded before the diagnosis of Bell's palsy is accepted—e.g., Lyme disease and sarcoidosis.

Melkersson-Rosenthal Syndrome

Melkersson-Rosenthal syndrome consists of the triad of peripheral facial nerve paralysis, noninflammatory swelling of the lips and face, and lingua plicata. The facial palsy is of a variable severity. A case report in association with pregnancy was published by Allen and Weil;[118] this syndrome does not appear to affect pregnancy, nor does pregnancy seem to affect the disease. Labor was rapid and uneventful with delivery of a viable infant.

Myoneural Junction Disorders

The primary disorder affecting the myoneural junction is myasthenia gravis. This condition is discussed in Chapter 11. There are other less common disorders affecting the myoneural junction. Myasthenic syndrome has been reported as being associated with pregnancy. In their review of drug-induced neurological disorders, Lane and Routledge[61] list drugs that have been reported to cause myasthenia gravis and myasthenic syndrome such as some aminoglycosides, phenytoin, and D-penicillamine. In addition, certain disorders such as amyotrophic lateral sclerosis or peripheral neuropathy may give an electrodiagnostic response similar to that seen with myasthenia gravis.[4]

Myopathies

Myopathy is usually suggested by a chief complaint of pelvic or shoulder girdle weakness. Exceptions are myotonic dystrophy and inclusion body myositis, which affect the distal muscles. Atrophy may be noted, and reflexes may be decreased late in the clinical course of the disease. Sensation is not affected.[4]

Myotonic Dystrophy

It has been said that to make the diagnosis of myotonic dystrophy, one should "always shake the hand of the pregnant patient with cataracts."[119] This statement succinctly summarizes the clinical characteristics of the pregnant patient with myotonic dystrophy. Myotonia refers to stiffness and difficulty in relaxing the grip. Cataracts are reported in 90% of patients. These are of the posterior subcapsular type and seldom interfere with vision. Menstrual irregularity and infertility are considered to be common but multiple reports discuss myotonic dystrophy and pregnancy. Other clinical features include wasting of the temporal muscles, ptosis of the eyelids, wasting and weakness of the neck muscles including the sternocleidomastoids that are described as strap-like, premature balding, weakness and atrophy of the small muscles of the hand, difficulty in swallowing, and respiratory muscle weakness. Smooth muscle involvement may be manifested by dysphagia, hoarseness, and nasal regurgitation.[120] Mental retardation is not uncommon.[121]

The disease is transmitted as an autosomal dominant trait and therefore males and females are affected equally.[121] The underlying problems in muscles have been variably described as a failure of the calcium adenosine triphosphate system[119] or as an abnormality of membrane chloride permeability. Myotonia has been treated with phenytoin (teratogenic potential must be considered), quinine, or procainamide, but the disease process itself cannot be altered. Quinine or procainamide shuld be avoided in patients with evidence of cardiac conduction disorders.

Most authors believe that pregnancy is uncommon in myotonic dystrophy. However, Webb and co-authors[121] report on the course and outcome of 23 pregnancies in six women affected by myotonic dystrophy and a seventh patient who had 14 pregnancies. A high rate of complications including polyhydramnios, premature onset of labor, postpartum hemorrhage, and neonatal death were noted. Direct observation of an atonic uterus at cesarean section suggests other evidence that uterine muscles may be affected. No change in muscular weakness and atrophy was noted in the one patient they followed throughout pregnancy. In one review, myotonic dystrophy worsened in 12 of 18 pregnant patients.[120] Deterioration usually occurred in the latter part of the second trimester and marked improvement was noted immediately postpartum. The authors postulated that an increase in the level of circulating progesterone adversely affected cell membranes, leading to functional deterioration. A few patients have been reported in which clinical features first become apparent during pregnancy.[122]

Prolonged labor has been described as a consistent complication of myotonic dystrophy. Shore[122] has summarized the findings of the three stages of labor. First stages between 24–51 hours have been reported. The second stage has been complicated by poor voluntary assistance because of severe weakness of the abdominal muscles. Excessive length of this stage has been associated with fetal stress and death. The failure of the uterus to contract normally has complicated the third stage of labor, resulting in postpartum hemorrhages. Manual removal of the placenta is sometimes necessary. Uterine inertia is responsive to oxytocin.[123] Shore[122] has also summarized the neonatal and infant complications associated with myotonic dystrophy. These include respiratory and feeding problems, and musculoskeletal dysfunction. Of 35 reported pregnancies[120] in one study, nine infants were either stillborn or died during the neonatal period of respiratory insufficiency.

Maternal deaths in pregnant patients with myotonic dystrophy are uncommon. The reported causes of death are cardiac failure and aspiration pneumonia.[120] Pre-existing respiratory impairment may be worsened during the course of pregnancy. Sedation used at delivery may further impair respiration, and temporary unresponsiveness after sedation has been reported.[124] It is acceptable to use local and regional anesthetics in myotonic dystrophy patients in labor. Electro-cardiographic monitoring should be done to detect any abnormality in cardiac conduction.

Genetic counseling is important since there is a 50% chance of myotonic dystrophy occurring in the offspring of affected family members.[125] Detection of a genetic marker would allow antenatal diagnosis of myotonic dystrophy and the consideration of selective abortion. Chromosomal localization techniques have identified chromosome 19 as the involved chromosome[126] and currently, Apolipoprotein C2[127] as the closest and most useful genetic marker. "Prenatal prediction is feasible in the first trimester of pregnancy using chorion villus biopsy."[125,128]

Myotonia Congenita

Myotonia congenita, or Thomsen's disease, is an autosomal dominant muscle disorder. The outstanding feature of this condition is myotonia and increased muscle bulk. Symptoms become evident by the time a child begins to walk. Limb muscles are more affected than cranial muscles, but all muscles may be involved with myotonia. Electromyographic evaluation reveals the presence of myotonic discharges.[129]

Three cases of pregnancy associated with congenital myotonia have been reported.[129,131] Myotonia worsened in the second half of pregnancy and improved after childbirth. In two cases, no obstetric problems were noted. The neurological examination of one of the infants has been reported, and although the child did not have clinical evidence of myotonia, electromyography on the sixth postnatal day showed some myotonic discharges.[129] In the third case, upon examination of the patient after initiation of labor, it was noted that the fetal heartbeat was absent. Uterine contractions were recorded during labor and were normal. Autopsy failed to reveal any abnormality to explain the intrauterine death of the fetus.[131]

Malignant Hyperpyrexia or Hyperthermia

Malignant hyperpyrexia has been associated with congenital myotonia.[132] Search of the medical literature has not revealed any reported cases of malignant hyperpyrexia associated with pregnancy or delivery. Sonenklar and Rendell-Baker[133] have stated that this may be due to the fact that muscle relaxants and halothane usage as anesthesia during pregnancy are probably the exception rather than the rule in the United States, and thus the numbers of patients exposed to this risk may be quite small.

Myophosphorylase Deficiency

Myophosphorylase deficiency (McArdle's disease) is a rare autosomal recessive myopathy characterized by symptoms of muscular fatigue and cramps during exercise. Myoglobinuria and elevation of serum creatinine phosphokinase can occur during exercise. Muscle biopsy reveals glycogen storage and the absence of phosphorylase activity. Symptoms can be alleviated by the administration of glucose and fructose. A case report[134] revealed that there was no exacerbation of symptoms during pregnancy. Uterine contractions during the first stage of labor were short and ineffective. Oxytocin was used, and the first stage was completed in 21 hours. Progress in the second stage was also slow because of the lack of a pushing reflex, felt to be secondary to the epidural analgesia used during the delivery. Delivery was assisted with forceps. A normal infant was delivered, and there were no complications to mother or child in the puerperium.

Polymyositis/Dermatomyositis

Polymyositis is a connective tissue disorder of muscle characterized by progressive muscle weakness. Involved muscles may be tender and histologically there is evidence of muscle destruction. Electromyographic studies reveal evidence of membrane instability, myopathic motor units, and bizarre high-frequency discharges. Thirty-one pregnant patients have been reported in the medical literature.[135–141] In all but three cases, dermatomyositis or polymyositis antedated the pregnancy. During pregnancy, the disease may exacerbate, improve, or remain unchanged. An infant mortality rate of 40% to 60% is reported.[136,138] If the disease remains quiescent during pregnancy, a successful outcome can be anticipated.[139] If exacerbation occurs, aggressive corticosteroid therapy may minimize fetal loss.[139]

Patients may be treated with immunosuppressive agents but the teratogenic potential is to be considered.[139,141]

Other Myopathies

Houston and Turner[142] reported a pregnant patient who had a jejunoileal bypass. She developed hypokalemic paralysis as well as severe hypocalcemia and hypomagnesemia. Muscle enzymes were elevated and normalized following correction of the hypokalemia. The paralysis developed during the 23rd week of pregnancy. The fetal condition seemed normal. The outcome of the pregnancy was not reported.

Stanton and Strong[143] report on an unusual myopathy that failed to respond to corticosteroid therapy; however, remissions occurred twice during pregnancy. Based on these observations, the patient was treated with high-dose estrogen and progesterone. Electrodiagnostic studies were compatible with myopathy. Etiology of the myopathy was not determined.

References

1. Ironside R: Discussion on neurological complications in pregnancy. *Proc Royal Soc Med* 321:588–595, 1939.
2. Aminoff MJ: Neurological disorders and pregnancy. *Am J Obstet Gynecol* 132:325–335, 1978.
3. Hilsinger RL Jr, Adour KK, Doty HE: Idiopathic facial paralysis, pregnancy, and the menstrual cycle. *Ann Otol Rhinol & Laryngol* 84:433–442, 1975.
4. Felsenthal G: An overview of the clincial application of electromyography and nerve conduction technique. *MD State Med J* 31:(Sept)59–61, (Oct)50–53, (Nov)60–62, 1982.
5. Graham JG: Neurological complications of pregnancy and anesthesia. *Clin Obstet Gynecol* 9:333–350, 1982.
6. Leontic EA: Respiratory diseases in pregnancy. *Med Clin North Am* 61(1):111–128, 1977.
7. Fast A, Shapiro D, Ducommun EJ, et al: Low-back pain in pregnancy. *Spine* 12:368–371, 1987.
8. McCall IW, Park WM, O'Brien JP: Induced pain referral from posterior lumbar elements in normal subjects. *Spine* 4:441–446, 1979.
9. Fast A, Weiss L, Parikh S, et al: Night backache in pregnancy: hypo-

thetical pathophysiological mechanisms. *Am J Phys Med* 68:227–229, 1989.

10. LaBan MM, Perrin JCS, Latimer FR: Pregnancy and the herniated lumbar disc. *Arch Phys Med Rehabil* 64:319–321, 1983.
11. Berg G, Hammar M, Moller-Nielsen J, et al: Low back pain during pregnancy. *Obstet Gynecol* 71:71–75, 1988.
12. Hagen R: Pelvic girdle relaxation from an orthopaedic point of view. *Acta Orthop Scand* 45:550–563, 1974.
13. LaBan MM, Meerschaert JR, Taylor RS, et al: Symphyseal and sacroiliac joint pain associated with pubic symphysis instability. *Arch Phys Med Rehabil* 59:470–472, 1978.
14. Barsony T, Polgar F: Osteitis condensans ilii, ein bisher nicht beschriebenes Krankheitsbild. *Fortschr Rontgenstr* 37:663–669, 1928.
15. Greenhill JP, Friedman EA: Orthopedic problems. In *Biological Principles and Modern Practice of Obstetrics*. Edited by JP Greenhill, EA Friedman. Philadelphia, PA. WB Saunders Company, 1974, pp. 507–511.
16. Beaulieu JG, Razzano CD, Levine RB: Transient osteoporosis of the hip in pregnancy. *Clin Orthop* 115:165–168, 1976.
17. Svancarek W, Chirino O, Schaefer G, et al: Retropsoas and subgluteal abscesses following paracervical and pudendal anesthesia. *JAMA* 237:892–894, 1977.
18. O'Connell JEA: Lumbar disc protrusions in pregnancy. *J Neurol Neurosurg Physchiary* 23:138–141, 1960.
19. Felsenthal G: Asymmetric hamstring reflexes indicative of L5 radicular lesions. *Arch Phys Med Rehabil* 63:377–378, 1982.
20. Weinreb JC, Wolbarsht LB, Cohen JM, et al: Prevalence of lumbosacral intervertebral disk abnormalities on MR images in pregnant and asymptomatic non-pregnant women. *Radiology* 170:125–128, 1989.
21. Holmes HE, Rothman RH: The Pennsylvania plan: an algorithm for the management of lumbar degenerative disc disease. *Spine* 4:156–162, 1979.
22. Simmons JW: An algorithmic approach to treatment of low back pain. *Orthop Rev* 11:81–84, 1982.
23. Tsairis P, Dyck PJ, Mulder DW: Natural history of brachial plexus neuropathy. *Arch Neurol* 27:109–117, 1972.
24. Taylor RA: Heredofamilial mononeuritis multiplex with brachial predilection. *Brain* 83:113–137, 1960.
25. Ungley CC: Recurrent polyneuritis in pregnancy and the puerperium affecting three members of a family. *J Neurol Psychopath* 14:15–26, 1933.
26. Geiger LR, Mancall EL, Penn AS, et al: Familial neuralgic amyotrophy: report of three families with review of the literature. *Brain* 97:87–102, 1974.
27. Redmond JMT, Cros D, Martin JB, et al: Relapsing bilateral brachial plexopathy during pregnancy. *Arch Neurol* 46:462–464, 1989.
28. Dumitra D, Liles RA: Postpartum idiopathic brachial neuritis. *Obstet Gynecol* 73:473–475, 1989.
29. King AB: Neurologic conditions occurring as complications of pregnancy. *Arch Neurol Psychiatry* 63:611–644, 1950.

30. Benson RC, Inman VT: Brachialgia statica dysesthetica in pregnancy. *West J Surg* 64:115–130, 1956.
31. Soferman N, Weissman SL, Haimov M: Acroparesthesias in pregnancy. *Am J Obstet Gynecol* 89:528–531, 1984.
32. Swift TR, Nichols FT: The droopy shoulder syndrome. *Neurology* 34:212–215, 1984.
33. Lord JW Jr, Rosati LM: Thoracic outlet syndromes. *Clin Symp* 23(2):1–32, 1971.
34. Simkin P: Intermittent brachial plexus neuropathy secondary to breast engorgement. *Birth* 15(2):102, 1988.
35. Hill EC: Maternal obstetric paralysis. *Am J Obstet Gynecol* 83:1452–1460, 1962.
36. Cole JT: Maternal obstetric paralysis. *Am J Obstet Gynecol* 52:372–385, 1946.
37. Whittaker WG: Injuries to the sacral plexus in obstetrics. *Can Med Assoc J* 79:622–636, 1958.
38. Brown JT, McDougall A: Traumatic maternal birth injury. *J Obstet Gynecol Br Emp* 64:431–435, 1957.
39. Goldstein PJ: The lithotomy position: surgical aspects. In *Obstetrics and Gynecology in Positioning in Anesthesia and Surgery*. Edited by I. Martin. Philadelphia, PA. WB Saunders Co., 1987, pp. 41–50.
40. Reif ME: Bilateral common peroneal nerve palsy secondary to prolonged squatting in natural childbirth. *Birth* 15(2):100–102, 1988.
41. Rosenblum J, Schwarz GA, Bendler E: Femoral neuropathy: a neurological complication of hysterectomy. *JAMA* 195:409–414, 1966.
42. Adelman JU, Goldberg GS, Puckett JD: Postpartum bilateral femoral neuropathy. *Obstet Gynecol* 42:845–850, 1973.
43. Warfield CA: Obturator neuropathy after forceps delivery. *Obstet Gynecol* 64:479–485, 1984.
44. Cohen H: Complications of regional anesthesia in obstetrics. *Clin Obstet Gynecol* 17:211–225, 1974.
45. King RA, Calhoun JH: Fourth cranial nerve palsy following spinal anesthesia. *J Clin Neuro-ophthal* 7:20–22, 1987.
46. O'Reilly DF, Brazis PW, Rubino FA: The misdiagnosis of unilateral presentation of amyotrophic lateral sclerosis. *Muscle Nerve* 5:725–726, 1982.
47. Levine MC, Michels RM: Pregnancy and amyotrophic lateral sclerosis. *Ann Neurol* 1(4):408, 1977.
48. Huston JW, Lingenfelder J, Mulder DW, et al: Pregnancy complicated by amyotrophic lateral sclerosis. *Am J Obstet Gynecol* 72:93–99, 1956.
49. Janiszewski DW, Caroscio JT, Wisham LW: Amyotrophic lateral sclerosis: a comprehensive rehabilitation approach. *Arch Phys Med Rehabil* 64:304–307, 1983.
50. Sivak ED, Gipson WT, Hanson MR: Long-term management of respiratory failure in amyotrophic lateral sclerosis. *Ann Neurol* 12:18–23, 1982.
51. Daw E, Chandler G: Pregnancy following poliomyelitis. *Postgrad Med J* 52:492–496, 1976.
52. Woollam CHM, Houlton MCC: Respiratory failure in pregnancy. *Anesthesia* 31:1217–1220, 1976.

53. Willson JR, Carrington ER: Disorders of the nervous system, the skin, and the bones and joints during pregnancy. In *Obstetrics and Gynecology*. Sixth Edition. Edited by JR Willson, ER Carrington. St. Louis, MO. CV Mosby Company, 1979, pp. 323–329.
54. Krieger HP: Neurologic complications. In *Medical, Surgical, and Gynecologic Complications of Pregnancy*. Second Edition. Edited by JJ Rovinsky, AF Guttmacher. Baltimore, MD. Williams & Wilkins, 1965, pp. 436–452.
55. Beline JH, Deming B: Charcot-Marie-Tooth disease and pregnancy: report of a case. *J LA State Med Soc* 125:393–395, 1973.
56. Pollock M, Nukada H, Kritchevsky M: Exacerbation of Charcot-Marie-Tooth disease during pregnancy. *Neurology* 32:1311–1314, 1982.
57. Porges RF, Axelrod FB, Richards M: Pregnancy in familial dysautonomia. *Am J Obstet Gynecol* 132:485–488, 1978.
58. McColl KEL, Moore MR, Thompson GG, et al: Treatment with haematin in acute hepatic porphryia. *Q J Med* 198:161–174, 1981.
59. Brodie MJ, Moore MR, Thompson GG, et al: Pregnancy and the acute porphyrias. *Br J Obstet Gynecol* 84:726–731, 1977.
60. Donaldson JO (ed): Neuropathy and muscle disease. In *Neurology of Pregnancy*. (Major Problems in Neurology Series, Volume 7). Philadelphia, PA. WB Saunders Company, 1978, pp.23–73.
61. Lane RJM, Routledge PA: Drug-induced neurological disorders. *Drugs* 26:124–147, 1983.
62. DeBenedetto M: Electrodiagnostic evidence of subclinical disease states in drug abusers. *Arch Phys Med Rehabil* 57:62–66, 1976.
63. Pearn J, Harvey P, DeAmbrosis W, et al: Ciguatera and pregnancy. *Med J Aust* 1:57, 1982.
64. Lawrence DN, Enriquez MB, Lumish RM, et al: Ciguatera fish poisioning in Miami. *JAMA* 244:254–258, 1980.
65. Nyland L, Brismar T, Lunell NO, et al: Nerve conduction in diabetic pregnancy: a prospective study. Diabetes Res Clin Pract 1:121–123, 1985.
66. White P: Diabetes mellitus in pregnancy. *Clin Perinatol* 1:331–347, 1974.
67. Donovan WH, Sumi SM: Diabetic amyotrophy: a more diffuse process than clinically suspected. *Arch Phys Med Rehabil* 57:397–403, 1976.
68. Waxman SG, Sabin TD: Diabetic truncal polyneuropathy. *Arch Neurol* 38:46–47, 1981.
69. Longsheath GF, Newcomer AD: Abdominal pain caused by diabetic radiculopathy. *Ann Intern Med* 86:166–168, 1977.
70. Scott AR, Tattersall RB, McPherson M: Improvement of postural hypotension and severe autonomic neuropathy during pregnancy. *Diabetes Care* 11:369–370, 1988.
71. Chaturachinda K, McGregor EM: Wernicke's encephalopathy and pregnancy. *J Obstet Gynecol Br Commonw* 75:969–971, 1968.
72. Karjalainen AO: Neurological disorders in pregnancy: mulitple sclerosis, gestational polyneuritis and meningitis. *Ann Chir Gynaecol Fenn* 54:453–461, 1965.
73. Duncan ME, Pearson JMH: Neuritis in pregnancy and lactation. *Int J Lepr* 50:31–38, 1982.

74. Asbury AK: Diagnostic considerations in Guillain-Barré syndrome. *Ann Neurol* 9(Suppl)1–5, 1981.
75. Hurwitz ES, Holman RC, Nelson DB, et al: National surveillance for Guillain-Barré syndrome: January 1978-March 1979. *Neurology* 33:150–157, 1983.
76. Bravo RH, Katz M, Inturrisi M, et al: Obstetric management of Landry-Guillain-Barré syndrome: a case report. *Am J Obstet Gynecol* 142(Pt 1):714–715, 1982.
77. Ahlberg G, Ahlmark G: The Landry-Guillain-Barré syndrome and pregnancy. *Acta Obstet Gynecol Scand* 57:377–380, 1978.
78. Ravn H: The Landry-Guillain-Barré syndrome: a survey and a clinical report of 127 cases. *Acta Neurol Scand Suppl* 30:1–64, 1967.
79. Elstein M, Legg NJ, Murphy M, et al: Guillain-Barré syndrome in pregnancy. *Anesthesia* 26:216–224, 1971.
80. Rudolph JH, Norris RH, Garvey PH, et al: The Landry-Guillain-Barré syndrome in pregnancy: a review. *Obstet Gynecol* 26:265–271, 1965.
81. Sudo N, Weingold AB: Obstetric aspects of the Guillain-Barré syndrome. *Obstet Gynecol* 45:39–43, 1975.
82. The Guillain-Barré Study Group: Plasmapheresis and acute Guillain-Barré syndrome. *Neurology* 35:1096–1104, 1985.
83. Parry GJ, Heirman-Patterson TD: Pregnancy and autoimmune neuromuscular disease. *Semin Neurol* 8:197–204, 1988.
84. Conomy JP, Braatz JH: Guillain-Barré syndrome: the physical therapist and patient care. *Phys Ther* 51:517–523, 1971.
85. Dalakas MC, Engel WK: Chronic relapsing (dysimmune) polyneuropathy: pathogenesis and treatment. *Ann Neurol* 9(Suppl):134–145, 1981.
86. McCombe PA, McManis PG, Frith JA, et al: Chronic inflammatory demyelinating polyradiculoneuropathy associated with pregnancy. *Ann Neurol* 21:102–104, 1987.
87. Novak DJ, Johnson KP: Relapsing idiopathic polyneuritis during pregnancy. *Arch Neurol* 28:219–223, 1973.
88. Calderon-Gonzalez R, Gonzalez-Cantu N, Rizzi-Hernandez H: Recurrent polyneuropathy with pregnancy and oral contraceptives. *N Engl J Med* 282:1307–1308, 1970.
89. Jones MW, Berry K: Chronic relapsing polyneuritis associated with pregnancy. *Ann Neurol* 9:413, 1981.
90. Schumacher HR, Dorwart BB, Korzeniowski OM: Occurrence of DeQuervain's tendinitis during pregnancy. *Arch Intern Med* 145:2083–2084, 1985.
91. Nygaard IE, Saltzman CL, Whitehouse MB, et al: Hand problems in pregnancy. *Am Fam Physician* 39(6):123–126, 1989.
92. Massey EW: Carpal tunnel syndrome in pregnancy. *Obstet Gynecol Surv* 33:145–148, 1978.
93. Dekel S, Papaioannou T, Rushworth G, et al: Idiopathic carpal tunnel syndrome caused by carpal stenosis. *Br Med J* 280:1297–1299, 1980.
94. Melvin JL, Burnett CN, Johnson EW: Median nerve conduction in pregnancy. *Arch Phys Med Rehabil* 50:75–80, 1969.
95. Felsenthal G: Comparison of evoked potentials in the same hand of

normal subjects and in patients with carpal tunnel syndrome. *Am J Phys Med* 57:228–232, 1978.

96. Felsenthal G, Spindler H: Palmar conduction time of median and ulnar nerves of normal subjects and patients with carpal tunnel syndrome. *Am J Phys Med* 58:131–138, 1979.

97. Voitk AJ, Mueller JC, Farlinger DE, et al: Carpal tunnel syndrome in pregnancy. *Can Med Assoc J* 128:277–281, 1983.

98. Nicholas GG, Noone RB, Graham WP: Carpal tunnel syndrome in pregnancy. *Hand* 3:80–83, 1971.

99. Gould JS, Wissinger A: Carpal tunnel syndrome in pregnancy. *South Med J* 71(2):144–154, 1978.

100. Tobin SM: Carpal tunnel syndrome in pregnancy. *Am J Obstet Gynecol* 97:493–498, 1967.

101. Gelberman RH, Weisman MH: Carpal tunnel syndrome. *J Bone Joint Surg* 62-A:1181–1184, 1980.

102. Byers CM, DeLisa JA, Frankel DL, et al: Pyridoxine metabolism in carpal tunnel syndrome, with and without peripheral neuropathy. *Arch Phys Med Rehabil* 64:512, 1983.

103. Hudson AR: Carpal tunnel syndrome in pregnancy. *Can Med Assoc J* 128:1348–1349, 1983.

104. Graham RA: Carpal tunnel syndrome: a statistical analysis of 214 cases. *Orthopedics* 6:1283–1287, 1983.

105. Simon JN, Mokriski BK, Malinow AM, et al: Reflex sympathetic dystrophy in pregnancy. *Anesthesiology* 69:100–102, 1988.

106. McLennon HG, Oats JN, Walstab JE: Survey of hand symptoms in pregnancy. *Med J Aust* 147:542–544, 1987.

107. Helm PA, Nepomuceno C, Crane CR: Tibial nerve dysfunction during pregnancy. *South Med J* 64:1493–1494, 1971.

108. Jones RK: Meralgia paresthetica as a cause of leg discomfort. *Can Med Assoc J* 111:541–542, 1974.

109. Keegan JJ, Holyoke EA: Meralgia paresthetica: an anatomical and surgical study. *J Neurosurg* 19:341–345, 1962.

110. Rhodes P: Meralgia paresthetica in pregnancy. *Lancet* 2:831, 1967.

111. Price GE: Meralgia paresthetica, recurring with repeated pregnancies. *Am Med J* 4:210–212, 1909.

112. Peterson PH: Meralgia paresthetica related to pregnancy. *Am J Obstet Gynecol* 64:690, 1952.

113. Pleet AB, Massey EW: Intercostal neuralgia of pregnancy. *JAMA* 243:770, 1980.

114. McGregor JA, Guberman A, Amer J, et al: Idiopathic facial paralysis in late pregnancy and the early puerperium. *Obstet Gynecol* 69:435–438, 1987.

115. Adour KK: Current concepts in neurology. *N Engl J Med* 307:348–351, 1982.

116. Walters BNJ, Reman CWG: Bell's palsy and cytomegalovirus mononucleosis in pregnancy. *J R Soc Med* 77:429–430, 1984.

117. Falco NA, Eriksson E: Idiopathic facial palsy and the puerperium. *Surg Gynecol Obstet* 169:337–340, 1989.

118. Allen JR, Weils TM, Shemwell RE: Melkersson-Rosenthal syndrome: report of a case in pregnancy. *South Med J* 65:1152–1153, 1972.
119. Cope I: Myotonic dystrophy and pregnancy. *Aust NZ J Obstet Gynecol* 21:240–241, 1981.
120. Hilliard GD, Harris RE, Gilstrap LC, et al: Myotonic muscular dystrophy in pregnancy. *South Med J* 70:446–452, 1977.
121. Webb D, Muir I, Faulkner J, et al: Myotonia dystrophica: obstetric complications. *Am J Obstet Gynecol* 132:265–270, 1978.
122. Shore RN: Myontonic dystrophy: hazards of pregnancy and infancy. *Develop Med Child Neurol* 17:356–361, 1975.
123. Sciarra JJ, Steer CM: Uterine contractions during labor in myotonic muscular dystropy. *Am J Obstet Gynecol* 82:612–615, 1961.
124. Gardy HH: Dystrophia myotonica in pregnancy. *Obstet Gynecol* 21:441–445, 1963.
125. Harper PS: The myotonic disorders. In *Disorders of Voluntary Muscle*. Edited by J Walton. Edinburgh. Churchill Livingstone, 1988, pp. 575–579.
126. Whitehead AS, Solomon E, Chambers S, et al: Assignment of the structural gene for the third component of human complement to chromosome 19. *Proc Nat Acad Sci USA* 79:5021–5025, 1982.
127. Shaw DJ, Meredith AL, Sarfarazi M, et al: The apolipoprotein CII gene: subchromosomal localization and linkage to the myotonic dystrophy locus. *Hum Genetics* 70:271–273, 1985.
128. Meredith AL, Huson SM, Lunt PW, et al: Application of a closely linked polymorphism of restriction fragment length to counseling and prenatal testing in families with myotonic dystrophy. *Br Med J* 293:1353–1356, 1986.
129. Hakim CA, Thomlinson J: Myotonia congenita in pregnancy. *J Obstet Gynecol Br Commonw* 76:561–562, 1969.
130. Gardiner CF: A case of myotonia congenita. *Arch Pediatr* 18:925–928, 1901.
131. Schwartz IL, Dingfelder JR, O'Tuama L, et al: Recessive congenital myotonia and pregnancy. *Int J Gynecol Obstet* 17:194–196, 1979.
132. King JO, Denborough MA, Zapf PW: Inheritance of malignant hyperpyrexia. *Lancet* 1:365–370, 1972.
133. Sonnenklar N, Rendell-Baker L: Hyperpyrexia during pregnancy. *Lancet* 2:43, 1972.
134. Cocrane P, Alderman B: Normal pregnancy and successful delivery in myophosphorylase deficiency (McArdle's disease). *J Neurol Neurosurg Psychiatry* 36:225–227, 1973.
135. Barnes AB, Link DA: Childhood dermatomyositis and pregnancy. *Am J Obstet Gynecol* 146:335–336, 1983.
136. Bauer KA, Siegler M, Lindheimer MA: Polymyositis complicating pregnancy. *Arch Intern Med* 139:449, 1979.
137. Tsai A, Lindheimer MD, Lamberg SI: Dermatomyositis complicating pregnancy. *Obstet Gynecol* 41:570–573, 1973.
138. Gutierrez G, Dagnino R, Mintz G: Polymyositis/dermatomyositis and pregnancy. *Arthritis Rheum* 27(3):291–294, 1984.

139. King CR, Chow S: Dermatomyositis and pregnancy. *Obstet Gynecol* 66:589–592, 1985.
140. England MJ, Permann T, Veriava Y: Dermatomyositis in pregnancy: a case. *J Reprod Med* 31:633–635, 1986.
141. Houck W, Melnyk C, Gast MJ: Polymyositis in pregnancy: a case report and literature review. *J Reprod Med* 32:208–210, 1987.
142. Houston BD, Turner T: Severe electrolyte abnormalities in a pregnant patient with a jejunoileal bypass. *Arch Intern Med* 138:1712–1713, 1978.
143. Stanton JB, Strong JA: Myopathy remitting in pregnancy and responding to high-dosage oestrogen and progestogen therapy. *Lancet* 2:275–277, 1967.

11

Myasthenia Gravis in Pregnancy

John T. Repke, M.D.

Introduction

Myasthenia gravis is a neuromuscular disease characterized by muscle weakness and fatigability. The disease was first described in 1672 by Thomas Willis and is a disease primarily of the voluntary muscles. Smooth muscles, including myometrium, are relatively unaffected. The similarities between myasthenia gravis and curare-like poisoning as well as the response of these patients to anticholinesterase drugs pointed to the neuromuscular junction as the probable site of abnormality. It is now clear that the site of abnormality is indeed at the neuromuscular junction, and that a decrease in the number of acetylcholine receptors at this junction results in the manifestations of the disease. This depletion of receptors is most likely secondary to an autoimmune phenomenon.[1]

Epidemiology

The prevalence of myasthenia gravis has been reported from 12 to 64 cases per million, with an overall prevalence of 40 cases per million population.[2] Myasthenia gravis affects both sexes, but in most large series, females exceed males by a ratio of approximately 2:1.

From Goldstein PJ, Stern BJ, (eds): *Neurological Disorders of Pregnancy. Second Revised Edition.* Mount Kisco NY, Futura Publishing Co., Inc., © 1992.

The peak incidence of the disease occurs in the third decade in females. The male peak incidence is in the seventh decade. A preponderance of nonwhite females are among those patients dying of their disease.[2] Genetic transmission of this disease has been hypothesized by several authors.[3,4] In a study by Namba,[4] an estimated familial incidence of 3.4% was obtained and the observation was made that the younger the patient at the onset of symptoms, the more likely a familial pattern of inheritance.

Pathophysiology

The basic defect in myasthenia gravis is at the neuromuscular junction. The neurotransmitter, acetylcholine, is primarily synthesized in the nerve terminals where it is stored in vesicles for eventual release. Hartzell[5] has postulated that each vesicle contains a quantum of acetylcholine consisting of approximately 10,000 molecules. Neurotransmission occurs when these quanta are released. The release sites are located in close proximity to the areas with the greatest concentration of acetylcholine receptors.[6] After acetylcholine and receptor combine, increased permeability to potassium and sodium occurs, resulting in electrical depolarization.[7] If sufficient quanta have been released, an action potential will be generated that will initiate muscle contraction. The muscular event is terminated when the acetylcholine that has been released diffuses away from the site or has been destroyed by the action of acetylcholinesterase. It had been originally postulated that the defect in myasthenia gravis was due to either a diminished number of acetylcholine molecules per quantum or a reduction in the number of acetylcholine receptors at the motor end plate. Although the receptor hypothesis was initially rejected, it was eventually confirmed when radioactively labeled α bungarotoxin became available making direct measurement of receptors possible. A reduction in receptors by 70% to 80% was noted in the muscles of myasthenic patients.[8,9] These findings have since been confirmed by both α bungarotoxin binding assays[10] and quantitative measurement of acetylcholine sensitivity.[11]

Immunopathology

Several investigators have independently proposed that myasthenia gravis is an autoimmune disease.[12-14] The favorable response of myasthenia gravis to thymectomy as well as the association of myasthenia gravis with other autoimmune diseases supports this hypothesis. Lindstrom found receptor binding antibodies in 87% of patients with myasthenia gravis.[15] The active immunoglobulin seems to be an IgG. Studies have demonstrated that myasthenic IgG alone will reduce the amplitude of the miniature end plate potentials, while also demonstrating that IgM had no such effect. Some studies have also demonstrated that the early part of the complement system (C-1 to C-3) seems to enhance the effect of the myasthenic IgG.[16]

However, serum concentrations of antibodies correlate poorly[17] with clinical severity of disease. Other factors that may be important in determining the severity of clinical illness have been sought. Drachman et al.[17] have observed that the quantitative extent of blockade of acetylcholine receptors by IgG and degradation of these receptors corresponded closely with the clinical severity of illness. This same study reconfirmed the lack of correlation between antibody titer and clinical illness, suggesting that it may be the functional activity of autoantibodies rather than absolute titer that is of major importance in determining severity of illness. In addition, some abnormality of T-cell regulation could theoretically result in a humoral autoimmune response that presents as myasthenia gravis.[18]

The clinical presentation of myasthenia gravis is extremely variable, which suggests that the autoimmune mechanism may also be variable in its effector expression. Equally interesting, is the role of the thymus gland in the expression of myasthenia gravis. As many as 75% of myasthenic patients have thymic abnormalities, and 85% of these patients exhibit thymic hyperplasia and the remainder demonstrate gross or microscopic thymomas. These facts support the association of thymic disease with the clinical expression of myasthenia gravis.[19,20] Also, the favorable results observed following thymectomy[21,22] provide additional evidence for the association of a thymic disorder and myasthenic disease.

Clinical Presentation and Diagnosis

Neuromuscular fatigue is the cardinal feature of myasthenia gravis. Due to the acetylcholine receptor abnormality, decremental muscular responses during repetitive nerve stimulation are seen in greater than 95% of myasthenic patients examined, if three or more different muscles are tested.[23] A relatively safe method of testing for the diagnosis of myasthenia gravis is by means of the drug edrophonium hydrochloride. By briefly interfering with the hydrolysis of acetylcholine at the neuromuscular junction, edrophonium hydrochloride allows for acetylcholine to remain available for neuromuscular action for a greater period of time. This results in transient improvement in patient strength and response to repetitive nerve stimulation. Edrophonium hydrochloride is best used as a diagnostic test when a clear-cut end point can be defined, such as resolution of dysconjugate gaze or ptosis. Edrophonium hydrochloride should be avoided in the patient with markedly impaired respirations or ability to handle oral secretions so as to avoid respiratory embarrassment.

Ischemic exercise can cause an apparent spread of weakness to other muscle groups.[24,25] This phenomenon has been attributed to the presence of lactate at the neuromuscular junction possibly interfering with neural acetylcholine release.[26,27]

It has also been demonstrated that antibody transfer can reproduce the symptoms of myasthenia gravis. Toyka[16] reported that serum from 94% of myasthenic patients produced hallmark features of the ddisease in reecipient mice. It is interesting to note that the abnormalities generally corresponded with the severity of the patient's disease from whom the serum was extracted. In trials of plasma exchange and plasmapheresis, the patient's clinical status seemed to correlate with the detectable serum levels of antibody.[28,29] Because the antibody is an IgG, which easily crosses the placenta, it is reasonable to assume that the neonatal myasthenia syndrome seen in approximately one of six infants born to mothers with myasthenia gravis is due to the implicated antibody.

General Clinical Considerations

The approach to the management of the pregnant patient with myasthenia gravis must include consideration not only for the effect of the disease process and its treatment on the mother and fetus, but also the risk attributable to pregnancy on the disease. Ideally, management should begin with preconception counseling and continue through the postpartum period with careful observation of the mother for development of myasthenic crises (see below) and careful observation of the neonate for the development of neonatal myasthenia gravis. Counseling prior to conception provides the couple with an opportunity to discuss with her physician the general risks that are involved in a prospective pregnancy for both the fetus and the mother. An informed decision about pregnancy can be made only after such a discussion.

Effect of Pregnancy on Myasthenia Gravis

The influence of pregnancy on the course of myasthenia gravis has been the subject of numerous reports.[30–40] Several points emerge that are accepted by most authors caring for large numbers of pregnant myasthenics. First, pregnancy does not predictably alter the course of the disease. Each pregnancy must be viewed as an isolated event during which the disease may remain stable, undergo partial or complete remission, or exacerbate. In addition, the course taken in a previous pregnancy cannot be used to predict the course in the current or future pregnancy.

Osserman's review[30] of 22 myosthenic patients having a total of 33 pregnancies revealed that one third of the patients showed a definite remission during pregnancy, one third showed a definite relapse associated with the pregnancy, and one third showed no change in the myasthenic state. All symptomatology patterns were usually established during the first trimester of pregnancy with little change during the second and third trimesters except in two cases. Viets and associates[31] found that a relapse occurred not uncommonly in the first trimester, with partial or complete remission often occurring at a later stage of the pregnancy, but again there was considerable variation in this respect.

In contradistinction to Osserman's and Viets' observations, Fraser's and Turner's review [32] of 12 patients with myasthenia gravis studied during 21 pregnancies found that a relapse was more likely to occur in the puerperium than during the pregnancy itself and recommended hospitalization for 3-weeks postpartum.

In an ongoing review of his experience with myasthenia gravis in pregnancy, Plauche[33,34] has reported on 164 pregnancies in 113 myasthenic mothers. Antepartum exacerbations occurred in 35.4% of these pregnancies, and postpartum exacerbations occurred in 35.4%. In this series, 14 spontaneous abortions, 14 therapeutic abortions, 12 perinatal deaths, and 6 maternal deaths occurred. Neonatal myasthenia gravis was definitely diagnosed in 22 infants and thought probable in an additional 4 cases for an overall incidence of 21% of live-born infants of myasthenic mothers developing neonatal myasthenia gravis.

Clearly, the effect of pregnancy on myasthenia gravis is unpredictable. Scott[35] reported that the mortality risk of myasthenic mothers bears an inverse relationship to the duration of the disease with the greatest risk in the first year and minimal risk after 7 years. He therefore feels that postponement of pregnancy is justified in newly diagnosed cases of myasthenia gravis. Although improvement of myasthenia gravis usually follows spontaneous abortions, this does not seem to occur with therapeutic abortions.[33,34,36–38] Therefore, myasthenia gravis is not an indication for termination of pregnancy. In fact, because the disease may exacerbate post abortion, therapeutic abortion should not be performed for this indication.[39] The decision concerning pregnancy for the woman with myasthenia gravis must be approached by the physician with a well planned management scheme that includes close monitoring for myasthenic crises as well as a firm patient education program.

Effect of Myasthenia Gravis on Pregnancy

To describe the effect of myasthenia gravis on pregnancy, one must consider how the disease affects the mother and the newborn, as well as the effect of drug therapy on both. This disease is not associated with infertility.[40] There is an apparent increase in the incidence of spontaneous abortion in myasthenia gravis patients.[41] There are no data to support or suggest either an increase in the prematurity rate or an increase in pregnancy-induced hypertension in pregnant myasthenics.

The effect of myasthenia gravis on the fetus and neonate can be described as the occurrence of the neonatal myasthenic syndrome and as the effect of maternal drug therapy. This will be described in a separate section.

Management of Myasthenia Gravis in Pregnancy

The management of myasthenia gravis in pregnancy is based on knowledge of the natural history of the disease and of the changes that occur during pregnancy. Two basic aspects of management need to be considered. First, the general management is aimed at obtaining the best possible outcome and least morbidity and mortality for both the mother and the fetus. This includes close surveillance and planning during the antepartum, intrapartum, and postpartum periods. The second aspect of management would aim to prevent and manage the special problems that the myasthenic could have during pregnancy. This would include anesthetic considerations, neonatal considerations, and the anticipation of myasthenic crises during the pregnancy. Patient counseling as well as early consultation among the obstetricians, pediatricians, anesthesiologists, neurologists, and labor and delivery personnel caring for the patient is an integral part of the management plan.

Antepartum Management

Antepartum management of the pregnant myasthenic includes close surveillance of the fetus and mother. A careful history of the course of the disease, the medications taken, and an assessment of the severity of the disease should be taken at the initial visit. Patient education as to what to expect during the pregnancy, intrapartum management, and the effect of myasthenia gravis on a pregnancy should be discussed in detail with the patient. Also, the patient needs to be made aware of the types of crises that could occur, because exacerbations that did not occur in the past may first present during the pregnancy.

There are numerous therapeutic modalities used in the treatment of myasthenia gravis. These include the use of anticholinesterases, corticosteroids, other immunosuppressants plasmapheresis, and thymectomy. At the time of initial presentation to the obstetrician, the patient may be on or have had any combination of these therapeutic modalities. Anticholinesterase medications remain the treatment of choice in the initial management of myasthenia gravis. Neostigmine 15 mg or pyridostigmine 60 mg may be given orally. Generally, improved neuromuscular transmission is noted within 15 to 30 minutes. Maximum muscle strength will be obtained in approximately 2 hours with the effect lasting for approximately 4 hours. Therefore, the dose of pyridostigmine or neostigmine is usually repeated every 4 hours during the time the patient is awake. If, during sleeping hours, respiratory embarrassment is a problem, delayed release forms of anticholinesterase drugs are available. Atropine sulfate in doses of 0.4 mg to 0.6 mg may also be administered in order to combat the annoying muscarinic side effects of these anticholinesterase medications. Excessive doses of anticholinesterase drugs should be avoided because this may worsen neuromuscular transmission, resulting in "cholinergic block". (It may occasionally be difficult to distinguish underdosage of drug from overdosage. In this situation, an injection of 2–10 mg of edrophonium chloride will improve strength if there is an underdosage; the strength remains the same or even decreases if an overdosage of anticholinesterase drugs has been given.) The majority of mild myasthenic patients may be maintained at a normal functional level with anticholinesterase medications alone. Up to 20% of patients will eventually have spontaneous remission of their disease, but the symptoms in some patients with more severe disease will require the addition of other therapeutic modalities to their anticholinesterase regime.[42]

There are three types of crises that may occur in a myasthenic patient under treatment. First is the myasthenic crisis, which is an exacerbation of the symptoms of myasthenia gravis: severe muscle weakness, increased fatigability, inability to swallow, and respiratory paralysis. Treatment includes increasing doses of anticholinesterase medications, the addition of other therapeutic modalities, and supportive care until the crisis has resolved. If respiratory function is compromised, the patient needs admission to a respiratory care unit and possibly intubation. The second crisis is the cholinergic crisis. This is caused by an excessive amount of anticholinesterase medication or decreased requirements. Symptoms of this crisis include nausea, vomiting, muscle weakness, abdominal pain, diarrhea, and increased salivation. Treatment includes withholding anticholinesterases, the administration of atropine, and supportive care. It is often difficult to distinguish the symptoms of a myasthenic crisis and a cholinergic crisis because the symptoms are often similar. A simple diagnostic test to distinguish the two crises is to inject edrophonium chloride (Tensilon®; [ICN Pharmaceuticals, Inc., Costa Mesa, CA, USA]). The intravenous injection of edrophonium chloride, a short-acting anticholinesterase, will briefly improve the weakness and fatigability in a myasthenic crisis but will decrease strength or have no effect in a cholinergic crisis. If there is improvement in strength, then more anticholinesterases are required.

The third and most severe type of crisis is the refractory crisis. The disease becomes refractory to the therapeutic modalities utilized. Ventilatory support is required until the resolution of this crisis. It is the refractory crisis that is often the cause of death in myasthenics. For severe refractory cases of myasthenia gravis, plasma exchange has been successfully used. The duration of improvement after plasma exchange remains controversial, but there is agreement that there is a place for this modality in selected cases. Although improvement may be expected in most cases, the hazards of plasma exchange, including thromboembolism, infection, hypotension, and death, would dictate that its use be confined to severe cases. In such cases, plasma exchange may effectively control symptoms, at least temporarily, while awaiting the results of other therapies.[43,44] Both the myasthenic crisis and the refractory crisis may be initiated by infection, emotional stress, and pregnancy. It is important to explain to the patient that increasing the dosage of an anticholinesterase above the optimal level will not increase muscle strength but can precipitate a cholinergic crisis.

Anticholinesterase medications in a pregnant myasthenic patient are administered in doses identical to those given to the nonpregnant myasthenic patient. Plauche[34] believes that myasthenic patients are best placed on a regimen of anticholinesterase medication and weaned from corticosteroid therapy before pregnancy is contemplated. If the disease remains stable, then pregnancy can be expected to progress with relative safety. Corticosteroids should be reserved for pregnant myasthenic patients unresponsive to anticholinesterase therapy.

A special problem is the initial diagnosis of myasthenia gravis in pregnancy. The hallmark of disease is weakness in specific muscle groups such as ocular or bulbar weakness. The diagnosis of myasthenia gravis requires a strong index of suspicion in any female complaining of intensifying weakness as the day progresses. Insidious ocular, bulbar, or generalized muscle weakness of voluntary muscle groups should be investigated. Neuromuscular symptoms may be transient, and the fact that physical and emotional stress may worsen subtle physical signs occasionally results in these patients being labeled as hypochondriacs. In the setting of pregnancy, these subtle signs may also be mistaken for simple pregnancy-related fatigue, so the clinician must be alert to the possibility that a neuromuscular diagnosis exists.[45] Confirming the diagnosis can easily be done with the intravenous test.

The use of edrophonium chloride during pregnancy may initiate premature labor or abortion, and the intramuscular injection of neostigmine bromide may be safely substituted for diagnostic purposes. One-half milligram of neostigmine is given and muscle strength is

Table I.
Drugs Requiring Caution in Myasthenia Gravis Patients

Antibiotics	
Tobramycin	Kanamycin
Gentamicin	Polymyxin group
Tetracycline	Bacitracin
Streptomycin	Colistin

Antiarrhythmics	
Quinine (tonic water)	Phenytoin
Quinidine	Procaine
Procainamide	

Anesthetics
Local: Procaine, xylocaine
General: Ether, chloroform

Muscle Rx
Curare, succinylcholine

Analgesics
Morphine sulfate, meperidine, benzodiazepines, chlorpromazine

Other	
Propranolol (and other β blockers)	
Magnesium sulfate	
Lithium	Tetanus antitoxin
Oral contraceptives	Corticosteroids
Calcium channel blockers	

reevaluated 30 minutes after injection. [39,46] Most mild myasthenics are maintained at a normal functional level using anticholinergic therapy. Minor stresses may require an increased dose of anticholinesterase medication and even the addition of steroids. The key to preventing exacerbation is to obtain as much rest as possible during the pregnancy, avoid infections, and aggressively treat any minor type of infection. In addition, certain drugs need to be avoided by the myasthenic patient to prevent exacerbation (Table I).

Intrapartum Management

The intrapartum period of the pregnancy requires a carefully planned and monitored approach with collaboration between neurology, anesthesiology, neonatology, and nursing. There are no indications for terminating pregnancy early. Cesarean section is not indicated unless there are obstetrical reasons. The course of labor is unchanged from the nonmyasthenic patient except for reported shortened labor due to generalized relaxation. [47] The use of outlet forceps has been recommended to shorten the second stage of labor, thereby minimizing muscle fatigue associated with expulsive efforts. [46] With regard to the conduct of labor, there may be a marked contrast between the strength of uterine contractions in the second stage and the general muscular weakness exhibited by the patient. [48]

The approach to the use of anticholinesterase therapy in labor is to substitute the oral dose of medication with an equivalent intramuscular or intravenous dose. Parenteral administration of anticholinesterases is preferred because of delayed gastric emptying and the desire for the patient to have an empty stomach. Neostigmine methyl

Table II.
Doses of Commonly Used Anticholinesterases

	IV	IM	Oral	Duration
Neostigmine (Prostigmin)	0.25–0.75 mg	0.5–1.5 mg	10–20 mg	2–3 hr
Pyridostigmine (Mestinon)	1–3 mg	3–5 mg	50–70 mg	3–4 hr

sulfate, 0.5 mg intramuscularly every 3 to 4 hours as indicated, is usually used (Table II). Narcotic analgesics, tranquilizers, and magnesium sulfate should be avoided.

Anesthesia Management of Myasthenia Gravis in Pregnancy

The pregnant patient with myasthenia gravis should be seen by an anesthesiologist early in the course of the pregnancy. For the patient, this will help allay anxiety and prepare her for the type of childbirth most acceptable to her. For the anesthesiologist, the preanesthetic assessment allows for determination of the severity of the disease and for obtaining the appropriate laboratory data in preparation for the intrapartum period. This might include a chest x-ray, an ECG, pulmonary function tests including spirometry and peak expiratory flow rate, thyroid function tests, and electrolytes. Evidence of restrictive lung disease can be further evaluated with arterial blood gas determinations. The electrocardiogram may be valuable in that alterations in T waves or ST segments may represent areas of focal myocardial necrosis associated with myasthenia gravis. Thyroid function studies should be obtained because autoimmune thyroid disease has been associated with myasthenia gravis.

Because respiratory compromise can present a severe problem to the obstetrician managing the myasthenic patient, narcotic analgesia is best avoided for the management of pain during labor. The respiratory depression that these drugs can cause may be potentiated by anticholinesterase medications. Regional anesthesia seems to be the method of choice for managing myasthenic patients during labor and delivery. Regional block via a spinal or epidural technique to a level of T-10 will frequently reduce the need for intravenous medication and facilitate outlet forceps delivery that will shorten the second stage of labor, thus preventing maternal exhaustion. Local anesthetics may be used, but large doses should be avoided because they may interfere with neuromuscular transmission. When regional techniques are used, it has been recommended that large doses of ester-type anesthetics be avoided. Because these drugs are hydrolyzed by cholinesterases, the presence of anticholinesterase drugs may impair this hydrolysis, producing maternal and fetal toxicity.

There is no evidence that amide-type drugs have altered metabolism in myasthenia gravis.

During the course of labor, it is very important to periodically assess these patients for any evidence of exhaustion or increasing muscular weakness. Serial vital capacities during labor may aid in this assessment. If progressive deterioration is noted after a series of three consecutive vital capacities have been taken, parenteral anticholinesterase therapy may require adjustment.

In the event that regional anesthesia is not possible and general anesthesia becomes necessary, either awake endotracheal intubation or rapid thiopental induction with cricoid pressure and immediate intubation is recommended for the obstetric patient with myasthenia gravis. Occasionally, muscle relaxants may be required in order to facilitate intubation. In the myasthenic patient, the use of curare-like compounds prior to the administration of succinylcholine should be avoided. Succinylcholine has a variable effect on myasthenia gravis with involved muscle groups being much more sensitive to its paralyzing effects. On the other hand, in patients with bulbar or respiratory disease, conduction anesthesia for cesarean section may be less safe than usual due to the high level of anesthesia required.[49]

Postpartum Management

The myasthenic patient may decompensate rapidly immediately after the infant is delivered. The first 3-weeks postpartum are particularly dangerous because a third of all patients will experience exacerbations that may be quite sudden and severe.[33,50] Whether the patient is delivered vaginally or by cesarean section, it is necessary to monitor the patient and to adjust the dose of anticholinesterase medications. In the postpartum period, the patient should be restarted on her previous antepartum dose of oral anticholinesterase medication; a slight increase in dose due to the increased activity and the stress of the delivery may be necessary. The development of postpartum endometritis, mastitis, respiratory tract infection, and urinary tract infection requires aggressive treatment. The patient should be encouraged to rest as much as possible.

Breast feeding is not contraindicated in mothers with myasthenia gravis, but the potential problems associated with breast feeding are multiple. Anticholinesterase medications and antiacetylcholine receptor antibodies may be found in maternal milk. Despite these facts, it is no longer generally thought that breast feeding adversely affects either the mother or the child.

The Management of Pregnancy-Induced Hypertension (Pre-Eclampsia) in the Myasthenic Pregnant Patient

The occurrence of pregnancy-induced hypertension in the patient with myasthenia gravis has been reported in three patients in the literature.[40,51] DeLara[52] states that the incidence of pre-eclampsia is not affected by myasthenia in pregnancy. The key point is that although magnesium sulfate is the drug of choice for the treatment of pregnancy-induced hypertension in most institutions in this country, its use is contraindicated in myasthenia gravis. Magnesium sulfate increases muscle weakness by decreasing acetylcholine release from the motor nerve terminal and by reducing the excitability of the postjunctional membrane.[53] The alternative is to use diazepam or phenobarbital in the management of pregnancy-induced hypertension requiring drug intervention. Phenytoin may also be used in this circumstance and appears to be a safe alternative.[54] We have suc-

---

Table III.
The Johns Hopkins Hospital, Division of Maternal-Fetal Medicine, Protocol for Phenytoin Administration in Preeclampsia

Patient Weight (kg)	Phenytoin Dose (mg)
< 50	1,000
50–70	1,250
> 70	1,500

A. Infusion rate not to exceed 25 mg/min—patients with serum albumin < 2.5 gm/L may benefit from slower infusion (12.5 mg/min).
B. After initial 750 mg, all patients should have infusion rate reduced to 12.5 mg/min.
C. Redosing may be necessary, depending on serum level after infusion.

cessfully used phenytoin in our institution for the management of routine pre-eclamptics (Table III).

Neonatal Myasthenia Gravis

Neonatal myasthenia gravis is a transient form of myasthenia gravis appearing in 12% of the babies born to myasthenic mothers. The neuromuscular symptoms of neonatal myasthenia gravis develop within the first 4 days of life; two thirds of cases develop at birth or within hours, and 80% of cases develop within the first postnatal day.[55–57] The average duration of symptoms of this self-limiting disorder is 3 weeks. The pathogenesis of neonatal myasthenia gravis is well explained by the fact that myasthenia gravis is an autoimmune disease caused by the immunopathological effect of specific antibodies directed against the acetylcholine receptor at the neuromuscular junction.[1] Neonatal myasthenia gravis is due to plancental transmission of antiacetylcholine receptor antibodies from mother to infant and a correlation exists between falling antibody titer in the infant and increasing muscular strength.[58,59] One explanation for the delay in the appearance of symptoms in the neonate is the protective effect of anticholinesterase drugs taken by the mother that are also transferred transplacentally. When the medication is no longer present, the neonatal myasthenia gravis syndrome can appear. Symptoms in the infant include lethargy, poor suck, feeble cry, generalized muscle weakness, and absent or weak Moro reflex. The infant may experience difficulty in swallowing and breathing. The diagnosis can be confirmed by using edrophonium chloride 0.05 cc to 0.1 cc subcutaneously. If there is improvement in symptomatology, then the diagnosis is confirmed and the infant needs to be treated with an anticholinesterase medication and supportive care.

It is of interest that the duration and severity of the disease in the mother is not associated with the development of neonatal myasthenia gravis. Usually, the pregnancy is normal. Term infants usually have normal Apgar scores. One provocative question pertains to the reason why all babies of myasthenic mothers do not develop neonatal myasthenia gravis syndrome. One hypothesis suggests that α-fetoprotein is protective. Another hypothesis proposes that blocking factors in the fetus alter the action of antiacetylcholine receptor antibodies on their target sites, thus preventing muscle weakness.[60]

The Johns Hopkins Hospital Experience

Over the past 8 years at the Johns Hopkins Hospital, we have treated nine patients with myasthenia gravis during pregnancy (Table IV). These patients represent a total of 16 deliveries. Five of our six patients had the diagnosis of myasthenia gravis confirmed clinically and serologically (Table V). Patient #6, the only patient delivered by cesarean section, was transferred from another institution and never had a diagnosis of myasthenia gravis confirmed at the Johns Hopkins Hospital. For this reason, this patient has been eliminated from the analyses of the data in calculating the mean gestational age, mean length of labor, and number of infants with confirmed neonatal myas-

Table IV.
Johns Hopkins Pregnancy Data

Patient	GA (wks)	Total Labor (hr)	Type of Delivery	BW (gm)	NMG	Parity
1a	39	$14\frac{1}{4}$	SVD	2870	+	1001
b	$39\frac{5}{7}$	$4\frac{1}{2}$	SVD	3040	−	2012
2a	$39\frac{5}{7}$	$20\frac{1}{2}$	ILF	2670	−	0000
b	$38\frac{1}{7}$	$4\frac{1}{2}$	SVD	3280	+	1011
c	$37\frac{2}{7}$	2	SVD	2880	−	2012
3	$39\frac{1}{7}$	$6\frac{1}{4}$	SVD	3480	−	0000
4	40	$5\frac{1}{2}$	SVD	3240	+	0030
5a	39	$9\frac{1}{2}$	SVD	2650	−	0000
b	42	$3\frac{1}{2}$	SVD	3180	−	1021
6*	35	0	LSTCS	2640	−	0020
7	39	$9\frac{1}{2}$	ILF	3229	−	0000
8a	$37\frac{6}{7}$	$13\frac{3}{4}$	SVD	2280	−	0010
	(twins)		ILF	2650	−	
b	$40\frac{5}{7}$	$12\frac{3}{4}$	SVD	3740	−	1012
c	40	10	SVD	3510	−	2013
9a	$39\frac{2}{7}$	$10\frac{1}{4}$	SVD	3220	+	0000
b	37	$7\frac{3}{4}$	ILF	3505	−	1001
MEAN	38.7	8.4	C/S% = 6.6	3063	$\frac{4}{17}$	

* Dx of M.G. never confirmed at JHH. GA = Gestational age; SVD = Spontaneous vaginal delivery; ILF = Indicated low forceps; LSTCS = Low segment transverse cesarean section; NMG = Neonatal myasthenia gravis; C/S = Cesarean section.

Table V.
Serologic Data

Patient	Range Ach Ab Levels	Thymic Status	ANA	RF	C3/C4	IgG	IgM	IgA
1	2.0×10^{-12} mol/mL to 4.6×10^{-12}	Thymectomy[+] Path-Lymphoid Hyperplasia CT—WNL	1:20	—	NA	WNL	WNL	WNL
2	2.26×10^{-12} to 407.0×10^{-12}		NA	NA	NA	NA	NA	NA
3*	3.5×10^{-12} to 23.93×10^{-12}	CT—WNL Thymectomy-Follicular Hyperplasia[+]	1:20	—	I/I	NA	NA	NA
4	13.05×10^{-12} to 260×10^{-12}	Thymectomy[+] Thymic Hyperplasia CT—WNL × 2	—	—	WNL	WNL	WNL	WNL
5	0×10^{-12} to 8.7×10^{-12}	WNL	1:20	NA	NA	WNL	WNL	WNL
6	0×10^{-12}	Thymectomy Follicular Hyperplasia	NA	NA	NA	NA	NA	NA
7	0×10^{9}		Neg	NA	NA	NA	NA	NA
8	0×10^{-12} to 0.66×10^{-12}	Thymectomy CT—WNL	NA	NA	NA	NA	NA	NA
9	9.5×10^{-12} to 76×10^{-12}	Thymectomy Follicular Hyperplasia	1:40	Pos	WNL	WNL	WNL	WNL

* This patient also had negative screens for thyroid, parietal, smooth muscle and mitochondrial antibodies. [+] All thymectomies preceded first delivery at JHH. NA = Not available; CT = Computed axial tomography; WNL = within normal limits.

thenia gravis. Although the literature is replete with statements about the reduced gestational age among infants delivered of myasthenics, our data demonstrate that the mean gestational age of our five patients' infants, representing nine deliveries, was 39.3 weeks. Our data do not support the proposition that myasthenics, possibly due to increased muscular relaxation, have shorter lengths of labor.

Although thymectomy has been shown to improve the condition of the myasthenic patient, the reproductive performance of those patients in our series who had undergone thymectomy did not seem to be any better than the reproductive performance of those patients who had not had thymectomy. Our data support the contention that the acetylcholine receptor antibody level does not necessarily correlate with either the clinical severity of disease or the occurrence of the neonatal myasthenic syndrome. All of our patients underwent vaginal delivery and none of them experienced significant exacerbations of their disease in the postpartum period except for patient #5. It is worthy to note that in her first delivery, patient #5 did not have the diagnosis of myasthenia gravis. However, 10 days after being discharged following a routine vaginal delivery and uneventful postpartum course, she was admitted to the medical intensive care unit with a myasthenic crisis requiring ventilatory assistance. All of our patients who received pharmacotherapy for their disease at the time of their deliveries displayed no apparent adverse neonatal effect. The mainstay of our therapy (Table VI) is pyridostigmine, which we usually start at 60 mg three times a day and titrate to individual needs. If respiratory difficulties are encountered during sleep, an extended release tablet of pyridostigmine may be used.

Occasionally, corticosteroid therapy is introduced. One approach is to start with prednisone 25 mg per day and increase this by 12.5 mg every third day to a maximum of 100 mg per day. Exacerbations may occur if large doses are initially used. A 3–month trial of corticosteroids is indicated prior to calling such therapy a failure. It may be necessary to titrate down the anticholinesterase drugs used during this period. If the patient presents with severe myasthenia gravis early in pregnancy, it is sometimes tempting to terminate the pregnancy due to the difficulty of treating these patients adequately. Termination of pregnancy does not necessarily lead to clinical improvement although improvement may follow spontaneous abortion in myasthenic patients who have experienced a relapse during pregnancy.[61]

When managing a patient in labor, one usually substitutes neos-

Table VI.
Pharmacological Data

	Patient		
	1	2	3
Medications at Delivery	A. Mestinon 60 mg p.o. tid B. Mestinon 60 mg p.o. bid	A. Mestinon 90 mg p.o. B. Mestinon 7a, 11a, 3p, 7p C. Timespan 180 mg p.o. at 11 p.m. Ephedrine 25 mg p.o. with each dose of Mestinon	A. Mestinon 60 mg p.o. tid

	Patient		
	4	5	6
Medications at Delivery	A. Mestinon 60 mg p.o. q5–6h	A. None B. Mestinon 60 mg p.o. bid	None

	Patient		9
	7	8	
Medications at Delivery	None	None	A. Mestinon 90 mg p.o. qid Mestinon Timespan 60 mg p.o. qhs B. Mestinon 90 mg p.o. qid Mestinon Timespan 60 mg p.o. qhs

A = 1st pregnancy; B = 2nd pregnancy; C = 3rd pregnancy.

tigmine for pyridostigmine once the patient has entered the active phase of labor. These drugs may be exchanged in a ratio of 60 mg of pyridostigmine being equal to approximately 1 mg of neostigmine. For example, if a patient were receiving 60 mg of pyridostigmine every 4 hours, then in the active phase of labor this could be replaced with neostigmine 1 mg mixed in 500 cc of crystalloid to run by continuous infusion pump over 4 hours. This method of management has worked very well at Hopkins.

Summary

Myasthenia gravis is an illness that poses potentially grave complications for both mother and infant. Maternal mortality may be as high as 3% to 4%, with a perinatal mortality being approximately five times higher than that seen in uncomplicated gestations. Because of these increased risks, it is extremely important that the patient and her obstetrician fully discuss the implications and requirements for the pregnancy to continue. Current treatment modalities consisting of anticholinesterase drugs, corticosteroids, thymectomy, plasmapheresis, immunosuppressive agents, or any combination thereof must be familiar to the obstetrician and discussed thoroughly with the patient. The patient with such a potentially grave disease should be carefully managed during labor and delivery at a facility equipped to deal with both maternal and neonatal needs. Close collaboration and communication among the obstetrician, neonatologist, anesthesiologist, and neurologist will result in an optimal outcome for mother and infant. Meticulous antepartum, maternal, and fetal surveillance combined with careful intrapartum management will maximize the possibility of a successful outcome.

References

1. Drachman DB: Myasthenia gravis. *N Engl J Med* 298:136–142, 1978.
2. Kurtzke JF: Epidemiology of myasthenia gravis. *Adv Neurol* 19:545, 1978.
3. Engle AA: Morphologic and immunologic findings in myasthenia gravis and EMG syndromes. *J Neurol Neurosurg Psychiatry* 43:477, 1980.
4. Namba T: Familial myasthenia gravis. *Arch Neurol* 25:49, 1971.
5. Hartzell HC, Kuffler SW, Yoshikami D: The number of acetylcholine molecules in a quantum, and the interaction between quanta at the subsynoptic membrane of the skeletal neuromuscular synapse. *Cold Spring Harbor Symp Quant Biol* 40:175–186, 1976.
6. Fertuck HC, Salpeter MM: Localization of acetylcholine receptor by ^{125}I-labeled alpha-bungarotoxin binding at mouse motor-endplates. *Proc Natl Acad Sci USA* 71:1376–1378, 1974.

7. Takeuchi A, Takeuchi N: On the permeability of end-plate membrane during the action of transmitter. *J Physiol (Lond)* 154:52–67, 1960.

8. Fambrough DM, Drachman DB, Satyamurti S: Neuromuscular junction in myasthenia gravis: decreased acetylcholine receptors. *Science* 182:293–295, 1973.

9. Drachman DB, Kao I, Pestronk A, et al: Myasthenia gravis as a receptor disorder. *Ann NY Acad Sci* 274:226–234, 1976.

10. Green DPL, Miledi R, Vincent A: Neuromuscular transmission after immunization against acetylcholine receptors. *Proc Royal Soc Lond (Biol)* 189:57–68, 1975.

11. Albuquerque EX, Rash JE, Mayer RF, et al: An electrophysiological and morphological study of the neuromuscular junctions in patients with myasthenia gravis. *Exp Neurol* 51:536–563, 1976.

12. Smithers DW: Tumors of the thyroid gland in relation to some general concepts of neoplasia. *J Fac Radiol* 10:3–16, 1959.

13. Simpson JA: Myasthenia gravis: a new hypothesis. *Scott Med J* 5:419–436, 1960.

14. Nastuk WL, Plescia OJ, Osserman KE: Changes in serum complement activity in patients with myasthenia gravis. *Proc Soc Exp Biol Med* 105:177–184, 1960.

15. Lindstrom JM, Seybold ME, Lennon VA, et al: Antibody to acetylcholine receptor in myasthenia gravis: prevalence, clinical correlates, and diagnostic valve. *Neurology* 26(11):1054–1059, 1976.

16. Toyka KV, Drachman DB, Griffin DE, et al: Myasthenia gravis: study of humeral immune mechanisms by passive transfer to mice. *N Engl J Med* 296:125–131, 1977.

17. Drachman DB, Adams RN, Josifek LF, et al: Functional activities of autoantibodies to acetylcholine receptors and the clinical severity of myasthenia gravis. *N Engl J Med* 307:769–775, 1982.

18. Greaves MF, Owen JJT, Roff MC: *T and B Lymphocytes: Origins, Properties and Roles in Immune Responses*. New York, NY. Excerpta Medica, 1974.

19. Castleman B: The pathology of the thymus gland in myasthenia gravis. *Ann NY Acad Sci* 135:496–503, 1966.

20. Namba T, Nakata Y, Grob D: The role of humoral and cellular immune factors in the neuromuscular block of myasthenia gravis. *Ann NY Acad Sci* 274:493–515, 1976.

21. Blalock A, Mason MF, Morgan HJ, et al: Myasthenia gravis and tumors of the thymic region: report of a case in which the tumor was removed. *Ann Surg* 110:544–561, 1939.

22. Simpson JA: An evaluation of thymectomy in myasthenia gravis. *Brain* 81:112–144, 1958.

23. Ozdemir C, Young RR: The results to be expected from electrical testing in the diagnosis of myasthenia gravis. *Ann NY Acad Sci* 274:203–222, 1976.

24. Walker MB: Myasthenia gravis: a case in which fatigue of forearm muscles could induce paralysis of extraocular muscles. *Proc Royal Soc Med* 31:722, 1938.

25. Walker MB: Some discoveries on myasthenia gravis: the background. *Br Med J* 2:42–43, 1973.

26. Patten BM: A hypothesis to account for the Mary Walker phenomenon. *Ann Intern Med* 82:411–415, 1975.
27. Munsat TL: A standardized forearm ischemic exercise test. *Neurology* 20:1171–1178, 1970.
28. Vincent A, Pinching AJ, Newsom DJ: Circulating antiacetylcholine receptor antibody in myasthenia gravis treated by plasma exchange. *Neurology* 27:364, 1977.
29. Dau PC, Lindstrom JM, Cassel CK, et al: Plasmapheresis and immunosuppressive drug therapy in myasthenia gravis. *N Engl J Med* 297:1134–1140, 1977.
30. Osserman KE: Pregnancy in myasthenia gravis and neonatal myasthenia gravis. *Am J Med* 19:718, 1955.
31. Viets HR, Schwab RS, Brazier MAB: The effect of pregnancy on the course of myasthenia gravis. *JAMA* 119:236, 1942.
32. Fraser D, Turner JWA: Myasthenia gravis and pregnancy. *Proc Royal Soc Med* 56:379, 1963.
33. Plauche WC: Myasthenia gravis in pregnancy. *Am J Obstet Gynecol* 88:404, 1964.
34. Plauche WC: Myasthenia gravis in pregnancy: an update. *Am J Obstet Gynecol* 135:691, 1979.
35. Scott JS: Immunologic diseases in pregnancy. *Prog Allergy* 23:371, 1977.
36. Hay DM: Myasthenia gravis and pregnancy. *Br J Obstet Gynaecol* 76:323, 1969.
37. Kitzmiller JL: Autoimmune disorders: maternal, fetal, and neonatal risks. *Clin Obstet Gynecol* 21:385, 1978.
38. Schlezinger WS: Pregnancy in myasthenia gravis and neonatal myasthenia gravis. *Am J Med* 19:718, 1955.
39. Perry CP, Hilliceral GD, Gilstrap LC, et al: Myasthenia gravis in pregnancy. *Ala J Med Sci* 12:219, 1975.
40. Duff GB: Preeclampsia and the patient with myasthenia gravis. *Obstet Gynecol* 54:355, 1979.
41. Foldes FF, McWall PG: Myasthenia gravis: a guide for anesthesiologists. *Anesthesiology* 23:837, 1967.
42. Bradley W, Adams N: NMJ disorders and episodic muscular weakness. In *Harrison's Principles of Internal Medicine*. 10th ed. Edited by KJ Isselbacher. New York, NY. McGraw Hill, Chap 372, 1981, pp. 2193.
43. Hawkey CJ, Newsom-Davis J, Vincent A: plasma exchange and immunosuppressive drug treatment in myasthenia gravis: no evidence for surgery. *J Neurol Neurosurg Psychiatry* 44:469, 1981.
44. Nielsen VK, Paulson OB, Rosenkvist J, et al: Rapid improvement of myasthenia gravis after plasma exchange. *Ann Neurol* 11:160, 1982.
45. Cameron LB, Kirsch JR: Myasthenia gravis: pharmacologic management. *Crit Care Rep* 1:157–163, 1989.
46. McNall PG, Jafarnier MR: Management of myasthenia gravis in the obstetrical patient. *Am J Obstet Gynecol* 92:518, 1965.
47. Chambers DC, Hall JE, Boyce J: Myasthenia gravis and pregnancy. *Obstet Gynecol* 29:597, 1967.

48. Aminoff MJ: Neurological disorders and pregnancy. *Am J Obstet Gynecol* 132:325, 1978.
49. James FM, Wheeler AS: *Obstetric Anesthesia: The Complicated Patient.* Philadelphia, PA. FA Davis, 1982, pp. 77.
50. Burkett G, Rodevique E: Acute myasthenia gravis in pregnancy. *West Indies Med J* 25:162, 1976.
51. Cohen BA, London RS, Goldstein PJ: Myasthenia gravis and preeclampsia. *Obstet Gynecol* 48:355, 1976.
52. DeLara M: Myasthenia gravis and pregnancy. *Acta Obstet Ginecol His Lusit* 21:1, 1973.
53. Ham J: Factors affecting administration of neuromuscular blocking agents: annual refresher course lectures. *Am Soc Anesthesiol* 1979.
54. Repke JT: Clinical dialogue: treating preeclampsia with phenytoin. *Contemp Ob/Gyn* 34:57–59, 1989.
55. Namba T, Brown SB, Grob D: Neonatal myasthenia gravis: report of 7 cases and review of the literature. *Pediatrics* 45:488, 1970.
56. Fenichel GM: Clinical syndromes of myasthenics in infancy and childhood. *Arch Neurol* 35:97, 1978.
57. Donaldson JO, Penn AS, Lisak RP, et al: Antiacetylcholine receptor antibody in neonatal myasthenia gravis. *Am J Dis Child* 135:222, 1981.
58. Kessey J, Lindstrom J, Cokely H, et al: Antiacetylcholine receptor antibody in neonatal myasthenia gravis. *N Eng J Med* 296:55, 1977.
59. Appel SH, Ellias SB: Antiacetylcholine receptor antibodies in myasthenia gravis. In *Plasmapheresis and the Immunobiology of Myasthenia Gravis.* Edited by PC Daw. Boston, MA. Houghton, Mifflin, 1979, pp. 52–59.
60. Abramsky O, Brenner T, Lisak RP, et al: Significance in neonatal myasthenia gravis on inhibitory effect of amniotic fluid on binding of antibodies to acetylcholine receptor. *Lancet* 1:1333, 1979.
61. Osserman KE: *Myasthenia Gravis.* New York, NY. Grune & Stratton, Inc, 1958.

12

Neurological Manifestations of Rheumatic Diseases in Pregnancy

John Meyerhoff, M.D.

Introduction

Neurological manifestations are common in many connective tissue diseases. Overall, there does not appear to be any consistent effect of pregnancy on the neurological manifestations of any of the rheumatologic diseases except rheumatoid arthritis (RA). Two excellent reviews are available that discuss those conditions not covered in this chapter.[1,2]

The etiologies of the rheumatologic diseases discussed in this chapter remain unknown. Attempts to find an infectious cause for RA and systemic lupus erythematosus (SLE) have been fruitless. Given the racial and sexual differences in the frequency of these diseases, it is clear that host factors play as important a role in the development of disease as does the etiologic event, if there is one. Mice of many strains develop lupus-like or vasculitic diseases without obvious exposure to an etiologic agent. It seems possible that some of these diseases are not caused by exogenous factors, but rather represent failures in self regulation of the immune system.

For many of the rheumatologic diseases, autoantibodies have

From Goldstein PJ, Stern BJ, (eds): *Neurological Disorders of Pregnancy. Second Revised Edition.* Mount Kisco NY, Futura Publishing Co., Inc., © 1992.

been described that are more common in individuals with a particular disease than in normals or patients with other connective tissue diseases. These autoantibodies may be present without disease ever occurring or disease can occur without detectable levels of autoantibodies (i.e., seronegative RA and antinuclear antibody (ANA)-negative SLE). These autoantibodies are neither necessary or sufficient to cause the development of the associated disease. In many of the rheumatologic diseases characterized by autoantibodies, multiple autoantibodies are the rule rather than the exception. As many as 68% of patients with RA have ANAs[3] and 30% of SLE patients have positive tests for rheumatoid factor (RF).[4]

The deposition of immune complexes containing self antigen and antibody to that self antigen (the autoantibody) is felt to be the pathogenic event in the autoimmune rheumatologic diseases. In RA, the self antigen is IgG and the IgM antibody directed against IgG is RF. This is in distinction to diseases such as myasthenia gravis or Graves' disease where the attachment of the autoantibody to a receptor site causes disease. The multitude of signs and symptoms of rheumatologic diseases are due to the differences between the physical characteristics of the particular antigen-antibody complex in each of these diseases, the different sites where these complexes deposit in the body, and how the humoral and cell-mediated immune systems (including complement) react to these antigens and antibodies.

One major effect of the rheumatologic disease on the fetus is an increased rate of fetal wastage in mothers with SLE.[5] A neonatal lupus syndrome characterized most often by skin lesions and/or heart block can be seen in the children of mothers with SLE and Sjögren's syndrome.[6] This syndrome can also occur in the children of asymptomatic women[7,8] and its occurrence seems to be strongly associated with certain HLA types.[9] The neonatal lupus syndrome seems to be related to the presence of an antibody known as the anti-Ro antibody. This antibody recognizes a group of small nuclear and cytoplasmic ribonucleoproteins (snRNP and scRNP).[10] Before the antigen was characterized, it was named the "Ro" antigen after the individual in whom it was found. (Some authors refer to this antigen as SSA for its initial association with Sjögren's syndrome. This association is much weaker than first supposed.) These RNPs have been found in the skin and cardiac conducting system of normal fetus.[11] It is presumed that the heart block and rash are due to the transplacental passage of anti-Ro antibodies into the fetus where they complex with the normally occurring RNA antigen. The resultant immune response leads to fibrosis of the conducting system and a rash. Some women with SLE have children who have transient symptoms of SLE due to the transplacental passage of other IgG antibodies which can last in the newborn's circulation for about six months.[12,13]

Rheumatoid Arthritis

Rheumatoid arthritis is two to three times more common in women than in men. The overall prevalence in women over the age of 18 is about 1%. The peak age of onset is between 35 and 45 years, but a wide range exists.[14–16]

The diagnosis of RA is based on the presence of an additive, symmetrical, inflammatory arthritis usually associated with a positive RF and characteristic radiological abnormalities. A recent revision of the criteria for RA has eliminated the use of adjectives such as "probable" in describing RA. This change recognizes that earlier criteria may have been overinclusive and that the use of adjectives did not help in classifying or treating RA.[17]

The most frequently associated autoantibody in RA is RF that is IgM directed against IgG. Approximately 90% of RA patients have RF in their serum. Of course the articular system is the most frequently affected organ in RA. Deposition of RF and its target antigen IgG with associated complement activation is the presumed pathogenesis of the inflammation seen in RA. Those patients who do not have detectable RF probably have IgG RF or very low levels of IgM RF. These patients may have a different pathological mechanism responsible for the initiation or continuation of the inflammatory process.[18]

Extra-articular manifestations of RA, presumably due to the deposition of immune complexes in extra-articular locations, are common.[19] Rheumatoid nodules are perhaps the most obvious of these manifestations, occurring in up to 35% of reported series. They usually occur over pressure points but may occur anywhere and sometimes produce symptoms due to their effect on the surrounding structures. Other organs that can be involved include the lungs with nodules and interstitial fibrosis, the muscles with an inflammatory myositis, the eyes with scleromalacia and episcleritis, the pleura and pericardium, and the exocrine glands with inflammation and fibrosis (Sjögren's syndrome). In Europe, amyloidosis occurs in patients with long-standing disease although it has rarely been reported in the United States.

Extra-articular manifestations of RA rarely occur at the same time as the onset of the arthritis. This is particularly true of the neurological complications of RA that are due either to instability of the cervical spine or vasculitis, both of which are usually late developments. Thus, without a history of previous RA or physical findings of such, RA should not be considered as a cause of neurological disease.

The neurological involvement in RA can be divided into compressive and vasculitic phenomena (Table I). Articular involvement in the cervical spine can lead to the destruction of the odontoid and/or the weakening of the spinal ligaments. The resultant instability of C-1 and C-2 can lead to compression of the spinal cord and a cervical myelopathy.[20] Presenting symptoms can include sensory or motor loss and bladder and bowel dysfunction. Joint swelling can lead to peripheral nerve entrapment. The carpal tunnel syndrome is the most common entrapment syndrome seen in RA.[21] Central nervous system rheumatoid nodules have been reported to compress nerves although they usually are asymptomatic.

Vasculitic involvement can result in a mild stocking-glove peripheral neuropathy that may be of varying severity and resolve spontaneously.[22] Although this neuropathy is due to a vasculitis,[23,24] it is a benign process that does not seem to affect prognosis. This vasculitis occurs in patients with long-standing RA (10- to 15-year duration) who have other signs of disease such as rheumatoid nodules.

A more serious vasculitic problem is the development of a mononeuritis multiplex. This usually presents as a motor neuropathy re-

---

Table I.
Neurological Features of Rheumatoid Arthritis

Compressive
  Spinal cord compression due to C1-C2 instability
  Peripheral entrapment (e.g., carpal tunnel syndrome)
Vasculitic
  Stocking-glove sensory neuropathy
  Mononeuritis multiplex

sulting in a foot or wrist drop. There is usually a vasculitis in other organ systems, and the full-blown form resembles polyarteritis no-dosa.[21,22] Pathological examination of the peripheral nerves shows a vasculitis of the vasa nervorum. This type of vasculitis has a poor prognosis and may result in death if not treated aggressively.[25] Central nervous system vasculitis and "rheumatoid meningitis" have been described.[26]

The beneficial effect of pregnancy on RA that has been reported since the 1930s continues to be confirmed by more recent reports.[27] This effect lasts only for the duration of pregnancy and patients will commonly relapse after delivery. Pregnancy is unlikely to affect the neurological manifestations outlined above. Most of the neurological events occur after 5 to 10 years of disease and by then the patient is usually out of the childbearing years. Additionally, the neurological manifestations are not necessarily due to currently active disease or may be so severe that the remittive effects of pregnancy are too mild to produce a response. Women who have juvenile onset rheumatoid arthritis may have had their disease long enough to develop neurological complications by the time they become pregnant. Patients with entrapment syndromes might get some relief from a reduction in joint swelling, but such patients might then be more likely to have a worsening of their entrapment syndrome due to the pregnancy alone.

Systemic Lupus Erythematosus

The development of serologic tests and a better understanding of the protean manifestations of SLE have made it obvious that this disease is more common and less deadly than initially reported. Prevalence rates in the general population of 15 to 50 cases per 100,000 individuals have been reported. There are striking age, sex, and racial prevalence differences. In one study, 15- to 44-year-old white, black, and Puerto Rican women had prevalence rates of 21.2, 80.9, and 56.9 cases per 100,000, respectively. The rates for males of the same ethnic groups were 5.0, 8.3, and 3.6 cases per 100,000, respectively. Since this study used hospital discharge summaries as its source, it clearly underestimates the frequency of SLE, but probably not the variation between racial groups.[28] Previous uncontrolled studies on pregnancy in SLE suggested that pregnancy would exacerbate SLE. More recent case controlled studies and better retrospective studies indicate that there is no consistent effect of pregnancy in SLE and that as many patients improve as worsen.[29-33]

The diagnosis of SLE is based on the appearance of typical symptoms (Table II) in association with positive serologic tests. The Amer-

---

Table II.
Signs and Symptoms of SLE

Cardiovascular	**Ocular**
Coronary vasculitis	Conjunctivitis
Libman-Sachs endocarditis	Cytoid bodies
Myocarditis	Episcleritis
Pericarditis	Sjögren's syndrome
Raynaud's phenomenon	**Pleuropulmonary**
Constitutional	Interstitial fibrosis
Anorexia	Pleural effusions
Fatigue	Pleurisy
Fever	Pneumonitis
Weight loss	**Renal**
Gastrointestinal	Glomerulonephritis
Abdominal pain	Interstitial nephritis
Dysphagia	Nephrotic syndrome
Hepatomegly	**Reticuloendothelial**
Mesenteric vasculitis	Lymphadenopathy
Xerostomia	Splenomegly
Hematologic	**Skin and Mucous Membranes**
Anemia of chronic disease	Alopecia
Circulating anticoagulants	Butterfly rash
Hemolytic anemia	Discoid lupus
Hypocomplementemia	Maculopapular rash
Leukopenia	Mouth ulcers
Thrombocytopenia	Periungual erythema
Musculoskeletal	Photosensitive rash
Myalgias	Rheumatoid nodules
Myositis	Vasculitis
Polyarthralgia	
Polyarthritis	
Tenosynovitis	
Neuropsychiatric	
Behavioral changes	
Migranous phenomena	
Peripheral neuropathy	
Psychosis	
Seizures	

Table III.
Sensitive Findings in SLE

Alopecia	Anti-DNA antibody
Arthritis	Antinuclear antibody
Pleurisy	Decreased complement
Proteinuria	LE cells

ican Rheumatism Association criteria applicable to SLE were developed to ensure that research on groups of patients with SLE in fact have SLE and not other diseases, specifically not RA.[4,34] They are not diagnostic criteria. A clinical diagnosis of SLE is based on finding a combination of those symptoms that are frequent enough in SLE to suggest that diagnosis (Table III, sensitive findings) and those that are uncommon enough in other rheumatologic diseases (Table IV, specific findings) to exclude those other diseases.[35]

An ANA is positive in about 90% of patients with SLE and therefore is a useful screening test. It is frequently positive in individuals with rheumatologic symptoms, other rheumatologic diseases and in relatives of patients with SLE.[36] In "normals" it is probably very rare; there is rarely a reason to get an ANA in a normal individual. To confirm a diagnosis of SLE in an ANA-positive individual, testing for antibodies to native (double-stranded) DNA or the Sm antigen should

Table IV.
Specific Findings in SLE

Discoid rash
Hemolytic anemia
Malar rash
Neuropsychiatric abnormalities
Oral ulcers
Pericarditis
Photosensitivity
Thrombocytopenia

Anti-DNA antibody
Anti-Sm antibody
LE cells
Serologic tests for syphilis

be done. The Sm antigen, found in a patient named Smith, is an extractable nuclear antigen (ENA). Both these antibodies are highly specific for SLE occurring in less than 1% of individuals with a false-positive ANA. They are diagnostic only if present. They do not rule out SLE if absent because the anti-DNA and the anti-Sm antibodies have a sensitivity of 50% and 40%, respectively.[37] Approximately 10% of patients with SLE do not have a positive ANA and thus have "ANA-negative SLE." Most of these patients do have some auto-antibodies other than an ANA.

One of the primary pathological events in SLE is thought to be the deposition of DNA-anti-DNA complexes in vascular structures resulting in the activation of the complement system. Patients may therefore develop skin rashes, vasculitis, glomerulonephritis, pericarditis, pleuritis, and arthritis. Additionally, antibodies to the red cells, white cells, and platelets can develop and cause destruction of these elements in the reticuloendothelial system. Lastly, antibodies specifically cytotoxic to cells or that induce cell-mediated cytolysis may develop.

Any or all of the pathological processes mentioned above may be present in a patient with neuropsychiatric (NP) lupus. Because usually pathological material is lacking except in those patients who die of SLE or in patients whose CNS event is not recent, a good correlation between symptoms and the pathology cannot always be made.[38] Immune complex deposition has been observed in the choroid plexus and such deposition is the likely cause of the vasculitis observed in the central and peripheral neurologic lesions.[39] Anti-platelet antibodies may be important because platelets and neurons both metabolize neurotransmitters, and abnormalities of platelet metabolism have been described in SLE.[40,41] Bluestein et al.[42] described cytotoxic antilymphocyte antibodies that cross-react with neurons and in experimental animals have caused neurological dysfunction. More recent studies have found various antineuronal and antineurofilament antibodies that may associate with neurological dysfunction.[43–45] Over the past 10 years the importance of antiphospholipid antibodies (including the lupus anticoagulant, anticardiolipin antibodies and the false-positive test for syphillis) has been recognized as a cause of thrombosis.[46] Some NP manifestations, particularly stroke, may be due to these antibodies and resultant CNS ischemic events.

Neuropsychiatric manifestations are thought to occur in one third

Table V.
Frequent Neuropsychiatric Manifestations in Systemic Lupus

Manifestation	Patients (52 total)
Psychiatric Illness/Organic Brain Syndrome	24
Seizures	17
Long Tract Signs	16
Cranial Nerve Abnormalities	16
Peripheral Neuropathy	15

to one half of patients with SLE although one recent study reported a frequency of 83%.[47-49] In only 5% of patients is NP disease the initial manifestation of SLE and in 90% of patients NP lupus occurs in the first 5 years. Patients may present with one or more of the findings listed in Table V.[47] Other reports have emphasized the presentation of CNS lupus with migraine-like symptoms, transverse myelopathy, multiple sclerosis, or Guillain-Barré-like illnesses.[50-53] Central nervous system involvement is now the leading direct disease-related cause of death in SLE patients.

Changes in mental status are the most common neurological manifestations in SLE. Other neurological findings can occur, most often seizures,[47,48] which are usually generalized motor events. Long tract and cranial nerve abnormalities are the next most frequent neurological findings and may occur as part of a diffuse process or stroke. A peripheral neuropathy may develop as a mild to moderate predominantly sensory polyneuropathy or as mononeuritis multiplex.

Migraine accompaniments such as fortification spectra, scotomas and flashing lights may occur either alone or in association with headache.[50,54] Rarely will headache be the sole CNS manifestation of SLE.

When NP manifestations occur along with signs and symptoms of active SLE, the diagnosis of NP is obvious. Other causes for the NP findings such as uremia and infections should be sought. In one study, 35% of the psychiatric symptoms in a group of patients were non-SLE related.[47]

There are no specific laboratory tests for NP SLE. The CSF is often abnormal with an elevated opening pressure, protein level, or white cell count. Elevated levels of antibodies to diverse neuronal components and oligoclonal bands have been detected in patients with NP lupus. These assays have rarely been done in patients without NP manifestations. Thus, while the frequency of these tests in patients with NP disease is known, the specificity of these tests (the frequency of negative tests in patients without NP manifestations) is not known. One cannot use a test to diagnose disease without knowing both the sensitivity and specificity of a test. A similar problem exists with the EEG (abnormal in up to 70% of patients) and MRI (abnormal in up to 66%). Magnetic resonance imaging scans are more likely to be abnormal in patients with neurological (rather than psychiatric) manifestations and in those with acute events. Until these assays and scans have been done in large numbers of lupus patients without past or current NP manifestations, their value in diagnosing active NP SLE remains speculative.

Scleroderma

Scleroderma (SD), or thickening and hardening of the skin, is a term used to describe a disease characterized by severe skin changes. Similar skin changes can occur in a number of diseases and can also be induced by drugs such as bleomycin and pentazocine and chemicals such as vinyl chloride.[55,56] Within the disease "scleroderma" there are two patterns: systemic sclerosis and the CREST syndrome.

In the full-blown form, SD may present with scleroderma, Raynaud's phenomenon, esophageal dysfunction, intersitial pulmonary fibrosis, pericarditis, wide mouth colonic diverticula, sclerosis of the bowel, and malignant hypertension. The CREST syndrome is characterized by calcinosis, Raynaud's phenomenon, esophageal dysfunction, sclerodactyly (scleroderma limited to the digits), and telangiectasias. There is clearly an improved survival with the CREST syndrome compared to systemic sclerosis. In an individual patient it may not always be possible to clearly characterize which group the patient belongs to. In this chapter, SD applies to both of these syndromes.

Scleroderma is a much rarer disease than SLE, occurring about only a tenth as often.[57] There is a 3:1 female to male ratio and a similar predominance among blacks. The median age of onset is between 40 and 50; the disease is rare below the age of 20 with only 9% of cases occurring below that age.[58] Thus, in the childbearing years, it is much rarer than RA and SLE.

The etiology and pathogenesis of SD is unknown. Antinuclear antibodies (ANA) frequently are found in patients, but clearly they are not specific to SD. Some more specific antinuclear antibodies have been discovered that may help differentiate systemic sclerosis from the CREST syndrome.[59,60] The pathogenesis of SD probably begins with injury to the vascular endothelial cells, followed by the release of substances such as platelet-derived growth factor from these and other cells, which in turn results in proliferative and fibrotic changes in the blood vessels and other tissues, primarily the skin.

Neurological involvement in SD is rare. Malignant hypertension with hypertensive encephalopathy may develop due to a proliferative vasculopathy in the kidney. The most frequent neurological complication is an isolated trigeminal sensory neuropathy.[61] This occurs in approximately 4% of patients and the mean age of onset is in the forties. Disease of the vascular supply of the nerve or nerve entrapment in sclerodermatous skin are the likely etiologies of the neuropathy. The symptoms may resolve spontaneously. No effective medical therapy is known for this problem. Recent reviews of SD and pregnancy suggest that there is no consistent effect of pregnancy on SD or its neurological manifestations.[62,63]

Sjögren's Syndrome

Sjögren's syndrome (SS) is characterized by symptoms of dry eyes (xerophthalmia) and dry mouth (xerostomia)—the sicca complex—due to lymphocytic and plasma cell infiltration of the exocrine glands.[64] Initial symptoms usually involve the mouth with complaints of dryness and excessive thirst or the eyes with grittiness or a foreign body sensation. Keratoconjunctivitis sicca occurs when the dryness results in the disruption of the corneal epithelium.

The sicca complex can occur as a primary disease or as a secondary phenomenon in association with other connective tissue diseases such as RA, SLE, and SD. The diagnosis is made by carefully questioning the patient about symptoms of dry eyes, dry mouth, increased dental caries, and symptoms of bronchitis or vaginal dryness that may occur when the exocrine glands in the bronchial tree or vagina are involved. The diagnosis is further suggested by finding dry eyes or mouth on examination. An ophthalmologist can do a Schirmer's test and slit lamp examination to further evaluate the eyes. The most definitive test is a minor salivary gland biopsy of the lip to look for characteristic pathological changes of cellular infiltration and fibrosis.

The frequency of SS is unknown because subclinical cases exist and few patients with sicca symptoms have a biopsy. In one study, only 18% of the patients with a complaint of dry eyes had both objective xerostomia and a positive biopsy.[65] These patients were all female. The mean age of onset of symptoms was 34 years. Frequencies of 100% of secondary SS in SLE and scleroderma have been reported when multiple methods of assessing exocrine function have been used and any one abnormal result was considered diagnostic of Sjögren's syndrome.[66,67] About one third of patients with SS will be positive for antibodies against the Ro antigen.

Neuropsychiatric manifestations occur in primary SS. The pathological basis is assumed to be an underlying vasculitis with associated complement activation.[68] Of 40 patients with NP SS, 27 had 51 various neurological findings and 25 had 60 different psychiatric manifestations.[69] CNS events included focal neurological deficits, seizures, movement disorders, cognitive dysfunction, and aseptic meningoencephalitis. Four patients had spinal cord dysfunction. Peripheral nervous system involvement was predominantly due to entrapment syndromes (16 of 22 events). A sensory polyneuropathy or neuronopathy can occur. Depression was the most common psychiatric diagnosis (19 patients) with personality disorders and somatization also occurring frequently (13 patients each).

As in SLE, many of these patients had abnormal CSF findings. An elevated IgG index and oligoclonal bands occurred in 10 patients each in this study. Given the multiplicity of neurological findings in these patients, such CSF findings could mistakenly lead to a diagnosis of multiple sclerosis if SS is not considered in the diagnosis. Magnetic resonance imaging scans have been reported to be abnormal in up to 75% of patients with active NP SS compared to only 9% of SS patients without NP manifestations.[70] The MRI was abnormal in 2 NP patients who had normal EEG, LP and evoked response testing and normal in 4 NP patients with one abnormality of the three other tests. There does not yet seem to be a single test that will determine if a clinical finding is or is not due to SS.

"Overlap" Syndromes

There are a number of patients who have features of several of the diseases discussed above. Some of the patients may have several features at the same time while others may evolve from one disease to another over time. Such patients are usually referred to as "overlap" patients.[71] The prognosis of these patients seems to relate to the type of organ involvement that is present at a particular time and patients should be treated on that basis.[72] Many of these patients would belong to the group of patients once defined as having "mixed connective tissue disease." These patients are not a homogeneous group of patients, but rather are a very heterogeneous group with different diseases and outcomes and should not be classified together.

Treatment

The drugs used in the rheumatologic diseases, the disease they are most used in, and the risk of fetal side effects are listed in Table VI. The neurological manifestations of RA, SLE, and SS do not respond to the less toxic agents such as the nonsteroidal antiinflammatory drugs (NSAIDs) or the antimalarials. The trigeminal neuropathy of SD may not respond to any therapy.

The treatment of rheumatoid arthritis begins with nonsteroidals and physical therapy. When additional therapy (traditionally referred to as "remittive" therapy) is needed, antimalarials, azulfidine, corticosteroids, D-penicillamine, gold (either IM or PO), and methotrexate are added. There is no agreement as to the order in which to use these, but there is more agreement on the need to treat the articular manifestations sooner and more aggressively with these agents than in the past. Azathioprine and cyclophosphamide would be the next drugs used. Lastly, experimental therapies such as various types of pheresis and total lymphoid irradiation have been tried.

The peripheral nervous system manifestations of RA are often treated with remittive agents if they are not already in use. If a patient

Table VI.
Antirheumatic Drugs

Name of Drug	Diseases Used In	Effective For Neurological Disease	Fetal Risk
Aspirin	RA, SLE, SD, SS	No	Low
Other NSAIDs	RA, SLE, SD, SS	No	Probably low
Antimalarials	RA, SLE	No	Occular risk
Corticosteroids	RA, SLE, SD, SS	Yes	Probably none
Gold	RA	Yes	Probably high
D-Penicillamine	RA, SD	Yes	Probably high
Methotrexate	RA	Yes	High
Cyclophosphamide	RA, SLE, SS	Yes	High
Azathioprine	RA, SLE, SS	Yes	High

Ra = Rheumatoid Arthritis; SLE = Systemic Lupus; SD = Scleroderma, SS = Sjögren's Syndrome.

develops "rheumatoid vasculitis" of the type which resembles po-lyarteritis, corticosteroids are added or increased for an immediate anti-inflammatory response. One of the "remittive" agents is usually also added if not already in use.

The treatment of SLE and SD depends on which manifestations are present in a particular patient. Many of the mucocutaneous, se-rosal and synovial symptoms of SLE can be treated with topical cor-ticosteroids, antimalarials or NSAIDs. Only when these therapies fail or other organ systems are involved are corticosteroids used. Scle-roderma and SS and approached similarly, only there is less agree-ment that treatment prevents progression of the underlying disease in either condition. Symptomatic treatment of nonvasculitic manifes-tations is the rule in these two diseases with steroids and cytotoxics reserved for vasculitic, myositic, nonentrapment neuropathies, and neuropsychiatric events.

The first agent usually used in patients with potentially treatable neurological disease is corticosteroids. The choice of dose, frequency, and route of corticosteroid dose is one that must be individualized from patient to patient. There are no double blind controlled trials of corticosteroids in the neurological complications of the diseases dis-cussed in this chapter.

Most rheumatologists would begin treatment with at least 60 mg of prednisone daily in a single dose with increases up to perhaps 100 mg daily in four divided doses. Some physicians will use up to 200 mg daily. It is clear that increasing doses, particularly above the equivalent of 100 mg of prednisone daily, bring increasing risks of opportunistic infections.[48] Other nonfatal complications of corticosteroids such as osteoporosis, diabetes, and adrenal suppression are also dose-dependent. Pulse therapy of 1,000 mg of IV methylprednisolone over 1 to 2 hours once a day for 3 days is being used increasingly for some patients with these diseases. These pulses may be the only corticosteroids given to some patients, while other patients may get the pulses in addition to moderate daily doses of corticosteroids. Also, this therapy has not been studied in a controlled fashion for CNS disease and while it may produce dramatic results, it does not seem to reduce the total corticosteroid dose.

Cytotoxic agents (azathioprine and cyclophosphamide) are also used when NP manifestations are present. Depending on the severity and nature of the neurological event, these agents may be started along with corticosteroids, or if corticosteroids do not produce a response. They are also used as corticosteroid-sparing agents in patients who respond to corticosteroids, but develop significant side effects. Cyclophosphamide is currently used more often than azathioprine, but is associated with the development of hemorrhagic cystitis and bladder carcinoma. Clearly, its use dictates a careful weighing of the risks and benefits involved.

Although it is clear that corticosteroids can induce fetal abnormalities in rats,[73] there is no evidence that these agents produce an increase in fetal abnormalities in humans.[74] Adrenal function in newborns exposed to corticosteroids in utero or in breast milk appears to be normal. Thus, this class of drugs appears to be as safe as any drugs can be in pregnancy.

All of the other drugs mentioned in this chapter, antimalarials, gold, D-penicillamine, methotrexate, azathioprine, and cyclophosphamide, are relatively contraindicated in pregnancy.[73–75] They are all teratogenic in animals at doses greater than those used in humans. Although there are case reports of normal children born to mothers on these agents, pregnancy should be continued in women who are given these agents only after a thorough discussion of the significant risk of fetal malformation. The risk of malformation is obviously greatest at the beginning of pregnancy and this fact should be taken into account in any decision to terminate or continue a pregnancy.

References

1. Cohen SB, Hurd ER: Neurological complications of connective tissue and other "collagen-vascular" diseases. *Semin Arthritis Rheum* 11:190–212, 1981.
2. Sigal LH: The neurologic presentation of vasculitis and rheumatologic syndromes. A review. *Medicine* 66:157–180, 1987.
3. Ritchie RF: The clinical significance of titered antinuclear antibodies. *Arthritis Rheum* 10:544–42, 1967.
4. Cohen AS, Reynolds WE, Franklin EC, et al: Preliminary criteria for the classification of systemic lupus erythematosus. *Bull Rheum Dis* 21:643–648, 1971.
5. Tozman EC, Urowitz MB, Gladman DD: Systemic lupus erythematosus and pregnancy. *J Rheumatol* 7:624–632, 1980.
6. Chameides L, Truex RC, Vetter V, et al: Association of maternal systemic lupus erythematosus with congenital complete heart block. *N Engl J Med* 297:1204–1207, 1977.
7. Scott JS, Maddison PJ, Taylor PV, et al: Connective-tissue disease, antibodies to ribonucleoprotein, and congenital heart block. *N Engl J Med* 309:209–212, 1983.
8. Lockshin MD, Bonfa E, Elkon K, et al: Neonatal lupus risk to newborns of mothers with systemic lupus erythematosus. *Arthritis Rheum* 31:697–701, 1988.
9. Watson RM, Lane AT, Barnett NK, et al: Neonatal lupus erythematosus: a clinical, serological and immunogenetic study with review of the literature. *Medicine* 63:362–378, 1984.
10. Wolin SC, Steitz JA: The Ro small cytoplasmic ribonucleoproteins: identification of the antigenic site and its binding site on the Ro RNAs. *Proc Natl Acad Sci USA* 81:1996–2000, 1984.
11. Lee LA, Harmon CE, Huff JC, et al: SSA (Ro) antigen expression in human, fetal and neonatal, and adult tissues. *Arthritis Rheum* 27:520, 1984.
12. Vetter VL, Rashkind WJ: Congenital complete heart block and connective-tissue disease. *N Engl J Med* 309:236–238, 1983.
13. Hess EW, Spencer-Green G: Congenital heart block and connective tissue disease. *Ann Intern Med* 91:645–646, 1979.
14. Hochberg MC, Arnett RC: Rheumatoid arthritis XII: epidemiology and genetics. *Md State Med J* 32:365–367, 1983.
15. Harris ED: The clinical features of rheumatoid arthritis. In *Textbook of Rheumatology*, 3rd edition. Edited by WN Kelley, ED Harris, S Sledge, et al. Philadelphia, PA. WB Saunders Company, 1989, pp. 943–974.
16. Masi AT, Medsger T: Epidemiology of the rheumatic diseases. In *Arthritis and Allied Conditions: A Textbook of Rheumatology*, 11th edition. Edited by DJ McCarty, Philadelphia, PA. Lea & Febiger, 1989, pp 16–54.

17. Arnett FC, Edworthy S, Bloch DA, et al: The American Rheumatism Association 1987 revised criteria for the classification of rheumatoid arthritis. *Arthritis Rheum* 31:315–324, 1988.
18. Alarcon GS, Koopman WJ, Acton RT, et al: Seronegative rheumatoid arthritis. A distinct immunogenetic disease? *Arthritis Rheum* 25:502–507, 1982.
19. Wigley FM: Rheumatoid arthritis II: systemic manifestations. *Md State Med J* 31:40–42, 1982.
20. Ball J, Sharp J: Rheumatoid arthritis of the cervical spine. *Med Trends Rheumatol* 2:117–138, 1971.
21. Pallis CA, Scott JT: Peripheral neuropathy in rheumatoid arthritis. *Br Med J* 1:1141–1147, 1965.
22. Hart FD, Golding JR: Rheumatoid neuropathy. *Br Med J* 1:1594–1600, 1960.
23. Beckett VL, Dinn JJ: Segmental demyelination in rheumatoid arthritis. Q J Med 41:71–80, 1972.
24. Conn DL, McDuffie FC, Dyck PJ: Immunopathologic study of sural nerves in rheumatoid arthritis. *Arthritis Rheum* 15:135–143, 1972.
25. Chamberlin MA, Bruckner FE: Rheumatoid neuropathy: clinical and electrophysiological features. *Ann Rheum Dis* 29:609–616, 1970.
26. Markenson JA, McDougal JS, Tsairis P, et al: Rheumatoid meningitis: a localized process. *Ann Intern Med* 90:786–789, 1979.
27. Persellin RH: The effect of pregnancy on rheumatoid arthritis. *Bull Rheum Dis* 27:922–927, 1976.
28. Masi AT: Clinical epidemiologic perspective of systemic lupus erythematosus. In *Current Topics in Rheumatology. Epidemiology of the Rheumatic Diseases.* Edited by RC Lawrence, LE Shulman. New York, NY. Gower Medical Publishing Limited, 1984, pp. 145–163.
29. Lochskin MD, Reinitz E, Druzin ML, et al: Lupus pregnancy: case-control prospective study demonstrating absence of lupus exacerbation during or after pregnancy. *Am J Med* 77:983, 1984.
30. Fine LG, Barnett EV, Danovitch GM, et al: Systemic lupus erythematosus in pregnancy. *Ann Intern Med* 94:667–677, 1981.
31. Tozman EC, Urowitz MB, Gladman DD: Systemic lupus erythematosus and pregnancy. *J Rheumatol* 7:624–632, 1980.
32. Lockshin MD. Pregnancy does not cause systemic lupus erythematosus to worsen. *Arthritis Rheum* 308:665–670, 1989.
33. Mintz G, Rodriguez-Alvarez E. Systemic lupus erythematosus. *Rheum Dis Clin* 15:255–274, 1989.
34. Tan EM, Cohen AS, Fries JF, et al: The 1982 revised criteria for the classification of systemic lupus erythematosus. *Arthritis Rheum* 25:1271–1277, 1982.
35. Meyerhoff J: Systemic lupus erythematosus VII: making the diagnosis. *Md State Med J* 33:42–45, 1984.
36. Richardson B, Epstein WV. Utility of the fluorescent antinuclear antibody test in a single patient. *Ann Intern Med* 95:333–338, 1981.
37. Meyerhoff J: Systemic lupus erythematosus VI: hematologic and sereologic abnormalities. *Md State Med J* 32:935–939, 1983.

38. Johnson RT, Richardson EP: The neurological manifestations of systemic lupus erythematosus: a clinical-pathological study of 24 cases and review of the literature. *Medicine* 47:337–369, 1968.
39. Atkins CJ, Knodon JJ, Quismoro FP, et al: The choroid plexus in systemic lupus erythematosus. *Ann Intern Med* 76:65–72, 1972.
40. Meyerhoff J, Dorsch CA: Decreased platelet serotonin in systemic lupus erythematosus. *Arthritis Rheum* 24:1495–1500, 1981.
41. Dorsch CA, Meyerhoff J: Mechanisms of abnormal platelet aggregation in systemic lupus erythematosus. *Arthritis Rheum* 25:966–973, 1982.
42. Bluestein HG, Williams GW, Steinberg AD: Cerebrospinal fluid antibodies to neuronal cells: association with neuropsychiatric manifestations of systemic lupus erythematosus. *Am J Med* 70:240–246, 1981.
43. Robbins ML, Kornguth SE, Bell CL, et al: Antineurofilament antibody evaluation in neuropsychiatric systemic lupus erythematosus. *Arthritis Rheum* 31:623–631, 1988.
44. Hanley JG, Rajaraman S, Behmann S, et al: A novel neuronal antigen identified by sera from patients with systemic lupus erythematosus. *Arthritis Rheum* 31:1492–1499, 1988.
45. Kelly MC, Denburg JA. Cerebrospinal fluid immunoglobulins and neuronal antibodies in neuropsychiatric systemic lupus erythematosus and related conditions. *J Rheumatol* 14:740–744, 1987.
46. Lockshin MD, Druzin ML, Goei S, et al: Antibody to cardiolipin as predictor of fetal distress or death in pregnant patients with systemic lupus erythematosus. *N Engl J Med* 313:152–156, 1985.
47. Feinglass EJ, Arnett FC, Dorsch CA, et al: Neuropsychiatric manifestations of systemic lupus erythematosus: diagnosis, clinical spectrum and relationship to other features of the disease. *Medicine* 55:323–339, 1976.
48. Sergent JS, Lockshin MD, Klempner MS, et al: Central nervous system disease in systemic lupus erythematosus. Therapy and prognosis. *Am J Med* 58:644–654, 1975.
49. Omdal R, Mellgren SI, Husby G. Clinical neuropsychiatric and neuromuscular manifestations in systemic lupus erythematosus. *Scand J Rheumatol* 17:113–117, 1988.
50. Brandt KD, Lessell S: Migrainous phenomenon in systemic lupus erythematosus. *Arthritis Rheum* 21:7–16, 1978.
51. Andrianakos AA, Duffy J, Suzuki M, et al: Transverse myelopathy in systemic lupus erythematosus: report of three cases and review of the literature. *Ann Intern Med* 83:616–624, 1975.
52. Fulford KWM, Catterall RD, Delhanty JJ, et al: A collagen disorder of the nervous system presenting as multiple sclerosis. *Brain* 95:373–386, 1972.
53. Rechthand E, Cornblath DR, Stern BJ, et al: Chronic demyelinating polyneruopathy in systemic lupus erythematosus. *Neurology* 34:1375–1377, 1984.
54. Brandt KD, Lessel S, Cohen AS: Cerebral disorders of vision in systemic lupus erythematosus. *Ann Intern Med* 83:163–169, 1975.
55. Rodnan GR: When is scleroderma not scleroderma? The differential diagnosis of progressive systemic sclerosis. *Bull Rheum Dis* 31:7–10, 1981.
56. Masi AT, Rodnan GR, Medsger TA, et al: Preliminary criteria for the

classification of systemic sclerosis (scleroderma). *Bull Rheum Dis* 31:1–6, 1981.

57. Stallones RA: The epidemiology of systemic slcerosis. In *Current Topics in Rheumatology. Epidemiology of the Rheumatic Diseases*. Edited by RC Larence, LE Shulman. New York, NY. Gower Medical Publishing Limited, 1984, pp. 169–172.

58. Tuffaneli DL, Winkelmann BK: Systemic scleroderma. A clinical study of 727 cases. *Arch Dermatol* 84:359–371, 1961.

59. Fitzler MJ, Kinsella TD, Garbutt E: The CREST syndrome: a distinct serologic entity with anticentromere antibodies. *Am J Med* 69:520–526, 1980.

60. McCarty GA, Rice JR, Bembe ML, et al: Anticentromere antibody: clinical correlations and association with favorable prognosis in patients with scleroderma variants. *Arthritis Rheum* 26:1–7, 1983.

61. Farrell DA, Medsger TA: Trigeminal neuropathy in progresive systemic sclerosis. *Am J Med* 73:57–62, 1982.

62. Black CM, Stevens WM: Scleroderma. *Rheum Dis Clin* 15:193–212, 1989.

63. Ballou SP, Morley JJ, Kushner I: Pregnancy and systemic sclerosis. *Arthritis Rheum* 27:295–298, 1984.

64. Strand V, Talal N: Advances in the diagnosis and concept of Sjögren's syndrome (autoimmune exocrinopathy). *Bull Rheum Dis* 30:1046–1052, 1979.

65. Forstot JZ, Forstot SL, Greer RO, et al: The incidence of Sjögren's sicca complex in a population of patients with keratoconjunctivitis sicca. *Arthritis Rheum* 25:156–160, 1982.

66. Alarcon-Segovia D, Ibanez G, Velazquez-Feoreo F, et al: Sjögren's syndrome in systemic lupus erythematosus: clinical and subclinical manifestations. *Ann Intern Med* 81:577–583, 1974.

67. Alarcon-Segovia D, Ibanex G, Hernandez-Ortiz J, et al: Sjögren's syndrome in progressive systemic slcerosis (scleroderma). *Am J Med* 57:78–85, 1974.

68. Alexander EL, Provost TT, Frank MM, et al: Serum complement activation in central nervous system disease in Sjögren's syndrome. *Am J Med* 85:513–518, 1988.

69. Malinow KL, Molina R, Gordon B, et al: Neuropsychiatric dysfunction in primary Sjögren's syndrome. *Ann Intern Med* 103:344–49, 1985.

70. Alexander EA, Beall SS, Gordon B, et al: Magnetic resonance imaging of cerebral lesions in patients with the Sjögren Syndrome. *Ann Intern Med* 108:815–823, 1988.

71. Alarcon-Segovia D: Mixed connective tissue disease: a decade of growing pains. *J Rheumatol* 8:535–540, 1981.

72. Hochberg MC, Dorsch CA, Feinglass EJ, et al: Survivorship in systemic lupus erythematosus. *Arthritis Rheum* 24:54–59, 1981.

73. Berkowitz RL, Coustan DR, Mochizuki TK: *Handbook for Prescribing Medications During Pregnancy*. Boston, MA. Little, Brown and Company, 1981.

74. Briggs GG, Bodendorfer TW, Freeman RK, et al: *Drugs in Pregnancy and Lactation: A Reference Guide to Fetal and Neonatal Risk*. Baltimore, MD. Williams and Wilkins, 1983.

75. *Physicians Desk Reference*. 44th ed. Oradell, NJ. Medical Economics Company, 1990.

13

Postpartum Depression

John B. Imboden, M.D.
Samuel E. Adler, M.D.

Introduction

The psychological significance of pregnancy is a highly individual and complicated matter, determined by a host of interacting variables. The patient's preexisting personality or character, the sum of her past experiences, and the concurrent life situation all help to determine what pregnancy and prospective motherhood mean to the individual woman.

For most women, the total experience of pregnancy and the puerperium is predominantly one of fulfillment and joy, but it is apparent that stresses associated with pregnancy are frequent and significant. In the postpartum period, emotional disturbances range from the extremely common but poorly understood "blues" that are mild and transient to the relatively infrequent (1–2 per 1,000 deliveries) postpartum psychoses, the latter being predominantly affective in type, and possibly requiring psychiatric hospitalization. There is no clear-cut evidence of a psychiatric disorder specific to pregnancy or to the puerperium. There is evidence, however, that the risk of psychiatric disorder is higher in the postpartum period than in non-postpartum periods of age-matched controls.

From Goldstein PJ, Stern BJ, (eds): *Neurological Disorders of Pregnancy. Second Revised Edition.* Mount Kisco NY, Futura Publishing Co., Inc., © 1992.

Postpartum "Blues"

Fifty percent or more of patients in the postpartum period experience a mild and transient feeling of depression, tearfulness, and lassitude.[1,2] This state is so common that it is considered almost a "normal" feature of the puerperium. Ordinarily, the "blues" last only a few hours or several days and require no specific management beyond the sympathetic attention, encouragement, and support of family and caregivers. The patient should, of course, be given adequate assistance in caring for her infant and for her other responsibilities and should be encouraged by her obstetrician to discuss any problems that concern her. It is important that the patient understand that her emotional state is a frequent occurrence and is usually transient.

While postpartum blues are extremely common, they nonetheless are not well understood. The factors postulated to be responsible generally fall into two groups: psychological and hormonal. Among the former, there is evidence that some mothers feel "let down" following delivery, as if the actual baby and the actual experience of holding and nursing the baby do not come up to the idealized anticipation of them. It is not unreasonable to postulate that the workload and responsibility of infant care, the change in lifestyle, and the loss of previous personal freedom because of the requirements of motherhood all "come home" quite vividly during the first several days after delivery. It is also possible that, for those women who found the experience of being pregnant especially fulfilling, the delivery is followed by a sense of loss or emptiness.

Dramatic changes in peripheral serum hormone concentrations occur in the first few days following delivery, so it is not surprising that in some way these changes have been implicated in the occurrence of postpartum "blues". Thus far, no firm conclusions have been reached by investigators in this field. Plasma levels of the precursors of serotonin and norepinephrine, namely tryptophan and tyrosine, may be altered by changes in steroid hormone production following parturition. Theoretically this could be linked to possible alteration in the central nervous system concentration of serotonin and norepinephrine that in turn could lead to disorder of mood in the postpartum period. Harris[3] has reported, however, that the administration of L-tryptophan, the precursor of serotonin, did not alleviate symptoms of postpartum blues. Others have suggested that postpartum blues could be correlated with alterations of progesterone,[4,5] prolactin,[6] or cortisol concentrations.[7] Kuevi et al.[8] measured plasma concentrations of follicle-stimulating hormone (FSH), prolactin, estrone, estradiol, progesterone, cortisol, norepinephrine, and epinephrine on postpartum days 2, 3, 4, and 5, and administered a self-rating mood scale on the same days. Approximately 50% of their 44 patients showed evidence of emotional lability or mood disturbance. These investigators were unable to show significant correlation between mood disturbance and the hormone plasma levels except for a significant reduction of catecholamine (norepinephrine and epinephrine) on the "peak" day of postpartum blues as compared with the preceding day or subsequent days.

Postpartum Depression

David et al.[9] tracked psychiatric admissions for all women under age 50 in Denmark who in a single year (1975) carried to term or had an induced abortion. Of the 71,378 women who gave birth during the year of study, 86 were admitted to a psychiatric hospital within 3 months of delivery for a rate of 12 per 10,000 women. This compares with a rate of 7.5 for all women for a comparable period of 3 months and a rate of 18.4 psychiatric admissions during the 3 months following abortion. Dean and Kendall[10] found that of 71 women who had psychiatric admissions within 3 months of delivery, 58 (82%) had affective disorders; 49 patients were diagnosed as having depressive disorders, and nine patients were diagnosed as having manic or hypomanic disorders.

It is important to note that these psychiatric disorders were severe enough to require psychiatric hospitalization. Depressive reactions that are much more serious than postpartum blues and which last for 6 weeks or longer but may not require hospitalization have been found by some investigators to occur in 10% to 12% of women following delivery.[11] Furthermore, Garvey et al.[12] found the rate of postpartum depression for pregnancies subsequent to an initial postpartum depression to be from 64% to 75%.

The reader is referred to the recent review of postpartum depression and other psychiatric syndromes in women associated with reproductive function by Gitlin and Pasnau.[13]

Clinical Features of Depression

In general, most studies have indicated that depression in the postpartum period does not differ in any essential way from depression that occurs at other times. However, some "organic signs" were noted in 7 of the 33 patients with severe depression reported by Dean and Kendell.[10] Organic signs include confusion, disorientation, and visual hallucinations. In the presence of such signs, it is important to rule out contributory conditions such as a postpartum infection. Drug side effects, particularly those with anticholinergic activity, may be associated with states of mental confusion.

A substantial number of patients with postpartum depression have a history of anxiety or depression during the pregnancy. Perhaps the most common symptom of depression is a subjective change in mood for which a number of different adjectives are commonly used, such as sad, blue, down-in-the-dumps, low, despondent, or simply depressed. Occasionally, an individual may be depressed without being aware of a mood change or without being able to describe her change in mood. Accompanying this change in mood, most patients report that life seems to be relatively pleasureless and nothing seems particularly interesting. The loss of capacity for pleasure (anhedonia) and loss of interest are commonly accompanied by a subjective feeling of having little or no energy so that the routine tasks of infant care or other responsibilities seem heavy, almost unaccomplishable. In severe depression, the patient may be visibly slower in verbal responses and motor behavior, the so-called psychomotor retardation. Some patients become restless or agitated.

In most instances of moderate or severe depression, the patient exhibits an attitude of self-deprecation. In its mild form, this may seem like an unremarkable variant of normal self-criticism. In severe depression, the self-deprecatory patient voices a conviction of being an inadequate person and often has feelings of being bad or guilty. In depressive psychosis, these self-deprecatory notions may be expressed in the content of auditory hallucinations in which the patient is accused or insulted. Somatic delusions may also appear.

The depressed patient frequently complains of insomnia. Awakening early in the morning is a common symptom. However, difficulty in falling asleep and fitful sleeping throughout the night also are frequent symptoms. Loss of appetite often occurs and, over a period of time, is accompanied by loss of weight.

The depressed patient may feel that her condition is hopeless and may wish to die. There is the danger that this wish to die may include the infant, being rationalized on the basis of not wanting to leave the infant motherless. In continuing depression, these passive wishes or fantasies of death may evolve into suicidal intentions and plans.

Etiology

The causes of depression are not fully known. The evidence to date favors a multifactorial model in which the principal factors can be grouped into three categories: psychological or psychosocial, humoral, and genetic.

The phenomenological similarity between mourning and depression has long been known and has been the point of departure for psychological theorizing by a number of investigators. Further, it is not rare for intense grief to evolve into depression. Additionally, careful investigation of the life situation of the depressed patient often reveals that some kind significant "loss" occurred shortly before onset of the illness.[5,14] In this context, loss refers not only to loss of loved ones by death, divorce, separation, or moving away but also to myriad experiences that result in loss of love, self-esteem, security, important sources of gratification, and so forth. It has also been observed that a person may become depressed on the anniversary of a loss, such as on the anniversary of an abortion.

Because of the symbolic function of the human mind, what signifies profound loss for one person may not for another. Thus, it is possible that the postpartum period itself with its expectation of infant care and the beginning of a new life may for some women represent a profoundly melancholic experience. It may arouse renewed feelings of being trapped in a miserable marriage or feelings of dismay and sadness in the setting of an unstable marital situation. The postpartum period may elicit a wish to undo the past and start life over again, but it may also elicit the futility of such a wish. The period can evoke the profound deficiencies of one's own mother, real or imagined, and with that the bitter feeling that one is expected to give what one never received or to be a good mother without having had a role model with which to identify. These are some of the possibilities that might be at work in those women who are observed to become depressed in the puerperium and who, as already noted, tend to repeat the depression with each successive delivery. Much research is needed to determine whether these and other possibilities are truly present and operative in these patients as compared with women who do not get depressed following delivery.

A currently favored humoral hypothesis suggests that depression may be associated with neurotransmitter deficiency in the central nervous system (CNS), specifically serotonin and/or norepinephrine. Investigators have observed that: (1) administration of the antihypertensive agent reserpine may be associated with depression and depletion of these neurotransmitters, and (2) isoniazid, an antituberculosis drug, raises central levels of these transmitters and was observed often to alleviate depression.[15–17] Presently available tricyclic antidepressants and monoamine oxidase inhibitors increase the availability of these biogenic amines, serotonin and norepinephrine, at receptor sites in the synaptic cleft, and this action may account for their efficacy in relieving depression.

Studies of the incidence of depression in the genetic relatives of depressed patients and of the concordance rates among monozygotic and dizygotic twins strongly suggest a hereditary predisposition to the illness.[18] It is possible that a "psychosomatic" model of depression best fits the currently available evidence. That is to say, in the hereditarily predisposed person, certain kind of psychic stress may somehow serve to induce neurochemical changes such as reduction in neurotransmitters which in turn is correlated with development of an affective disturbance. It is clear that at the present time, the mechanism by which psychological stress induces changes in the CNS function is unknown.

Diagnosis

The diagnosis is readily made if the patient exhibits the characteristic symptoms of the depressive syndrome. The patient may appear sad or gloomy or have a relatively immobile facies and, when asked, will usually admit to feeling depressed. Several or all of the following symptoms occur in varying degrees: lack of pleasure or interest; low energy or feelings of tiredness; crying; feelings of being sluggish or slowed down; restlessness or agitation; insomnia, especially early morning awakening; anorexia and weight loss; feelings of being inadequate; guilt feelings; in severe depression there may be mood-congruent hallucinations and delusions; feelings of hopelessness; suicidal thoughts and feelings.

As already noted, some investigators have reported signs of organicity in a substantial minority of women with postpartum depression. If one does find evidence of "organicity," such as disorientation, incoherent speech, memory or other cognitive impairment, or visual hallucination, the physician should search diligently for an underlying organic condition such as an unrecognized vascular, neoplastic, or infectious process. Drugs with anticholinergic side effects may contribute to the development of an organic brain syndrome.

Other psychiatric disorders may occur in the postpartum period, though less frequently than depression. The manic state is differentiated from depression without difficulty. In mania, the patient is usually elated, with accompanying irritability in varying degrees. The manic patient typically is full of energy, talks a great deal, and may be inclined to get involved in activities that reflect a grandiose self-image and poor judgment.

In schizophrenic disorders the patient may display inappropriate or flat effect, tend to be withdrawn, and may have a variety of hallucinatory and/or delusional experiences with a clear sensorium. A discussion of these and other psychiatric conditions is well developed in a recent comprehensive textbook.[19]

Management

Management begins in the antepartum period with the careful assessment of the risk of postpartum depression in the individual patient. As noted by several observers, the patient who develops a serious depression in the postpartum period often has manifested evidence of anxiety or depression during the pregnancy.[10] The patient whose marriage is troubled or who cannot count on a stable and supportive relationship with the father of the unborn child may be more apt to become depressed in the postpartum period. Further, with a past history of depression in the postpartum period or a history of recurrent depressive episodes, the patient should be considered to be at increased risk of developing postpartum depression.

The practitioner then will carefully assess the patient's emotional state during the period of prenatal care to assess the presence or absence of anxiety, depression, and significant problems in the patient's life situation, particularly problems of special relevance to the security and support essential to the emotional well being of the mother and the newborn child. The mother will be encouraged to express her feelings about being pregnant, being a mother, the commitment involved in raising a child, the delivery itself, and relevant significant problems in her life, including the effect of parenthood on the infant's father. It is most important for the expectant mother to be able to express her feelings of ambivalence about any aspect of the pregnancy experience or the anticipated experience of childcaring if she has such feelings. Educational classes and other group experiences may be helpful in achieving a sense of competence and confidence concerning the delivery and infant care. However, it is possible for such experiences to unintentionally intensify the guilt of the ambivalent expectant mother who may feel that she is monstrously wrong to have anything but feelings of pure joy at the prospect of having a baby. The expectant mother who is ambivalent and feels guilty needs an opportunity to begin to work through these feelings prior to delivery. It seems that there are no empirical studies demonstrating the preventive efficacy of this psychotherapeutic approach to the emotionally troubled pregnant patient. It also seems reasonable to predict that such an approach would help the patient adjust to her situation in the postpartum period.

In some instances, the obstetrician may elect to refer the patient to a specialist for psychotherapy particularly if, as a result of exploratory interview(s), he/she judges that the patient has evidence of emotional problems or conflicts that may necessitate relatively long-term or intensive psychotherapy. Psychotherapy during the prenatal period for the patient who is judged to be at risk for postpartum depression not only has the possible advantage of helping to prevent or moderate later depression but also establishes the patient in a relationship with the therapist in the event of later need.

With regard to management of the mother who has become seriously depressed in the postpartum period, several important management decisions have to be addressed. The first one concerns the issue of hospitalization versus outpatient therapy. It is important to make a judgment concerning the risk of suicide, possible harm to the infant, or both. Most depressed patients, indeed almost all, have at least a passing thought that death would be a welcome release, and the possibility of suicide commonly occurs to the patient. However, continuing or recurrent preoccupation with death or suicide or the intention of committing suicide, the development of a plan, the preparation for leaving by putting one's affairs in order, or any other indicators of grave suicidal danger necessitate psychiatric consultation and hospitalization. The physician should ask the patient directly about suicidal thoughts and intentions if they are suspected to be present. Other indications for hospitalization are related to the possible need for relieving the patient of home and infant care responsibilities from which, by virtue of depression and/or unsettling ambivalence toward the baby, the patient needs to be temporarily relieved. In the event that the patient feels intellectually or emotionally unprepared to care for the infant, she can be gradually and supportively reintroduced to the mothering role in a hospital setting. This may be particularly useful for the mother who is frightened of her own hostile feelings toward the baby.

Whether psychiatric treatment is conducted on an outpatient basis or in an inpatient setting, a decision must be made concerning the use of antidepressant drugs in postpartum depression. Generally speaking, in cases of moderately severe to severe depression, chemotherapy is indicated, particularly when the patient experiences insomnia with early awakening, anorexia with weight loss, psychomotor retardation or agitation, excessive guilt, and a history of the depression being worse in the morning.

Antidepressant drugs for the nursing mother present a problem because these drugs do appear in breast milk. Because the effect of these drugs on the suckling infant is not known, it may be best to defer chemotherapy. If chemotherapy cannot be deferred, then the baby should be weaned prior to instituting antidepressant medication.

If there is a past history of mania, it is advisable to obtain psychiatric consultation. In such cases, the administration of a lithium salt with or without the concomitant administration of a tricyclic antidepressant may be indicated because of the possible precipitation of a manic episode by the use of an antidepressant drug. Lithium

Table I.
Side Effects Commonly Encountered with Cyclical Antidepressants

	Drowsiness (see text)
Anticholinergic action, peripheral	Impaired visual accommodation, increased intraocular pressure in patients with closed angle glaucoma, dry mouth, tachycardia, constipation, urinary retention.
Anticholinergic action, central	Mental confusion or delirium
α-Adrenergic blocking	Orthostatic hypotension.
Interference with impulse conduction in the heart	QRS prolongation, ST-T wave abnormalities.
Drug interaction	Interference with antihypertensive effect of certain drugs such as guanethidine and clonidine. Cyclical antidepressants should not be administered concomitantly with monoamine oxidase inhibitors.
Dopamine-blocking activity associated with amoxapine	Extrapyramidal symptoms; possibility of tardive dyskinesia.

salts do appear in the milk of the nursing mother and therefore breast feeding should be discontinued prior to their use.

When prescribing cyclic antidepressant drugs, as with any potent agent, it is essential to be familiar with the side effects of the drug.[20] Some important common side effects of cyclic antidepressants are listed in Table I. Drowsiness is commonly encountered, especially in the initial period of treatment, and the CNS depressant effect of alcohol may be enhanced.

The newer antidepressant drug, fluoxitine, seems not to have significant anticholinergic activity but it is associated with other side effects such as restlessness, insomnia, nausea and mild weight loss. It is possible that the side effects associated with fluoxitine mentioned may be lessened or avoided by prescribing the medication every other day for the first several doses.

The doses listed in Table II are those which are considered effective for most people; however, some individuals may require more, others less.

It is wise to begin treatment with a dose equal to about one fourth of the anticipated therapeutic dose (with the exception of fluoxitine)

Table II.
Average Dosage for Antidepressants

Generic Name	Commercial Name	Average Dose (mg/day)
Amitriptyline	Elavil™	150
Amoxapine	Asendin™	200
Desipramine	Norpramine™, Pertofrane™	125
Doxepin	Sinequan™, Adapin™	150
Fluoxetine	Prozac™	20
Imipramine	Tofranil	150
Maprotiline	Ludiomil™	150
Nortriptyline	Aventyl™	100
Protriptyline	Vivactil™	20
Trazodone	Desyrel™	200

and increase in quarterly increments every several days as tolerated by the patient. Generally, response to treatment is gradual over a period of several weeks. Not infrequently the depressed patient manifests behavioral improvement observed by those around her before she feels a corresponding improvement in subjective sense of well being. In instances of serious suicidal danger, electroconvulsive treatment (ECT) may well be indicated. Electroconvulsive treatment should be jointly administered by an anesthesiologist and a psychiatrist experienced in this form of treatment.

The prognosis for an acute episode of depression is good. Even without treatment, a substantial percentage of depressed patients, including those who require hospitalization, experience significant or complete remission of symptoms in about a year or less. with treatment, marked improvement occurs much more quickly, i.e., in a matter of weeks. About 70% to 80% of acutely depressed patients respond to treatment.

References

1. Pitt B: "Maternity blues." *Br J Psychiatry* 122:431–433, 1973.
2. Robin AM: Psychological changes of normal parturition. *Psych Quarterly* 36:129–150, 1962.

3. Harris B: Prospective trial of L-tryptophan in maternity blues. *Br J Psychiatry* 137 233–235, 1980.
4. Nott PN, Franklin M, Armitage C, et al: Hormonal changes and mood in the puerperium. *Br J Psychiatry* 128:379–383, 1976.
5. Paykel E, Myers J, Dienett M, et al: Life events and depression: a controlled study. *Arch Gen Psychiatry* 21:752, 1969.
6. George AJ, Copeland JRM, Wilson KCM: Prolactin secretion and postpartum blues syndrome. *Br J Pharmacol* 70:102, 1980.
7. Handley SL, Dunn TL, Baker JM, et al: Mood changes in puerperium and plasma tryptophan and cortisol concentrations. *Br Med J* ii:18–22, 1977.
8. Kuevi V, Canson R, Dixson AF, et al: Plasma amine and hormone changes in "postpartum blues". *Clin Endocrinol* 19:39–46, 1983.
9. David HP, Rasmussen NK, Holst E: Postpartum and postabortion psychotic reactions. *Fam Plann Perspect* 13:88–92, 1981.
10. Dean C, Kendell RE: The symptomatology of puerperal illness. *Br J Psychiatry* 139:128–133, 1981.
11. Braverman J, Roux JF: Screening for the patient at risk for postpartum depression. *Obstet Gynecol* 52:731–736, 1978.
12. Garvey MJ, Tuason VB, Lumry AE, et al: Occurrence of depression in the postpartum state. *J Affective Disord* 5:97–101, 1983.
13. Gitlin MJ, Pasnau RO: Psychiatric syndromes linked to reproductive function in women: a review of current knowledge. *Am J Psychiatry* 146:1413, 1989.
14. Thompson KC, Hendrie H: Environmental stress in primary depressive illness. *Arch Gen Psychiatry* 26:130, 1972.
15. Bladessarini RJ: *Biomedical Aspects of Depression and its Treatment.* Washington, DC, American Psychiatric Press, Inc., 1983.
16. Maas J: Biogenic amines and depression. *Arch Gen Psychiatry* 32:1357, 1975.
17. Schildkraut JJ: The catecholamine hypothesis of affective disorders: a review of supporting evidence. *Am J Psychiatry* 122:509, 1965.
18. Schlesser MA, Altschuler KZ: The genetics of affective disorder, data, theory, and clinical applications. *Hosp Community Psychiatry* 34:415, 1983.
19. Kaplan HI, Sadock BJ (eds): *Comprehensive Textbook of Psychiatry.* Volumes 1 and 2, Edition 4. Baltimore, MD. Williams and Wilkins, 1985.
20. *Physicians' Desk Reference.* Edition 44. Oradell, NJ, Medical Economics Company, 1990.

14

Sex Hormone Effects on Excitable Membranes

Sanjay Datta, M.D.
Andrew M. Malinow, M.D.

Introduction

Sex hormones have long been suspected of having a significant impact on the excitability of the central and peripheral nervous system. The complete specific role of these hormones is not fully understood at the present time. However, observations from both clinical practice and from basic science experiments suggest that these hormones have a definite effect on nerve tissue and certain smooth muscles. This chapter will deal with current information regarding the role of these hormones in affecting the excitability of neural membranes and smooth muscles and the consequent physiological implications. Additionally, some anesthetic practice considerations will be highlighted. This chapter will not consider in detail the complex and elegant neurohormonal interactions among various nuclear anatomical sites.

Central and Peripheral Nervous System

Clinical Evidence

Bromage[1] reported a wider dermatomal spread of epidural analgesia in pregnant patients and urged clinicians to use smaller doses

From Goldstein PJ, Stern BJ, (eds): *Neurological Disorders of Pregnancy. Second Revised Edition.* Mount Kisco NY, Futura Publishing Co., Inc., © 1992.

of local anesthetics in parturients than in nonpregnant patients. Bromage's observation was confirmed by Hehre and colleagues.[2] Bromage suggested that the volume of the epidural space was decreased because of distention of the epidural veins caused by partial obstruction of the inferior vena cava by the gravid uterus. Indeed, acute obstruction of the inferior vena cava in dogs has been shown to enhance the spread of epidural injected contrast media.[3]

However, Fagareus et al.[4] observed that the wider dermatomal spread of local anesthetic drugs in the epidural spaces existed as early as the first trimester of pregnancy. This very early pregnancy finding could not be explained on the basis of mechanical factors. These authors advanced other potential causative factors, including direct biochemical and hormonal changes. Gianetti and Cerimele[5] reported that progesterone and estrogen alter the permeability of the intracellular matrix of connective tissue in rats. Therefore, it is plausible that sex hormones can, in some way, increase the local anesthetic diffusion across the nerve membrane and increase its effect.

Kendrick and Drewett[6] reported a 50% increase in the refractory period of central nervous system neurons in rats following castration. Recording from single hypothalamic neurons subjected to antidromic stimulation, they tested the minimum interval between successive conducted action potentials. The increase in refractory period was reversed by 16 or more days of administration of testosterone propionate and was restricted to hypothalamic neurons shown by prior lesion studies to be essential to expression of sexual behavior. The effect of castration was restricted to the pathway known on other grounds to be involved in the control of sexual behavior, and must have been due to the removal of testosterone because it was reversed by testosterone injections. The authors concluded that testosterone must affect these neurons directly, because the refractory period is altered. A change in the refractory period implies a membrane change.

Erulkar et al.[7] studied the neural control of a clasp reflex in male amphibians (*Xenopus laevis*) using anatomical, electrophysiological, and biochemical techniques. Neurons in the spinal segments of two castrated males accumulated radioactivity after injection of 3H-dihydrotestosterone. By recording from the nerve to the appropriate muscle in an isolated spinal cord preparation from a castrated male, the authors were able able to show increased activation of the neurons in response to neural stimulation after addition of dihydrotestosterone to the bath.

Another interesting study supports a hormonal influence on the modulation of excitable membranes.[8] The electric organ of mormyrid fish has a highly characteristic and repeatable discharge waveform. Bass and Hopkins[8] used a species where the waveform showed sexual specificity in that it was of longer duration in the male. Female fish in aquaria were bathed in 17 α methyltestosterone dissolved in stream water. A progressive shift from the brief discharge waveform was measured with a duration nearly twice as long. The shift was detectable on the first day and was complete in about a week. No changes were found in the motorneurons driving the electric organ that led them to conclude that the changes in waveform and duration produced by testosterone were localized to the electric organ itself. The authors considered two sites of action of the gonadal hormones and their metabolites: the peripheral electrolytes themselves or the central motor pathway controlling electric organ excitation. They found that the central command is nearly identical for specimens with electrical organ discharges of differing form and duration. The general properties of the spinal command signal were unchanged in testosterone-treated females. This proved that hormonal effects appear to be distal to the command signal generator, at the level of the electric organ. Gonadal hormones can, of course, affect the spontaneous activity and refractory period of central neurons. There are different ways in which testosterone can exert its effects in such situations: (1) it can change the physiology of the synapse between the electromotorneurons and the electrolyte's stalk; (2) it may alter the cable properties of the electrolyte; (3) it may change the distribution of magnitude of different ion channels in the electrolyte's excitable membranes.

Pfaff and McEwan,[9] in an elegant review of estrogen and progesterone action on nerve cells, distinguish between relatively long-term and short-term effects. Citing the well known specificity of steroid hormone localization in the brain, they summarize much of what is known about neural functional alterations. For example, estrogen changes the rate of firing of highly specific hypothalamic neurons. In addition, estrogen receptors are localized in various cellular nuclei in the brain. Cytosol, as well as nuclear receptor sites, are also found in highly specific brain locations. Of special interest are the acute electrical activity changes noted. Several authors report decreased thresholds for electrical stimulation in estrogen-treated animals. Others report changes that probably occur on the basis of a classic steroid induction of nucleotides with manufacture of peptides that become, in fact, neurotransmitters. But a few reports suggest a different mechanism: direct alterations of cell membrane. Even in vitro experiments demonstrate an acute membrane effect.[10]

Datta et al.[11] compared the onset of conduction blockade in the vagus nerve of pregnant and nonpregnant rabbits, utilizing an in vitro sheathed nerved preparation. The times required for 50% depression of the action potential elevation (AP) of A, B, and C vagal fibers from five pregnant and six nonpregnant animals were determined after the application of bupivacaine (0.35 mL). The onset of conduction blockade occurred faster in all three fiber types of the nerves of pregnant animals compared to nonpregnant animals (Table 1). This difference in sensitivity exists even in the lower concentrations (0.1 mL–0.3 mL).[11] Using a similar nerve preparation, Flanagan et al.[12] plotted dose response curves using log incur plots of the reduction of peak compound action potential amplitude of A, B, and C fibers as a percent of control at 30 minutes after varying doses of bupivacaine. Regression analysis recorded a significantly increased sensitivity to bupivacaine of fibers from pregnant animals for A and C fibers with an insignificant but similar shift for B fibers. However, the study failed to correlate progesterone levels with the degree of conduction blockade. Because progesterone levels are five to seven times higher in pregnant than in nonpregnant rabbits, the authors suggested that the

Table I.
Time in Minutes for 50% Block with 0.35 mM Bupivacaine HCl in Hepes Liley's Solution

Nerve Fibers (N = 6)	Pregnant Animal	Nonpregnant Animal	P
A	11.2 ± 0.4	19.4 ± 3.7	0.001
B	6.7 ± 2.8	17.9/	0.03
C	12.1 ± 5.2	31.6/	0.001

* Statistical method employed does not yield a standard deviation in these two instances.
Median ± robust estimation of the standard deviation.
Used with permission.[11]

increase in progesterone in pregnant animals was responsible for the differences in sensitivity between the nerve fibers. To observe the specific effect of progesterone on the neural sensitivity, these same authors injected 30 mg/kg of exogenous progesterone to ovariectomized rabbits for 4 days.[13] Exogenous progesterone administered chronically made the action potential of the vagus nerve more sensitive to bupivacaine compared to the control group. Finally, to observe the acute progesterone effect, the same authors exposed 200 mg/mL of progesterone to the isolated rabbit vagus nerves directly in the bath. Progesterone did not have any acute effect on neural blockade and subsequent exposure of these tissues to bupivacaine demonstrated no increased membrane sensitivity. Time-dependent uptake of radioactive progesterone by neural tissue was measured using radio-labeled progesterone.[14] These experiments suggest that chronic exposure of progesterone is necessary to induce the changes in neural sensitivity to bupivacaine.

Datta et al.[15] have also measured the cerebrospinal fluid (CSF) progesterone concentration in nonpregnant, term parturient, and immediate postpartum patients. Progesterone concentration in the CSF was ten times and three times greater in pregnant and postpartum patients, respectively (Fig. 1). Because progesterone has a direct effect on neuronal sensitivity, continuous bathing of the spinal cord by high-progesterone concentration might be an explanation of the increased dermatomal spread in parturients and immediate postpartum patients than in nonpregnant patients using the same amount of local anesthetics.

Sheth et al.[16] have suggested that the temporal pattern of CSF protein reduction in early pregnancy, term pregnancy, and early postpartum match the same period of pregnancy-related increase in potency of local anesthetic. A reduced protein content can affect the potency of the local anesthetics in two ways. First, it would decrease buffering capacity. Reduced buffering capacity may allow local anesthetic to remain as a salt for a longer time, allowing wider dermatomal spread. Second, decreased protein binding allows a higher concentration of unbound local anesthetic for action in the subarachnoid space.

Butterworth et al.[17] have investigated the effects of pregnancy on the sensitivity to local anesthetics in pregnant and nonpregnant human volunteers. Median nerve block at the wrist was done with 1% lidocaine HCl. Sensory nerve action potential amplitude (SNAP)

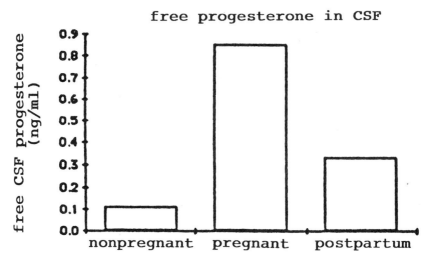

Figure 1: Cerebrospinal fluid (CFS) progesterone concentration in nonpregnant, term parturient, and immediate postpartum patients.

and compound motor action potential (CMAP) were recorded to quantitate inhibition of median nerve, α sensory, and motor fibers, respectively. Additionally, inhibition of median nerve C fibers was assessed by measuring the increase in skin temperature (ST) and decrease in median (relative to ulnar) galvanic skin potential (GSP) amplitude.

Lidocaine inhibited SNAP to a greater extent in pregnant than in nonpregnant women over the 20 minute postinjection study period. The CMAP amplitude declined significantly after lidocaine injection in a time-related fashion. Although between group differences at any time were not significantly different, pregnant women achieved a steady-state level of CMAP reduction more quickly than nonpregnant women.

Skin temperature increased more rapidly and to a higher degree in nonpregnant women. The ratio of median to ulnar galvanic skin potential did not achieve statistical significance in pregnant subjects as compared to nonpregnant women, although there again was a tendency towards a faster decline of the GSP in pregnant subjects.

Butterworth et al.[17] have, thus, presented preliminary in vitro evidence that pregnancy renders mammalian peripheral nerves more susceptible to local anesthetics, and indeed, confirm the earlier in vivo work of Datta[11] and Flanagan.[12,13] Butterworth et al.[22] speculate that either progesterone (or some other pregnancy-related hormone) alters the local anesthetic binding site in the Na^+ channel producing increased affinity for the local anesthetic molecules, or alternately, pregnancy alters the myelination of peripheral nerve decreasing the neural anesthetic concentration needed to inhibit conduction via myelinated fibers.

Central Nervous System

Selye[18] as early as 1941, observed that steroid hormones such as progesterone, androgens, and estrogens cause general anesthesia in various experimental animals. Of these agents, progesterone was found to be most potent. He also observed that the anesthetic effect of all steroid hormones is more marked in female than in male animals. Spaying did not alter the sensitivity of females but castration raised the responsiveness of males to the female level. The anesthetic effect of the steroid hormones is greatly increased after partial hepatectomy in both sexes and probably related to reduced detoxification by the liver. He also reported a true potentiation of the action of volatile anesthetics, such as ether or chloroform, when administered simultaneously with a steroid anesthetic such as progesterone.

One of the most impressive findings has been that the intramsucular injection of progesterone before initiation of an agenized zein diet, which ordinarily produced seizures in all control animals, protected one half of the dogs against convulsion.[19] In a study on cats, progesterone with a plasma concentration of 40 mg/dL depressed spontaneous interictal spikes produced by the application of penicillin to the cerebral cortex. In fact, progesterone therapy for epileptic patients has been suggested (see Chapter 2).

Merryman et al.[20] induced sleep in women by giving large daily doses of intravenous progesterone. Additionally, Palahniuk et al.[21] reported decreased requirement for inhaled anesthetic agents using minimal alveolar concentration as the variable.

Datta et al.[22] studied the relationship between progesterone and the minimum alveolar concentration (MAC) of halothane required to achieve an adequate level of anesthesia. The results indicated that in ovariectomized rabbits, pretreatment with progesterone for 8 days, resulting in progesterone blood levels ranging from 10 to 50 ng/mL, significantly decreased the MAC for halothane from control values of 1.6–1.8 to values of 1.4 (p < O.05) and was negatively correlated to the MAC required for an adequate level of anesthesia. These findings indicate that sex hormones, specifically progesterone, have modulator actions on excitable cells of the CNS as well as the peripheral nerves. If the axon-based theory of general anesthesia is correct, then the neural effects of progesterone might unify the increased susceptibility of the pregnant woman to both local as well as general anesthetics.[23]

Smooth and Cardiac Muscles

The effects of hormones on the function of smooth muscle have long been recognized. Most evidence suggests that the hormones affect muscle cell excitability. For example, Datta et al.[24] reported diminished mechanical response of the mouse ileum to a variety of stimuli in pregnancy compared to the nonpregnant state.

This effect on gut smooth muscle was tested by giving acetylcholine or potassium chloride or by electrical stimulation. Whether in vivo or in vitro, the gut muscle, specifically the ileum, was modified by progesterone. The hormone seems to alter the muscle plasma membrane or the cellular contractile apparatus. In any case, whether tested in ileum derived from pregnant animals or subjected to exogenous progesterone, muscular activity was diminished.

Changes in intestinal propulsion are observed in humans and can probably be explained by the changes in responsiveness of the gut to progesterone in vitro. Furthermore, the effects of pregnancy on intestinal propulsion in the human are not due to mechanical effects, such as increased abdominal pressure, but likely are also associated with diminished response of the ileum to stimuli. It is probable that the high circulating concentrations of progesterone are responsible for this phenomenon.

Csapo[25] reported that the transmembrane potential of single smooth muscle cells of the rabbit uterus, as assayed by microelectrode penetration, was influenced by endocrine regulation during pregnancy. They showed that the "resting" potential of the myometrial cell in the parturient rabbit is about 50 mV. Mechanical activity of such a uterus in vitro is infrequent. By increasing the membrane potential slightly, spontaneous activity is abolished, whereas reducing the membrance potential gradually, as with excess potassium, increases contractile activity stepwise. Activity becomes maximal at a "critical" potential of about 30 mV and further depolarization only leads to sustained contracture. This observation is evidence that the uterus obeys the "threshold relation," as generally do other excitable tissues. It is also evident that decreased spontaneous mechanical activity is a function of the membrane potential excess over a critical value, and that the contractile system of the uterus is so balanced that activity prevails unless rest is enforced by processes that impose upon the cell a membrane potential excess.

The role of estrogen on the control of the synthesis of the smooth muscle contractile system is unclear. Experiments show that estrogen

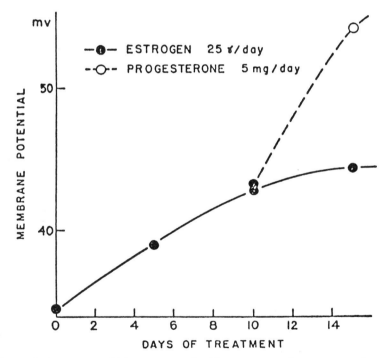

Figure 2: Immature rabbits are treated with estrogen and estrogen and progesterone, respectively, and the membrane potentials of the excised uteri determined. Note the increment in membrane after several days of estrogen treament and a further increment on treatment with progesterone. (Used with permission.[18])

treatment of the immature animal brings the membrane potential of the myometrial cell into the "firing range," which is a prerequisite of normal excitability as well as pharmacological response (Fig. 2). It is well known that the removal or functional elimination of endocrine glands supplying progesterone during gestation terminates pregnancy, whereas effective progesterone replacement therapy secures the maintenance of gestation. Studies with respect to the action of progesterone in controlling human pregnancy show the involvement of hyperpolarization of the membrane or a block of conduction, respectively (Fig. 3). The progesterone-dominated uterus in contrast to that dominated by estrogen does not propagate the excitation wave set up at one end of a uterine strip. Studies of propagated activity of the rabbit uterus during early and late pregnancy revealed two types of block. Along the whole length of the uterus, it is uniform except

THE EFFECT OF PREGNANCY ON THE MEMBRANE POTENTIAL OF THE MYOMETRIAL CELL

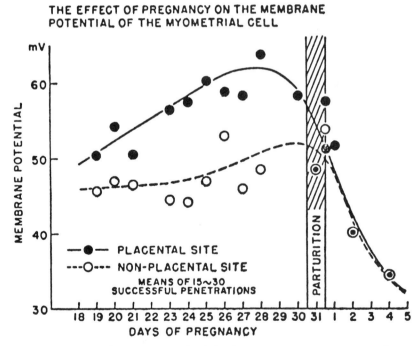

Figure 3: The membrane potential of the late pregnant, parturient, and postpartum rabbit uterus at placental and nonplacental sites. Note the higher membrane potential at placental uterine portions and the drop in membrane potential during and after delivery. (Used with permission.[18])

over the placenta. At the placenta, the block appears to be segmented. The first type is explained by the systemic progesterone effect, and the second by the "local" effect of the placenta. In addition, the membrane potential is high, about 60 mV, as compared to the estrogen-dominated uterus, and is higher at placental than at interplacental uterine portions.

Ryan and Pellecchia[26] pretreated adult male guinea pigs with 2 mg/kg of progesterone and examined the in vitro contractile response of gallbaldder strips to acetylcholine and to an octapeptide of cholecystokinin, comparing this response to those obtained from untreated control animals. Progesterone pretreatment produced an apparent decrease in the potencies to elicit tension of both hormones. These decrements were also accompanied by significant decrease in the maximal contractile response. The serum progesterone levels were within the range reported for the guinea pig estrus cycle, but were considerably greater than normally occur in male animals (Figs. 4 and 5).

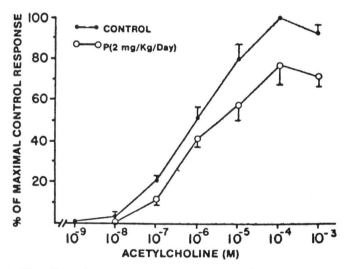

Figure 4: The effect of progesterone pretreatment on the in vitro contractile response of gallbladder smooth muscle to acetylcholine stimulation. Solid circles represent the response from untreated control animals and open circles represent the response from progesterone-pretreated animals. Each point is expressed as a percent of the maximal contractile response obtained from the control animals. The data points represent the mean and standard error of the results obtained on 10 muscle strips from 10 animals. (Used with permission.[19])

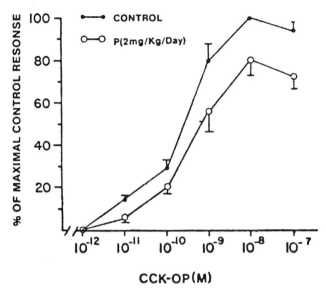

Figure 5: The effect of progesterone pretreatment on the in vitro contractile response of gallbladder smooth muscle to CCK-OP stimulation. The symbols are the same as in Figure 4. Each point is expressed as a percent of the maximal response to CCK-OP in the control group. The data points represent the mean and standard error of the results obtained on 10 muscle strips from 10 animals. (Used with permission.[19])

Cardiac Muscle

Morishima et al.[27] observed that significantly lower doses of bupivacaine were required to produce cardiovascular collapse in the pregnant ewe when compared with nonpregnant animals (Fig. 6). The enhanced cardiac toxicity in pregnant animals was not due to a greater uptake of drug by the myocardium. The cardiac tissue/blood contraction ratio of bupivacaine was approximately the same in pregnant and nonpregnant ewes. The authors speculated that the enhanced cardiotoxicity was most probably related to a greater sensitivity of the myocardium during, at least, the late stage of pregnancy. Another interesting finding in this respect is in the presence of progesterone receptors in baboon cardiovascular tissue that might suggest that progestins can directly influence cardiovascular tissue function.[28]

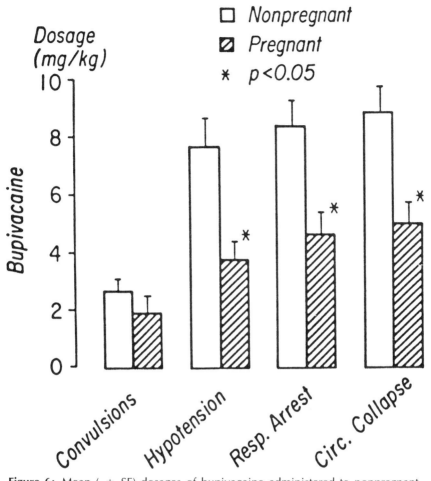

Figure 6: Mean (± SE) dosages of bupivacaine administered to nonpregnant and pregnant ewes up to the onset of each toxic manifestation. * Significantly different from nonpregnant ewes. (Used with permission.[20])

Moller et al.[29] have investigated effects of local anesthetics on pregnant cardiac tissue. These authors observed the effect of local anesthetic on transmembrane action potentials from progesterone pretreated ovariectomized rabbits. Bupivacaine at 1 and 3 mcg/mL suppressed V_{max} significantly more in cardiac tissues from progesterone treated animals than from nonprogesterone treated animals.

At 1 mcg/mL bupivacaine, V_{max} was depressed an average of 30% in 7 vehicle-treated animals (control), while the same concentration in progesterone treated animals depressed V_{max} an average of 65%. Interestingly, lidocaine showed no difference in its effect upon this parameter between progesterone and nonprogesterone treated animals.

Summary

There is a large body of evidence that demonstrates great variation in target-tissue responses that take place with the administration of steroid hormones.[30] The female sex steroids such as progesterone can exert regulatory effects on the synthesis, activity, and possibly even the degradation of tissue enzymes and structural proteins. These responses seem to be dependent on the synthesis of nuclear RNA.

These reports concerning the effect of sex hormones, particularly those occurring during pregnancy, on smooth muscles and excitable membranes at either peripheral or central sites are interesting. However, the mechanisms of action are not clear at present. Although many questions remain, it is clear from basic science reports that pregnancy alters neural sensitivity. Whether the specific mechanism is by changes in excitable membranes, cellular proteins, or cellular environment, the evidence is clear that the pregnant female is a "different" person from her nonpregnant sister.

References

1. Bromage PR: Continuous lumbar epidural analgesia for obstetrics. *Can Med Assoc J* 85:1136–1140, 1961.
2. Hehre FW, Moyes ZA, Senfield RM, et al: Continuous lumbar peridural anesthesia in obstetrics II. Use of minimal amounts of local anesthetics during labor. *Anesth Analg* 44:89–93, 1965.
3. Hehre FW, Yules RB, Hipona FA: Continuous lumbar epidural anesthesia in obstetrics III. Attempts to produce spread of contrast media by acute vena caval obstruction in dogs. *Anesth Analg* 45:551–556, 1966.
4. Fagareus L, Urban BJ, Bromage PR: Spread of epidural analgesia in early pregnancy. *Anesthesiology* 58:184–187, 1983.
5. Gianetti A, Cerimele D: Effects of steroid hormones on the matrix of the dermis of the rat. In *Chemistry and Molecular Biology of the Intercellular Matrix*. Vol III. Edited by EA Balaz. London. Academic Press, Inc, Ltd., 1970, pp. 1821–1827.

6. Kendrick KM, Drewett RF: Testosterone reduces refractory period of Stria terminalis neurons in the rat brain. *Science* 204:877–879, 1979.
7. Erulkar SD, Kelley DB, Jurman ME, et al: Modulation of the neural control of the clasp reflex in male xenopus levels by androgens: a multidisciplinary study. *Proc Natl Acad Sci* 78:5856–5880, 1981.
8. Bass AH, Hopkins CD: Hormonal control of sexual differentiation changes in electric organ discharge wave form. *Science* 220:971–973, 1983.
9. Pfaff DW, McEwen BS: Actions of estrogens and progestins on nerve cells. *Science* 219:808–814, 1983.
10. Dufy B, Vincent JD, Fleury H, et al: Membrane effects of thyrotropin-releasing hormone and estrogen shown by intracellular recording from pituitary cells. *Science* 204:509–511, 1979.
11. Datta S, Lambert DH, Gregus J, et al: Differential sensitivities of mammalian nerve fibers in pregnancy. *Anesth Analg* 62:1070–1072, 1983.
12. Flanagan HL, Datta S, Lambert DH, et al: Effect of pregnancy on bupivacaine induced conduction blockade in isolate rabbit vagus nerve. *Anesth Analg* 66:123–126, 1987.
13. Flanagan HL, Datta S, Moller RA, et al: Effects of exogenously administered progesterone in susceptibility of rabbit vagus nerves to bupivacaine (abstract). *Anesthesiology* 69:A676, 1988.
14. Bader AM, Datta S, Moller RA, et al: Effects of acute progesterone treatment on bupivacaine-induced conduction blockade in the isolated rabbit vagus nerve. *Anesth Analg* 71(5):545–548, 1990.
15. Datta S, Hurley RJ, Naulty JS, et al: Plasma and cerebrospinal fluid progesterone concentrations in pregnant and nonpregnant women. *Anesth Analg* 65:950–954, 1986.
16. Sheth AP, Dautenhahn DL, Campbell SD, et al: Decreased CSF protein during pregnancy as a mechanism facilitating the spread of spinal anesthesia (abstract). *Soc Obstet Anesth Perinatol* p. 83, 1985.
17. Butterwodh JF, Walker FD, Lyzak SZ: Pregnancy increases median nerve susceptibility to lidocaine. *Anesthesiology* 72:962–965, 1990.
18. Selye H: Studies concerning the anesthetic action of steroid hormones. *J Pharmacol Exp Ther* 73:127–141, 1941.
19. Landgren S, Backstrom T, Kahsratov G: The effect of progesterone on the spontaneous interictal spike evoked by the application of penicillin to the cat's cerebral cortex. *J Neurol Sci* 36:119–133, 1978.
20. Merryman W, Boiman R, Barnes L: Progesterone "anesthesia" in human subjects (correspondance). *J Clin Endocrinol Metab* 14:1567–1569, 1954.
21. Palahniuk FJ, Shnider SM, Eger EL: Pregnancy decreases the requirement for inhaled anesthetic agents. *Anesthesiology* 41:82–83, 1974.
22. Datta S, Mighozzi RP, Flanagan HL, et al: Chronically administered progesterone decreases halothane requirements in rabbits. *Anesth Analg* 68:46–50, 1989.
23. Butterworth JF, Raymond SA, Roscoe RF: Effects of halothane and enflurane in firing threshold of frog myelinated axons. *J Physiol (Lond)* 411:493–516, 1989.
24. Datta S, Hey VM, Pleury BJ: Effects of pregnancy and associated hormones in mouse intestine in vivo and vitro. *Pflugers Arch* 346:85–87, 1974.

25. Csapo A: The in vivo and in vitro effects of estrogen and progesterone on the myometrium. In *Mechanism of Action of Steroid Hormones*. Edited by C Ville, LI Engel. New York, NY. Pergamon Press, 1961.
26. Ryan PJ, Pellechhia D: Effect of progesterone pretreatment on guinea pig gall bladder motility in vitro. *Gastroenterology* 83:81–83, 1982.
27. Morishima HO, Pedersen H, Finister M, et al: Bupivacaine toxicity in pregnant and nonpregnant ewes. *Anesthesiology* 63:134–139, 1985.
28. Liu AL, McGill HG, Shain SA: Hormone receptors by the baboon cardiovascular system: biochemical characterization of aortic and myocardial cytoplasmic progesterone receptors. *Circ Res* 50:610–616, 1982.
29. Moller RA, Datta S, Fox J, et al: Progesterone induced increase in cardiac sensitivity to bupivacaine (abstract). *Anesthesiology* 69:A675, 1988.
30. O'Malley BW, Means AR: Female steroid hormones and target cell nuclei. *Science* 183:610–620, 1974.

Index

Abducens nerve palsy, 238
Abscess
  epidural, 134–135
  retropsoas or subgluteal, from
    anesthetic agents, 230–231
Acetaminophen, affecting fetus, 120
Acetylcholine receptors, in myasthenia
    gravis, 270
Acetylsalicylic acid
  affecting fetus, 120
  in rheumatic diseases, 306
Acromegaly, in pituitary tumors, 86
  treatment of, 90
Acroparesthesia, 235
ACTH
  safety in pregnancy, 176
  secretion by pituitary tumors, 86
Acyclovir, in herpes encephalitis,
    139–140
Adenomas, pituitary, 86–91
AIDS. *See* HIV infection
Air embolism, strokes in, 63
Akathisia, 196
Alcohol intake
  and cerebrovascular disease, 67
  and tremor suppression, 189
α-fetoprotein levels, maternal, and
    neural tube defects in fetus, 39
Amantadine, in Parkinson's disease,
    191
Amenorrhea-galactorrhea syndrome,
    in pituitary tumors, 86
  treatment of, 90
Amikacin, safety in pregnancy, 154
Aminoglycosides, safety in pregnancy,
    154
Amitriptyline
  affecting fetus, 120
  in postpartum depression, 323
Amniocentesis, in detection of neural
    tube defects, 39
Amoxapine, in postpartum
    depression, 323
Amoxicillin, in Lyme disease, 133
Amphotericin B
  in cryptococcal meningitis, 148
  in fungus infections, 136

safety in pregnancy, 155
Ampicillin, safety in pregnancy, 155
Amyotrophic lateral sclerosis, 238–239
Amyotrophy
  diabetic, 245
  neuralgic, 234
Anesthesia
  in autonomic dysreflexia, 213–214,
    217
  in craniotomy, 100–101
  dermatomal spread of epidural
    agents in, 325–326
  in intracranial lesions, 99–100
  in myasthenia gravis, 280–281
  and peripheral nerve sensitivity to
    local agents in pregnancy,
    329–331
  retropsoas or subgluteal abscess
    from, 230–231
Aneurysmal subarachnoid
    hemorrhage, 55–58
  risk periods for, 69
Ankle jerk, in lumbosacral
    intervertebral disc syndromes,
    231, 232
Antibiotics
  interaction with oral contraceptives,
    174–175
  in pregnancy, 154–156
    risk factor categories for, 152–153
Anticholinergic agents, in dystonia,
    192, 193
Anticoagulants
  in cardiogenic embolism, 64–54
  in cerebrovascular disease, 70
  in intracranial venous thrombosis,
    60
Anticonvulsants
  in eclampsia, 9–17
  in epilepsy. *See* Epilepsy,
    antiepileptic drugs in
  in glial tumors, 95–96
  in intracranial venous thrombosis,
    60
  teratogenicity of, 36–41, 95–96
Antidepressants, 321–323

Dihydroergotamine, in migraine, 119
Disc syndromes, intervertebral,
    231–233
  cervical, 233
  lumbosacral, 231–233
Diuretics, in pseudotumor cerebri, 99
L-Dopa. *See* Levodopa
Doxepin, in postpartum depression,
    323
Droopy shoulder syndrome, 235
Droperidol, neuroleptic malignant
    syndrome from, 197
Drug abuse
  cerebrovascular disease in, 67–68
  and chorea from cocaine, 187
Drug-induced conditions
  chorea, 186–187
  dystonia, 192
  fetal disorders in
    from heparin, 64
    from mannitol, 70
    from meperidine, 120
    from tetracyclines, 130, 133, 155
  in magnesium toxicity, 10–11
  myasthenic syndrome, 255–256
  neuroleptic malignant syndrome,
    196–197
  neuropathy, 244
  teratogenic effects. *See*
    Teratogenicity
  tremor, 189
Dysautonomia, familial, 242
Dysesthesias, 234–236
Dyskinesia, tardive, drug-induced,
    186–187
Dysreflexia, autonomic, in spinal cord
    injury, 211–214
Dystonia, 192–193
Dystrophy
  myotonic, 256–258
  reflex sympathetic, with carpal
    tunnel syndrome, 251

Echocardiography, in cardiogenic
    emboli, 64
Eclampsia, 1–21
  cerebral pathology in, 5–8, 68
    risk periods for, 69
  clinical course of, 8
  convulsions in, 33
    etiology of, 3
  diagnosis of, 4
  differential diagnosis of, 8

electroencephalography in, 5–6, 16
hypertension in, 4
  management of, 15–16
incidence of, 1, 20
labor and delivery in, 17–18
laboratory findings in, 5
magnesium sulfate in, 9–14
  dosage of, 9–10
  and EEG findings, 12
  mechanism of action, 11–12
  toxic effects of, 10–11
management of, 9–17
and outcome of pregnancy, 19–21
pathophysiology of, 1–4
phenytoin in, 14–15
Edema of brain, in glial tumors, 92
  corticosteroids in, 92, 95
Edrophonium test in myasthenia
    gravis, 272, 276, 277
Electroconvulsive therapy, in
    postpartum depression, 323
Electroencephalography
  in eclampsia, 5–6, 16
    magnesium sulfate affecting, 12
  in epilepsy, 27, 28
Electromyography, 225–226
Embolism
  air, strokes in, 63
  cardiogenic
    risk periods in, 69
    strokes in, 62–65
  fat, strokes in, 63, 66
  paradoxical, strokes in, 62–63
  in transient aortoarteritis, 62
Emetine, safety in pregnancy, 156
Encephalitis
  cytomegalovirus, 140
  equine, 141
    vaccine for, 153
  herpes, 139–140
    chorea in, 184
    in HIV infection, 145, 147
  parkinsonism after, 191
  toxoplasmosis, in HIV infection, 147
Encephalomyelitis, experimental
    allergic, pregnancy affecting,
    170
Encephalopathy in HIV infection,
    145–146
Endocarditis
  infective, meningitis in, 127
  nonbacterial thrombotic
    cerebral embolism in, 63
    risk periods in, 69

Multiple sclerosis (*cont.*)
etiology of, 167
fertility in, 168
genetic factors in, 172, 173
labor and delivery in, 175–176
management of, 174–175
pregnancy affecting, 169–171
pregnancy counseling in, 174–177
relapse in postpartum period, 169,
171, 173
reproductive counseling in, 172
tremor in, 190
Mumps meningitis, 139
Muscle-contraction headache, 112–114
Myasthenia gravis, 255–256, 269–288
anesthesia in, 280–281
crisis in, 276–277
diagnosis of, 272
experience in Johns Hopkins
Hospital, 284–288
pharmacologic data in, 287
serologic data in, 285
hypertension in, 282–283
immunopathology of, 270–271
incidence of, 269–270
management of, 275–283
antepartum, 275–279
intrapartum, 279–280, 286–288
postpartum, 281–282
and neonatal myasthenic syndrome,
272, 283
pathophysiology of, 270
pregnancy affecting, 273–274
thymectomy in, 271, 286
thymus gland in, 271
Mycobacterial infection, 127–129
Myelopathy
cervical, in rheumatoid arthritis,
296
vacuolar, in HIV infection, 151
Myoclonus, 195
Myoneural junction disorders,
255–256
Myopathy, 256–260
compared to neuropathy, 224–226
in HIV infection, 151
unusual causes of, 260
Myophosphorylase deficiency, 259
Myotonia congenita, 258
and malignant hyperpyrexia,
258–259
Myotonic dystrophy, 256–258

Nafcillin, safety in pregnancy, 155
Neostigmine in myasthenia gravis
diagnostic use of, 278–279
therapeutic use of, 276, 286–287
Nerve conduction studies, 226
Netilmycin, safety in pregnancy, 154
Neural tube defects, detection of, 39
Neuralgia, intercostal, 253
Neuritis, brachial plexus, 234
Neuroacanthocytosis, 188
Neuroleptics
chorea from, 186–187
malignant syndrome from, 196–197
Neuropathy, 240–249
compared to myopathy, 224–226
diabetic, 244–245
hereditary, 241–242
in HIV infection, 149–151, 249
idiopathic, 247–249
infectious, 246
in leprosy, 246
in lupus erythematosus, 301
metabolic, 242–243
nutritional, 245–246
in rheumatoid arthritis, 296
in scleroderma, 303
toxic, 244
Neurosyphilis, 129–130
in HIV infection, 149
Niclosamide, safety in pregnancy, 156
Norfloxacin, safety in pregnancy, 155
Nortriptyline, in postpartum
depression, 323
Nutritional factors
in migraine, 119
in neuropathy, 245–246

Obstetric palsies, maternal, 236–238
Obturator nerve compression, 236, 238
Ofloxacin, safety in pregnancy, 155
Oligodendrogliomas. *See* Glial tumors
Osteitis condensans ilii, 229
Osteoporosis of hip, transient, 230
Overlap syndromes, 305
Oxacillin, safety in pregnancy, 155

Pain
in back, 228–233
in peripheral nervous system
disorders, 224
and sensitive structures in
headache, 107